D0154015

DATE DUE

DEMCO, INC. 38-2971

Healthy Herbs

Healthy Herbs

FACT VERSUS FICTION

Myrna Chandler Goldstein
and Mark A. Goldstein, MD

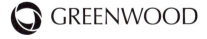

GREENWOOD

AN IMPRINT OF ABC-CLIO, LLC
Santa Barbara, California • Denver, Colorado • Oxford, England

COLLEGE OF THE SEQUOIAS
LIBRARY

Copyright 2012 by ABC-CLIO, LLC

All rights reserved. No part of this publication may be reproduced, stored in a retrieval system, or transmitted, in any form or by any means, electronic, mechanical, photocopying, recording, or otherwise, except for the inclusion of brief quotations in a review, without prior permission in writing from the publisher.

Library of Congress Cataloging-in-Publication Data

Goldstein, Myrna Chandler, 1948–
    Healthy herbs : fact versus fiction / Myrna Chandler Goldstein and Mark A. Goldstein.
        p. cm.
    Includes bibliographical references and index.
    ISBN 978-0-313-39780-6 (hardcopy : alk. paper) — ISBN 978-0-313-39781-3 (ebook)   1. Herbs—Therapeutic use.   2. Alternative medicine.   I. Goldstein, Mark A. (Mark Allan), 1947–   II. Title.
    RM666.H33G64   2012
    615.3'21—dc23   2011049149

ISBN: 978-0-313-39780-6
EISBN: 978-0-313-39781-3

16   15   14   13   12   1   2   3   4   5

This book is also available on the World Wide Web as an eBook.
Visit www.abc-clio.com for details.

Greenwood
An Imprint of ABC-CLIO, LLC

ABC-CLIO, LLC
130 Cremona Drive, P.O. Box 1911
Santa Barbara, California 93116-1911

This book is printed on acid-free paper ∞

Manufactured in the United States of America

This book discusses treatments (including types of medication and mental health therapies), diagnostic tests for various symptoms and mental health disorders, and organizations. The authors have made every effort to present accurate and up-to-date information. However, the information in this book is not intended to recommend or endorse particular treatments or organizations, or substitute for the care or medical advice of a qualified health professional, or used to alter any medical therapy without a medical doctor's advice. Specific situations may require specific therapeutic approaches not included in this book. For those reasons, we recommend that readers follow the advice of qualified health care professionals directly involved in their care. Readers who suspect they may have specific medical problems should consult a physician about any suggestions made in this book.

We dedicate this book with love to our grandchildren:
Aidan Zev
Payton Maeve
Milo Adlai
Erin Abigail

Contents

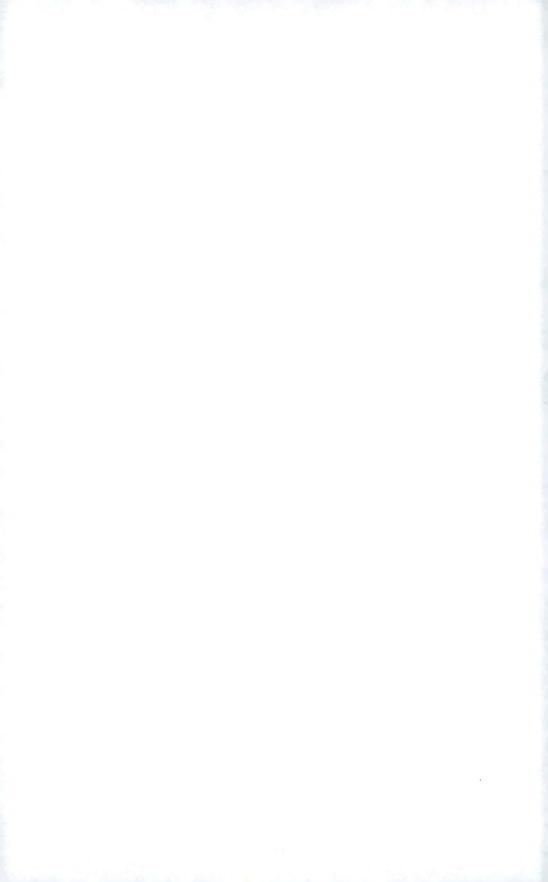

List of Entries

Introduction

As the costs associated with health care and medications continue to rise, many people look for alternative ways to meet their health care needs. They may also want more natural, time-tested products that come with fewer, if any, side effects. And, so, in recent years, perhaps because of the advice of a magazine article, a newspaper story, or the recommendation of a television or radio personality, some have turned to herbs, or plants with leaves, seeds, or flowers. Readily available in stores and online, herbs are certainly less expensive than most medications. But, are they effective? Are they useful for only minor problems? Are they able to address more serious concerns? Are they safe?

The goal of this book is to examine actual research studies on 50 different herbs. This is not as easy as it might initially appear to be. The research conducted on many herbs is actually quite limited, or the studies might be too esoteric for the needs of the typical reader. So, while there were scores of herbs on our initial list, many had to be eliminated. Still, the book is comprehensive and somewhat unique. We have been unable to locate a similar work.

An important point must be noted. Just because herbs are more natural than conventional medications, do not assume that they are always safe. For example, it is not uncommon for herbs to interact with medications; sometimes, that interaction may have serious and undesirable consequences. And, just because an herb may be healthful in small or moderate amounts, do not assume that it is also safe when consumed in larger amounts or in supplementation. Moreover, women who are pregnant, may become pregnant, or are breastfeeding should not use many herbs. In fact, before beginning an herbal regime, it is a good idea to discuss your intentions with your health care provider.

A

Acai

Grown in the Amazon jungle for thousands of years, the acai berry is a truly ancient medicinal herb. However, it has been recognized by the Western world for only a relatively short period of time. Still, acai berry, which is scientifically known as *Euterpe oleracea,* has been said to address a vast number of medical concerns. For example, acai is believed to support cardiovascular health and improve memory, sleep, energy, vision, and immunity. Some think acai is useful for weight loss, reducing inflammation, and eliminating toxins from the body.[1] It is important to review what researchers have learned.

Cardiovascular Health

In a study published in 2010 in *Nutrition,* researchers based in Brazil investigated the ability of acai to increase antioxidants and lower cholesterol levels in rats fed a standard or high-cholesterol diet. The researchers divided their rats into four groups. Two groups consumed the standard rat diet; the other two groups were fed a high-fat diet containing 25% soy oil and 1% cholesterol. In addition, the rats in one standard diet group and one high-fat group were also fed 2% acai pulp. After six weeks, the researchers noted that the rats in the high-fat group experienced increases in total cholesterol and decreases in high-density lipoprotein (HDL) ("good") cholesterol. These changes were attenuated in the rats fed high-fat and acai diets. The researchers concluded that their findings "suggest that the consumption of acai improves antioxidant status and has a hypocholesterolemic effect in an animal model of dietary-induced hypercholesterolemia."[2]

In a study published in 2011 in *Atherosclerosis,* researchers from Arkansas and Washington conducted two similar trials on mice bred to have high serum lipid levels. In the first trial, for 20 weeks, they fed one group of 15 mice a regular rodent diet and a second group of 15 mice a rodent diet plus 5% freeze-dried acai juice powder. The second trial was similar, but it was conducted for only 5 weeks. The researchers found that the mice that also consumed acai had fewer atherosclerotic lesions. Apparently, acai imparted a degree of protection against the development of atherosclerosis.[3]

In an open-label pilot study published in 2011 in *Nutrition Journal,* researchers from California evaluated supplementing the diets of healthy but overweight subjects with acai fruit pulp. The cohort consisted of 10 overweight adult men and women; they were assigned to take 100 mg of acai pulp twice daily before meals for one month. When compared to their baseline values, the researchers found that by the end of the trial the participants experienced a lowering of several markers of cardiovascular risk, such as a significant reduction in total cholesterol and borderline significant reductions in low-density lipoprotein (LDL) ("bad") cholesterol and the ratio of total cholesterol to HDL cholesterol. The researchers commented that further studies were needed.[4]

Pain Reduction
In a pilot study published in 2011 in the *Journal of Medicinal Food,* researchers from Oregon and Washington wanted to learn if acai could help people dealing with pain. The cohort consisted of 14 people between the ages of 44 and 84 who had range of motion (ROM) limitations and pain. For 12 weeks, the study participants consumed "120 mL MonaVie Active® fruit juice, predominantly containing acai pulp." The participants were evaluated at baseline and at 2, 4, 8, and 12 weeks. The researchers found that the juice consumption "resulted in significant pain reduction, improved ROM measures, and improvement in ADLs [activities of daily living]."[5]

Kills Esophageal Cancer Cells
In a study published in 2010 in *Pharmaceutical Research,* researchers from Columbus, Ohio, compared the ability of different types of berries, including acai, to prevent the formation of chemically induced esophageal cancer cells in rats. The researchers began by treating rats for five weeks with a carcinogen that fosters esophageal cancer. The rats were then placed on

diets containing 5% acai and other berries, such as black and red raspberries and strawberries. The researchers determined that all the berry types were about equally effective in inhibiting the growth of cancer. Still, the researchers noted that "the data are preliminary in that the berries were tested at only a single dose level (5%) in the diet."[6]

Antiaging Properties

In a study published in 2010 in *Experimental Gerontology,* researchers from Baltimore, Maryland, and Washington evaluated the role that acai could play on the life span of female fruit flies. The researchers began by establishing two models. The first would test acai's ability to mitigate a poor diet and the second would study acai's ability to promote longevity.

In the first study, the researchers divided fruit flies into two groups. Both groups were fed a high-fat diet that would reduce longevity by 19%. But, one of these groups was also fed 2% acai supplementation. While the flies fed only the high-fat diet did indeed have a reduction in life span, the flies fed acai had a 22% increase in longevity.

In the second model, the researchers used fruit flies that had been genetically mutated so that an enzyme that repairs cells and reduces the damage caused by free radicals failed to function properly. Unable to repair their oxidative damage, the fruit flies were forced to remain in a constant state of oxidative stress. But, while one group was fed a normal diet, the second group was also fed a normal fly diet that included 2% acai pulp. When compared to the flies fed only the normal diet, the flies fed the diet plus acai had an 18% longer life span. So, one of the ways that acai extends the life span is by reducing oxidative stress. The researchers concluded that acai "has the potential to antagonize the detrimental effect of fat in the diet and alleviate oxidative stress in aging."[7]

Protective Effect against Emphysema in Cigarette Smokers

In a truly innovative piece of research that was published in 2011 in *Food and Chemical Toxicology,* researchers from Brazil wanted to compare the lung damage in mice caused by 60 days of chronic inhalation of regular cigarette smoke to that caused by the inhalation of cigarette smoke containing 100 mg of hydroalcoholic extract of acai berry stone. They began by dividing their mice into three groups. The first group of mice became the control. They were "sham-smoked—exposed to ambient air using a smoking chamber." The mice in the second group were exposed to smoke from "12 commercially-obtained full-flavor . . . filtered Virginia cigarettes." The mice in the third group were exposed to the same cigarette smoke, but their cigarettes also contained acai berry stone, which was injected into each cigarette. At the end of the trial, the mice were sacrificed so that the researchers could examine their lungs.

While the mice in the control group had normal lungs, the mice in the cigarette-smoking group had evidence of emphysema. Meanwhile, the lungs of the cigarette-smoking and acai group were not the same as the lungs of the mice in the control group. But, they "appeared less affected by emphysema than did the lungs of the mice in the CS [cigarette-smoking] group." So, adding acai to cigarettes has the potential to reduce the many deleterious effects associated with the smoking of cigarettes.[8]

Is Acai Beneficial?

Acai is certainly an intriguing herb that may well be useful for a wide variety of medical concerns. It will be interesting to see what future studies on this herb learn.

Notes

1. Acai Berry. www.acaiberry.org.
2. De Souza, M.O., M. Silva, M.E. Silva, et al. July–August 2010. "Diet Supplementation with Acai (*Euterpe oleracea* Mart.) Pulp Improves Biomarkers of Oxidative Stress and the Serum Lipid Profile in Rats." *Nutrition* 26(7–8): 804–810.
3. Xie, C., J. Kang, R. Burris, et al. June 2011. "Açai Juice Attenuates Atherosclerosis in ApoE Deficient Mice through Antioxidant and Anti-Inflammatory Activities." *Atherosclerosis* 216(2): 327–333.
4. Udani, J.K., B.B. Singh, V.J. Singh, and M.L. Barrett. May 2011. "Effects of Acai (*Euterpe oleracea* Mart.) Berry Preparation on Metabolic Parameters in a Healthy Overweight Population: A Pilot Study." *Nutrition Journal* 10(1): 45.
5. Jensen, Gitte S., David M. Ager, Kimberlee A. Redman, et al. July–August 2011. "Pain Reduction and Improvement in Range of Motion after Daily Consumption of an Açai (*Euterpe oleracea* Mart.) Pulp-Fortified Polyphenolic-Rich Fruit and Berry Juice Blend." *Journal of Medicinal Food* 14(7–8): 702–711.
6. Stoner, G.D., L.S. Wang, C. Seguin, et al. June 2010. "Multiple Berry Types Prevent *N*-Nitrosomethylbenzylamine-Induced Esophageal Cancer in Rats." *Pharmaceutical Research* 27(6): 1138–1145.
7. Sun, Xiaoping, Jeanne Seeberger, Thomas Alberico, et al. March 2010. "Açai Palm Fruit (*Euterpe oleracea* Mart.) Pulp Improves Survival of Flies on a High Fat Diet." *Experimental Gerontology* 45(3): 243–251.

8. De Moura, Roberto Soares, Karla Maria Pereira Pires, Thiago Santos Ferreira, et al. April 2011. "Addition of Açai (*Euterpe oleracea*) to Cigarettes Has a Protective Effect against Emphysema in Mice." *Food and Chemical Toxicology* 49(4): 855–863.

References and Resources

Magazines, Journals, and Newspapers

De Moura, Roberto Soares, Karla Maria Pereira Pires, Thiago Santos Ferreira, et al. April 2011. "Addition of Açai (*Euterpe oleracea*) to Cigarettes Has a Protective Effect against Emphysema in Mice." *Food and Chemical Toxicology* 49(4): 855–863.

De Souza, M.O., M. Silva, M.E. Silva, et al. July–August 2010. "Diet Supplementation with Acai (*Enterpe oleracea* Mart.) Pulp Improves Biomarkers of Oxidative Stress and the Serum Lipid Profile in Rats." *Nutrition* 26(7–8): 804–810.

Jensen, Gitte S., David M. Ager, Kimberlee A. Redman, et al. July–August 2011. "Pain Reduction and Improvement in Range of Motion after Daily Consumption of an Açai (*Euterpe oleracea* Mart.) Pulp-Fortified Polyphenolic-Rich Fruit and Berry Juice Blend." *Journal of Medicinal Food* 14(7–8): 702–711.

Stoner, G.D., L.S. Wang, C. Seguin, et al. June 2010. "Multiple Berry Types Prevent *N*-Nitrosomethylbenzylamine-Induced Esophageal Cancer in Rats." *Pharmaceutical Research* 27(6): 1138–1145.

Sun, Xiaoping, Jeanne Seeberger, Thomas Alberico, et al. March 2010. "Açai Palm Fruit (*Euterpe oleracea* Mart.) Pulp Improves Survival of Flies on a High Fat Diet." *Experimental Gerontology* 45(3): 243–251.

Udani, J.K., B.B. Singh, V.J. Singh, and M.L. Barrett. May 2011. "Effects of Acai (*Euterpe oleracea* Mart.) Berry Preparation on Metabolic Parameters in a Healthy Overweight Population: A Pilot Study." *Nutrition Journal* 10(1): 45.

Xie, C., J. Kang, R. Burris, et al. June 2011. "Açai Juice Attenuates Atherosclerosis in ApoE Deficient Mice through Antioxidant and Anti-Inflammatory Activities." *Atherosclerosis* 216(2): 327–333.

Website

Acai Berry. www.acaiberry.org.

Aloe Vera 🌿

Aloe vera was esteemed by the ancient Greeks as a universal panacea. The ancient Egyptians thought it was the plant of immortality. In fact, the word aloe comes from the Arabic word *alloeh,* which means "shinning bitter substance," and, in Latin, the word *vera* means "true."[1]

Historically, aloe vera was used for a wide variety of medical problems, such as the treatment of soldiers' wounds, skin irritations, and constipation. Still, aloe vera was also used for general skincare, overall health, beauty, and well-being. Today, it is primarily used as a skin-care product.[2] But, what have the researchers learned?

Burns

In a study published in 2009 in *Surgery Today,* Iranian researchers investigated the treatment of second-degree burns with either aloe vera cream or silver sulfadiazine (SSD), a sulfur medicine used to prevent and treat bacterial and fungal infections. Their cohort consisted of 30 patients with second-degree burns on two different sites of their bodies. Each subject had one site treated with aloe vera cream and the other site treated with SSD. The researchers found that the site that was treated with aloe vera healed significantly faster than the site treated with SSD. "The sites treated with aloe were completely healed in less than 16 days versus 19 days for the sites treated with SSD. These results clearly demonstrated the greater efficacy of aloe cream over SSD cream for treating second-degree burns."[3]

Another study on burns was published in 2008 in the journal *Burns.* In this trial, Australian researchers examined the use of aloe vera, saliva, a tea tree oil impregnated dressing (Burnaid), or nothing (the control) on burns made under anesthesia on the flank skin of eight-week-old pigs. Though the researchers initially hoped to collect a sufficient amount of pig saliva, and since that effort was fruitless, they used saliva from a human volunteer. After the burns were created, the researchers applied the 20-minute weekly treatments for 6 weeks. They noted that while all three treatments reduced the subdermal temperature, "they did not decrease the microflora or improve the re-epithelialisation [regrowth of epithelium over surface of a wound], scar strength, scar depth or cosmetic appearance of the scar." As a result, the researchers concluded that the treatments they tested "cannot be recommended for the first aid treatment of partial thickness burns."[4]

In an article published in 2007 in *Burns,* Thai researchers reported on their systematic review of four controlled clinical trials in which aloe vera was used for the treatment of burns. In total, the studies included 371 patients. The researchers determined that the wounds treated with aloe vera healed, on average, 8.79 days shorter than those treated with a control. Yet, because there were "differences of products and outcomes measures," the researchers thought that these results should be viewed with at least some degree of caution. Nevertheless, they added that "cumulative evidence tends to support that aloe vera might be an effective intervention used in burn wound healing for first to second degree burns."[5]

Psoriasis

In a randomized, double-blind, eight-week clinical study published in 2010 in the *Journal of the European Academy of Dermatology and Venereology,* Thai researchers randomly treated 80 people with mild to moderate psoriasis with either a 70% aloe vera cream or 0.1% triamcinolone acetonide, a topical steroid medication. The researchers found that the people treated with the aloe vera cream had a greater reduction in the Psoriasis Area and Severity Index (PASI). Although the findings were not statistically significant, the researchers noted that the aloe vera cream "may be more effective than 0.1% TA [triamcinolone acetonide] cream in reducing the clinical symptoms of psoriasis; however, both treatments have similar efficacy in improving the quality of life of patients with mild to moderate psoriasis."[6]

On the other hand, a double-blind, placebo-controlled Danish study published in 2005 in the *Journal of the European Academy of Dermatology and Venereology* came to different conclusions. This study included a two-week washout period that was followed by a four-week treatment period with two daily applications of commercial aloe vera gel or a placebo. There were also two follow-up visits—after one month and after two months. The findings are noteworthy. "Aloe vera-treated sites compared with 82.5% of the placebo-treated areas from week 0 to week 4, which was statistically significant in favour of the placebo treatment." Moreover, 55% of the 40 participants who completed the study reported side effects, primarily a drying of the skin on the test areas. The researchers concluded that "the effect of this commercial Aloe vera gel on stable plaque psoriasis was modest and not better than placebo."[7]

Skin Inflammation

In a randomized, double-blind, placebo-controlled study published in 2008 in *Skin Pharmacology and Physiology,* German researchers investigated the use of highly concentrated aloe vera gel, a placebo gel, or three different types of corticosteroids, on skin that was inflamed from exposure to ultraviolet light. The researchers found that after 48 hours the aloe vera gel "displayed some anti-inflammatory effects superior to those of 1% hydrocortisone in a placebo gel." However, the "1% hydrocortisone in cream was more efficient than A. vera gel [aloe vera gel]."[8]

Oral Health

In an in vitro study published in 2009 in *General Dentistry,* researchers acknowledged that there has been disagreement concerning the ability of aloe vera tooth gel to eliminate pathogenic oral microflora or disease-causing bacteria in the mouth. So, they compared the ability of aloe vera gel to fight germs in the mouth to two commercially popular toothpastes. The researchers found that the aloe vera gel and the toothpastes were equally effective against some disease-causing bacteria, and aloe vera gel was more effective in one particular type of bacteria—*Streptococcus mitis*. Why is this important? Commercially available toothpastes often contain abrasive elements that may be too harsh for people with sensitive teeth or gums.[9] So, aloe vera may be a suitable substitute.

Kidney Stones

Two separate studies published in 2006 in the *Journal of the Medical Association of Thailand* show an association between the intake of aloe vera and the possible prevention of kidney stone formation. (Kidney stones can develop when a substance, such as calcium oxalate, and chemicals in urine form crystals that stick together.) One study included 31 healthy male medical students between the ages of 18 and 23. After consuming 100 g of fresh aloe gel twice a day for seven consecutive days, the subjects experienced changes in the chemical composition of their urine and decreases in their excretion of oxalate. According to the researchers, these changes have the potential to prevent kidney stone formation in adults.[10] When the same study was conducted on 13 healthy boys between the ages of 9 and 13, their urine was found to have significant increases in the concentration of citrate. The researchers noted that the moderately high citrate content of aloe vera may be useful in the prevention of kidney stones.[11]

Is Aloe Vera Beneficial?

Aloe vera seems to be useful for a number of skin conditions. And, it also may be beneficial when taken by mouth. However, when consumed, aloe vera may cause cramps and diarrhea. And, because it may lower blood glucose levels, people with diabetes or other illnesses subject to low blood sugar should probably not take aloe vera internally.

Notes

1. Surjushe, Amar, Resham Vasani, and D. Saple. October–December 2008. "Aloe Vera: A Short Review." *Indian Journal of Dermatology* 53(4): 163–166.
2. Surjushe, Amar, Resham Vasani, and D. Saple. October–December 2008. "Aloe Vera: A Short Review." *Indian Journal of Dermatology* 53(4): 163–166.
3. Khorasani, Ghasemali, Seyed Jalal Hosseinimehr, Mohammad Azadbakht et al. July 2009. "Aloe versus Silver Sulfadiazine Creams for Second-Degree Burns: A Randomized Controlled Study." *Surgery Today* 39(7): 587–591.
4. Cuttle, Leila, Margit Kempf, Olenea Kravchuk et al. December 2008. "The Efficacy of Aloe Vera, Tea Tree Oil, and Saliva as First Aid Treatment for Partial Thickness Burn Injuries." *Burns* 34(8): 1176–1182.
5. Maenthaisong, R., N. Chaiyakunapruk, S. Niruntraporn, and C. Kongkaew. September 2007. "The Efficacy of Aloe Vera Used for Burn Wound Healing: A Systematic Review." *Burns* 33(6): 713–718.
6. Choonhakarn, C., P. Busaracome, B. Sripanidkulchai, and P. Sarakarn. February 2010. "A Prospective, Randomized Clinical Trial Comparing Topical Aloe Vera with 0.1% Triamcinolone Acetonide in Mild to Moderate Plaque Psoriasis." *Journal of the European Academy of Dermatology and Venereology* 24(2): 168–172.
7. Paulsen, E., L. Korsholm, and F. Brandrup. May 2005. "A Double-Blind, Placebo-Controlled Study of a Commercial Aloe Vera Gel in the Treatment of Slight to Moderate Psoriasis Vulgaris." *Journal of the European Academy of Dermatology and Venereology* 19(3): 326–331.
8. Reuter, J., A. Jocher, J. Stump et al. 2008. "Investigation of the Anti-Inflammatory Potential of Aloe Vera Gel (97.5%) in the Ultraviolet Erythema Test." *Skin Pharmacology and Physiology* 21(2): 106–110.
9. George, Dilip, Sham S. Bhat, and Beena Antony. May–June 2009. "Comparative Evaluation of the Antimicrobial Efficacy of Aloe Vera Tooth Gel and Two Popular Commercial Toothpastes: An In Vitro Study." *General Dentistry* 57(3): 238–241.
10. Kirdpon, Sukachart, Wichit Kirdpon, Wanchai Airarat et al. 2006. "Effect of Aloe (*Aloe vera*) on Healthy Adult Volunteers: Changes in Urinary Composition." *Journal of the Medical Association of Thailand* 89(Supplement 2): S9–S14.
11. Kirdpon, Sukachart, Wichit Kirdpon, Wanchai Airarat et al. 2006. "Changes in Urinary Compositions among Children after Consuming Prepared Oral Doses of Aloe (*Aloe vera* Linn)." *Journal of the Medical Association of Thailand* 89(8): 1199–1205.

References and Resources

Magazines, Journals, and Newspapers

Choonhakarn, C., P. Busaracome, B. Sripanidkulchai, and P. Sarakarn. February 2010. "A Perspective, Randomized Clinical Trial Comparing Topical Aloe Vera with 0.1% Triamcinolone Acetonide in Mild to Moderate Plaque Psoriasis." *Journal of the European Academy of Dermatology and Venereology* 24(2): 168–172.

Cuttle, Leila, Margit Kempf, Olena Kravchuk, et al. December 2008. "The Efficacy of Aloe Vera, Tea Tree Oil, and Saliva as First Aid Treatment for Partial Thickness Burn Injuries." *Burns* 34(8): 1176–1182.

George, Dilip, Sham S. Bhat, and Beena Anthony. May–June 2009. "Comparative Evaluation of the Antimicrobial Efficacy of Aloe Vera Tooth Gel and Two Popular Commercial Toothpastes: An In Vitro Study." *General Dentistry* 57(3): 238–241.

Khorasani, Ghasemali, Seyed Jalal Hosseinimehr, Mohammad Azadbakht, et al. July 2009. "Aloe versus Silver Sulfadiazine Creams for Second-Degree Burns: A Randomized Controlled Study." *Surgery Today* 39(7): 587–591.

Kirdpon, Sukachart, Wichit Kirdpon, Wanchai Airarat, et al. 2006. "Changes in Urinary Compositions among Children after Consuming Prepared Oral Doses of Aloe (*Aloe vera* Linn.)." *Journal of the Medical Association of Thailand* 89(8): 1199–1205.

Kirdpon, Sukachart, Wichit Kirdpon, Wanchai Airarat, et al. 2006. "Effect of Aloe (*Aloe vera* Linn.) on Healthy Adult Volunteers: Changes in Urinary Composition." *Journal of the Medical Association of Thailand* 89(Supplement 2): S9–S14.

Maenthaisong, R., N. Chaiyakunapruk, S. Niruntraporn, and C. Kongkaew. September 2007. "The Efficacy of Aloe Vera Used for Burn Wound Healing: A Systematic Review." *Burns* 33(6): 713–718.

Paulsen, E., L. Korsholm, and F. Brandrup. May 2005. "A Double-Blind, Placebo-Controlled Study of a Commercial Aloe Vera Gel in the Treatment of Slight to Moderate Psoriasis Vulgaris." *Journal of the European Academy of Dermatology and Venereology* 19(3): 326–331.

Reuter, J., A. Jocher, J. Stump, et al. 2008. "Investigation of the Anti-Inflammatory Potential of Aloe Vera Gel (97.5%) in the Ultraviolet Erythema Test." *Skin Parmacology and Physiology* 21(2): 106–110.

Surjushe, Amar, Resham Vasani, and D. Saple. October–December 2008. "Aloe Vera: A Short Review." *Indian Journal of Dermatology* 53(4): 163–166.

Website

International Aloe Science Council. www.iasc.org.

Arnica 🐾

Scientifically known as *Arnica montana,* arnica has been considered a medicinal herb since at least the 1500s. The Europeans and Native Americans used arnica to sooth muscle aches, heal wounds, and reduce inflammation. Today, arnica is thought to be effective for many conditions, such as bruises, sprains, muscle aches, wound healing, superficial phlebitis, inflammation from insect bites, and the swelling caused by a fracture. Arnica is now available as a topical cream, ointment, liniment, salve, tincture, or as an extremely diluted orally administered homeopathic remedy. Native to the mountains of Europe and Siberia, arnica is cultivated in many North American locations.[1] But, as with the other herbs in this book, it is important to review what researchers have learned about arnica.

Osteoarthritis

In a randomized, double-blind study published in 2007 in *Rheumatology International,* researchers from Switzerland compared the effectiveness of two different gels—one containing ibuprofen (nonsteroid anti-inflammation medication) and the other arnica—on treating people with radiologically confirmed osteoarthritis of the hands. At the beginning of the investigation, the cohort consisted of more than 200 people. The participants were instructed to rub the gel over the affected joints three times a day for three weeks. And, they were asked to refrain from washing their hands for one hour after each application. The researchers found that both gels improved pain and function in hand osteoarthritis. They noted that they observed similar results "with regard to [the] number of painful joints, severity and duration of morning stiffness, as well as perceived efficacy by patients and doctors."[2]

Postoperative (Tonsillectomy) Pain Relief

In a study published in 2007 in *Homeopathy,* researchers from the United Kingdom examined the use of arnica for the postsurgical pain from a tonsillectomy (removal of the tonsils). The cohort consisted of 190 patients over the age of 18. They were randomized to receive either arnica or an identical placebo—two tablets six times in the first postoperative day, and then, two tablets twice a day for the next seven days. The researchers found that the patients taking arnica "had a significantly larger drop in pain score from day one to day 14 . . . compared to the placebo group." They concluded that "the results of this trial suggest that *Arnica montana* given after tonsillectomy proves a small, but statistically significant, decrease in pain scores compared to placebo."[3]

Healing of Skin Bruising

In a blinded, randomized, controlled trial published in 2010 in the *British Journal of Dermatology,* researchers from Northwestern University in Chicago compared the skin bruise–healing properties of four substances—20% arnica, 5% vitamin K, 1% vitamin K combined with 0.3% retinol, and white petrolatum (control). Using a 595-nm pulsed-dye laser, the researchers created 4 standard bruises on the arms of each of the 16 healthy volunteers. Then, the bruises were treated with one of the agents, twice a day for two weeks. A dermatologist not involved with the project rated the bruises for their degree of healing. The dermatologist found that the bruises treated with 20% arnica experienced more healing than the bruises treated with the combination of vitamin K and retinol and the white petroleum. However, the improvement with arnica "was not greater than with 5% vitamin K cream." The researchers concluded that "higher concentrations of topical arnica ointment appear to be effective in reducing laser-induced bruises."[4]

Different results were obtained by researchers in Tucson, Arizona, in a prospective, placebo-controlled, double-blind trial published in 2010 in *Ophthalmic Plastic and Reconstructive Surgery.* Thirty men who had undergone eyelid surgery (upper eyelid blepharoplasty) were recruited to take four days of postsurgical arnica tablets or placebos. On postsurgical days three and seven, the men were evaluated for the degree of bruising (ecchymosis). The researchers found no statistical difference between the amount of bruising on the men taking arnica and the amount of bruising on those taking the placebo. They concluded that there was "no evidence that homeopathic *A. montana,* as used in this study, is beneficial in the reduction or the resolution of ecchymosis after upper eyelid blepharoplasty."[5]

Recovery from Bunion Removal Surgery

In a randomized, double-blind, parallel-group study published in 2008 in *The Journal of Alternative and Complementary Medicine,* researchers from

Frankfurt, Germany, compared the bunion removal surgery wound healing efficacy of arnica to diclofenac, a commonly used nonsteroidal antiinflammatory, antipain medication. The cohort consisted of 88 patients. For the first four days after surgery, they took either arnica D4 (D4 denotes the dilution of arnica) at a dose of 10 pills, three times per day, or diclofenac sodium, 50 mg three times per day. The researchers found that arnica and diclofenac reduced about the same amount of the wounds' redness, swelling, and inflammation. Still, the patients on arnica had increased mobility and those on diclofenac had better pain relief. But, it is important to note that the patients had fewer problems with arnica than with diclofenac. Nine patients taking diclofenac (20.45%) and two taking arnica (4.5%) reported intolerances.[6] From these findings, it appears that arnica may well be able to play a role in postsurgical treatments.

Treatment for Lumbago

In a placebo-controlled, double-blind trial published in 2010 in *Phytotherapy Research,* researchers from Brazil examined the effect that Brazilian arnica had on lumbago, nonspecific lower back pain. The researchers assembled two groups of people with lower back pain. Both groups administered a gel on their lower backs twice daily for 15 days. One group of 10, between the ages of 19 and 44, used a gel containing Brazilian arnica. The second group of 10, between the ages of 18 and 37, used a gel containing a placebo. The people using arnica reported that it was "effective in treating lumbago and increasing lumbar function." The researchers noted that arnica "had a marked analgesic effect in the treatment of lumbago compared with placebo dosages when applied to the skin as a gel." And, the researchers concluded that their findings "contribute to the evaluation of Brazilian arnica as a medicinal plant useful in the treatment of lumbago."[7]

Muscle Pain

Meanwhile, a randomized, double-blind, placebo-controlled trial published in 2010 in *The Annals of Pharmacotherapy* found that arnica was unable to resolve muscle pain. The Texas researchers began by recruiting 55 male and female adult volunteers. Each volunteer received two containers: one was labeled "left" and the other was labeled "right." One container contained arnica and the other had a placebo. The subjects had no way to determine which container actually contained arnica and which had the placebo. All the subjects followed a protocol for performing calf raises that would induce muscle soreness. After completing the exercises, the participants applied the appropriate cream to each leg. They were instructed to leave the cream undisturbed for one hour. About 48 hours later, they returned to the research site for an evaluation. Fifty-three of the original 55 volunteers completed the study. The findings were dramatic and unexpected. According to the researchers, the arnica failed to diminish the pain associated with the exercises. In fact, the researchers found that the legs treated with arnica had greater levels of pain. They noted that they had "no compelling explanation" for their results.[8]

Is Arnica Beneficial?

While most of the research on arnica appears to show that it is useful for a number of health problems, there are studies that have found that arnica offers limited or no health benefits. At the same time, there is a vast array of anecdotal reports describing how arnica helped deal with a medical problem. It may be that arnica works better in some people than in others. Or, different brands may be more effective than others. Because arnica is so inexpensive and readily available, for people dealing with some of the problems noted early in this entry, it may well be worth trying.

Notes

1. University of Maryland Medical Center Website. www.umm.edu.
2. Widrig, Reto, Andy Suter, Reinhard Saller, and Jorg Melzer. April 2007. "Choosing between NSAID and Arnica for Topical Treatment of Hand Osteoarthritis in a Randomized, Double-Blind Study." *Rheumatology International* 27(6): 585–591.
3. Robertson, A., R. Suryanarayanan, and A. Banerjee. January 2007. "Homeopathic *Arnica montana* for Post-Tonsillectomy Analgesia: A Randomised Placebo Control Trial." *Homeopathy* 96(1): 17–21.
4. Leu, S., J. Havey, L. E. White, et al. September 2010. "Accelerated Resolution of Laser-Induced Bruising with Topical 20% Arnica: A Rater-Blinded Randomized Controlled Trial." *British Journal of Dermatology* 163(3): 557–563.
5. Kotlus, B. S., D. M. Heringer, and R. M. Dryden. November–December 2010. "Evaluation of Homeopathic *Arnica montana* for Ecchymosis after Upper Blepharoplasty: A Placebo-Controlled, Randomized, Double-Blind Study." *Ophthalmic Plastic and Reconstructive Surgery* 26(6): 395–397.
6. Karow, J. H., H. P. Abt, M. Fröhling, and H. Ackermann. January–February 2008. "Efficacy of *Arnica montana* D4 for Healing of Wounds after Hallux Valgus Surgery Compared to Diclofenac." *The Journal of Alternative and Complementary Medicine* 14(1): 17–25.

7. Da Silva, A.G., C.P. de Sousa, J. Koehler, et al. February 2010. "Evaluations of an Extract of Brazilian Arnica (*Solidago chilensis* Meyen, Asteraceae) in Treating Lumbago." *Phytotherapy Research* 24(2): 283–287.
8. Adkison, J.D., D.W. Bauer, and T. Chang. October 2010. "The Effect of Topical Arnica on Muscle Pain." *The Annals of Pharmacotherapy* 44(10): 1579–1584.

References and Resources

Magazines, Journals, and Newspapers

Adkison, J.D., D.W. Bauer, and T. Chang. October 2010. "The Effect of Topical Arnica on Muscle Pain." *The Annals of Pharmacotherapy* 44(10): 1579–1584.

Da Silva, A.G., C.P. de Sousa, J. Koehler, et al. February 2010. "Evaluation of an Extract of Brazilian Arnica (*Solidago chilensis* Meyen, Asteraceae) in Treating Lumbago." *Phytotherapy Research* 24(2): 283–287.

Karow, J.H., H.P. Abt, M. Fröhling, and H. Ackermann. January–February 2008. "Efficacy of *Arnica montana* D4 for Healing of Wounds after Hallux Valgus Surgery Compared to Diclofenac." *The Journal of Alternative and Complementary Medicine* 14(1): 17–25.

Kotlus, B.S., D.M. Heringer, and R.M. Dryden. November–December 2010. "Evaluation of Homeopathic *Arnica montana* for Ecchymosis after Upper Blepharoplasty: A Placebo-Controlled, Randomized, Double-Blind Study." *Ophthalmic Plastic and Reconstructive Surgery* 26(6): 395–397.

Leu, S., J. Havey, L.E. White, et al. September 2010. "Accelerated Resolution of Laser-Induced Bruising with Topical 20% Arnica: A Rater-Blinded Randomized Controlled Trial." *British Journal of Dermatology* 163(3): 557–563.

Robertson, A., R. Suryanarayanan, and A. Banerjee. January 2007. "Homeopathic *Arnica montana* for Post-Tonsillectomy Analgesia: A Randomised Placebo Control Trial." *Homeopathy* 96(1): 17–21.

Widrig, Reto, Andy Suter, Reinhard Saller, and Jorg Melzer. April 2007. "Choosing between NSAID and Arnica for Topical Treatment of Hand Osteoarthritis in a Randomised, Double-Blind Study." *Rheumatology International* 27(6): 585–591.

Websites

Drugs.com. www.drugs.com.

University of Maryland Medical Center. www.umm.edu.

Ashwagandha 🌿

Scientifically known as *Withania somnifera,* ashwagandha is an ancient Ayurvedic herb that has been used for thousands of years for a wide variety of medical problems. These include stress, strain, fatigue, diabetes, gastro-intestinal issues, rheumatoid arthritis, and osteoarthritis. It is also thought to kill cancer cells, quell anxiety, and support the central nervous system.[1] Is ashwagandha really effective for all these disparate medical concerns? It is important to review what researchers have learned.

Kills Cancer Cells

In a study published in 2010 in *Immunological Investigations,* researchers from India and Libya tested the ability of ashwagandha to kill colon cancer in mice. The researchers began by injecting azoxymethane in Swiss albino mice once a week for 28 days. This caused the mice to develop colon cancer. The mice were then treated orally with 400 mg/kg body weight of ashwagandha extract once a week for four weeks. At the end of the trial, when the mice were sacrificed, the researchers found that the ashwagandha was killing cancer cells. They concluded that ashwagandha "could be useful in the treatment of colon cancer."[2]

Reduces Blood Sugar Levels

In a study published in 2010 in *Plant Foods for Human Nutrition,* researchers from India and Korea examined the ability of extracts of ashwagandha roots and leaves to lower elevated blood glucose levels in diabetic rats. The researchers began by designating six rats to serve as controls. Then, they used a compound (alloxan) to induce diabetes in 36 rats, and they subdivided the rats into various groups. Over the course of eight weeks, the rats received different amounts of ashwagandha; one group took an oral medication for diabetes—glibenclamide. The researchers found that both forms of ashwagandha as well as glibenclamide lowered the elevated sugar levels to a normal range. And, they concluded that their findings presented evidence that ashwagandha "may play a vital role in reduction of blood glucose level in alloxan-induced diabetic rats."[3]

Improve Cognitive Functioning

In a study published in 2010 in the *Indian Journal of Biochemistry and Biophysics,* researchers from India investigated the ability of ashwagandha to ease the cognitive problems rats have when exposed to propoxur, a commonly used insecticide. The researchers began by dividing rats into four groups of eight rats. The rats in the first group served as the control. They were treated with olive oil. The rats in the second group were treated with propoxur dissolved in olive oil. The rats in the third group were treated with propoxur and ashwagandha. And, the rats in the fourth group were treated only with ashwagandha. The researchers found that ashwagandha gave the rats a degree of defense against the cognitive damage caused by propoxur. And, they concluded that "it may be suggested that *W. somnifera* [ashwagandha] has a neuroprotective effect."[4]

Improvement in Symptoms from Parkinson's Disease

In a study published in 2009 in the *Journal of Ethnopharmacology,* researchers from Tamilnadu, India, noted that ashwagandha has been proven to help "neural growth and locomotor function." So, they wondered if it might be useful for people dealing with the symptoms of Parkinson's disease. The researchers began by dividing mice into three groups of six mice. The mice in the first group received no treatment; they served as the control. The mice in the second group were injected with a compound (1-methyl-4-phenyl-1,2,3,6-tetrahydropyridine; MPTP) to induce Parkinson's disease. And, the mice in the third group were injected with MPTP and were treated with ashwagandha. The researchers found that ashwagandha improved the symptoms associated with Parkinson's disease, and they noted that ashwagandha could be considered a potential drug for treating this debilitating disorder.[5]

Reduces Anxiety

In a study published in 2009 in *PLoS ONE,* researchers from Canada wanted to learn if ashwagandha could play a role in the treatment of anxiety. The researchers randomly assigned people who have experienced moderate to severe anxiety for longer than six weeks to receive one of two forms of treatment. One group, which included 40 participants, received standardized psychotherapy, training in deep-breathing techniques, and a placebo; the members of the other group, which included 41 participants, had ashwagandha supplementation, dietary counseling, training in deep-breathing relaxation techniques, and multivitamins. The researchers followed the 75 participants (93%) who completed the trial for eight or more weeks.

The participants in both forms of therapy had significant lowering of their levels of anxiety. However, when the two groups were compared, the researchers found "a significant decrease in anxiety levels in the NC group [naturopathic care—the group that included ashwagandha supplementation] over the PT group [standardized psychotherapy intervention]." Furthermore, "significant improvements in secondary quality of life measures were also observed in the NC group compared to PT."[6]

Kidney Protection

In a study published in 2009 in *Renal Failure,* researchers from India tested the ability of ashwagandha to protect rat kidneys harmed by gentamicin, a broad-spectrum antibiotic. The researchers began by dividing rats into several different groups. Rats in the first group served as the control. Rats in groups two to four were, respectively, administered three different doses of ashwagandha (250, 500, and 750 mg/kg) for 14 days. Rats in the fifth group were treated with gentamicin. Then, rats in groups six through eight were first, respectively, treated with 250, 500, and 750 mg/kg of ashwagandha for 14 days. That was followed by 8 days of treatment with gentamicin. Though the gentamicin-treated rats had evidence of kidney toxicity, the rats treated with 500 mg/kg ashwagandha experienced significant reverses in these changes. The researchers concluded that ashwagandha protects kidney cells, "which could be by enhancing antioxidant activity with natural antioxidants and scavenging the free radicals."[7]

Effects on Physical Performance and Cardiorespiratory Endurance

In a study published in 2010 in the *International Journal of Ayurveda Research,* researchers from India investigated the ability of ashwagandha and another herb (arjuna) to improve physical performance and cardiorespiratory endurance. The researchers randomly divided 40 men and women, between the ages of 18 and 25, into one of four groups. Ten volunteers, who served as controls, received capsules with flour. One group of 10 took ashwagandha supplements; one group of 10 took arjuna supplements; and, a final group of 10 took both supplements. At the end of eight weeks, the researchers found that ashwagandha was useful for "generalized weakness and to improve speed and lower limb muscular strength and neuromuscular coordination."[8]

Enhancing Immunity

In a study published in 2009 in *The Journal of Alternative and Complementary Medicine,* researchers from Portland, Oregon, tested the ability of ashwagandha to enhance immunity. The researchers began by taking blood samples from five healthy volunteers—three female and two male—with a mean age of 26. This enabled the researchers to establish a baseline for immune cell level. For the next four days, the volunteers consumed two teaspoons of an alcohol and water extract of ashwagandha in eight ounces of cow's milk twice daily. In order to detect differences in the cells, bloods were drawn after 24 hours and again after 96 hours. The researchers found a statistically significant overall increase in the level of white blood cell activation, which means the body experienced enhanced immunity. The researchers concluded that their findings "suggest that Ashwagandha stimulates a clinically relevant augmentation of the immune response by increasing the activation state and population of certain immune effector cells. The mechanisms reported herein suggest clinical benefits including prophylaxis and treatment of infectious disease, especially against viruses and other intracellular parasites."[9]

Is Ashwagandha Beneficial?

From a review of the research (primarily on animal models), there is some good evidence that ashwagandha may well be effective for a wide variety of health concerns. Indeed, there are countries, such as India, in which it is widely used. Ashwagandha may be an herb to discuss with medical providers.

Notes

1. Memorial Sloan-Kettering Cancer Center Website. www.mskcc.org.
2. Muralikrishnan, G., A. K. Dinda, and F. Shakeel. 2010. "Immunomodulatory Effects of *Withania somnifera* on Azoxymethane Induced Experimental Colon Cancer in Mice." *Immunological Investigations* 39(7): 688–698.
3. Udayakumar, R., S. Kasthurirengan, A. Vasudevan, et al. June 2010. "Antioxidant Effect of Dietary Supplement *Withania somnifera* L. Reduce Blood Glucose Levels in Alloxan-Induced Diabetic Rats." *Plant Foods for Human Nutrition* 65(2): 91–98.
4. Yadav, C. S., V. Kumar, S. G. Suke, et al. April 2010. "Propoxur-Induced Acetylcholine Esterase Inhibition and Impairment of Cognitive Function: Attenuation by *Withania somnifera*." *Indian Journal of Biochemistry and Biophysics* 47(2): 117–120.
5. RajaSankar, S., T. Manivasagam, V. Sankar, et al. September 2009. "*Withania somnifera* Root Extract Improves Catecholamines and Physiological Abnormalities Seen in a Parkinson's Disease Model." *Journal of Ethnopharmacology* 125(3): 369–373.

6. Cooley, K., O. Szczurko, D. Perri, et al. August 2009. "Naturopathic Care for Anxiety: A Randomized Controlled Trial ISRCTN78958974." *PLoS ONE* 4(8): e6628.

7. Jeyanthi, T. and P. Subramanian. 2009. "Nephroprotective Effect of *Withania somnifera*: A Dose-Dependent Study." *Renal Failure* 31(9): 814–821.

8. Sandhu, Jaspal, Biren Shah, Shweta Shenoy, et al. July–September 2010. "Effects of *Withania somnifera* (Ashwagandha) and *Terminalia arjuna* (Arjuna) on Physical Performance and Cardiorespiratory Endurance in Healthy Young Adults." *International Journal of Ayurveda Research* 1(3): 144–149.

9. Mikolai, Jeremy, Andrew Erlandsen, Andrew Murison, et al. April 2009. "*In Vivo* Effects of Ashwagandha (*Withania somnifera*) Extract on the Activation of Lymphocytes." *The Journal of Alternative and Complementary Medicine* 15(4): 432–430.

References and Resources

Magazines, Journals, and Newspapers

Cooley, K., O. Szczurko, D. Perri, et al. August 2009. "Naturopathic Care for Anxiety: A Randomized Controlled Trial ISRCTN78958974." *PLoS ONE* 4(8): e6628.

Jeyanthi, T. and P. Subramanian. 2009. "Nephroprotective Effect of *Withania somnifera*: A Dose-Dependent Study." *Renal Failure* 31(9): 814–821.

Mikolai, Jeremy, Andrew Erlandsen, Andrew Murison, et al. April 2009. "In Vivo Effects of Ashwagandha (*Withania somnifera*) Extract on the Activation of Lymphocytes." *The Journal of Alternative and Complementary Medicine* 15(4): 423–430.

Muralikrishnan, G., A.K. Dinda, and F. Shakeel. 2010. "Immunomodulatory Effects of *Withania somnifera* on Azoxymethane Induced Experimental Colon Cancer in Mice." *Immunological Investigations* 39(7): 688–698.

RajaSankar, S., T. Manivasagam, V. Sankar, et al. September 2009. "*Withania somnifera* Root Extract Improves Catecholamines and Physiological Abnormalities Seen in a Parkinson's Disease Model Mouse." *Journal of Ethnopharmacology* 125(3): 369–373.

Sandhu, Jaspal, Biren Shah, Shweta Shenoy, et al. July–September 2010. "Effects of *Withania somnifera* (Ashwagandha) and *Terminalia arjuna* (Arjuna) on Physical Performance and Cardiorespiratory Endurance in Health Young Adults." *International Journal of Ayurveda Research* 1(3): 144–149.

Udayakumar, R., S. Kasthurirengan, A. Vasudevan, et al. June 2010. "Antioxidant Effect of Dietary Supplement *Withania somnifera* L. Reduce Blood Glucose Levels in Alloxan-Induced Diabetic Rats." *Plant Foods for Human Nutrition* 65(2): 91–98.

Yadav, C.S., V. Kumar, S.G. Suke, et al. April 2010. "Propoxur-Induced Ace-tylcholine Esterase Inhibition and Impairment of Cognitive Function: Attenu-ation by *Withania somnifera*." *Indian Journal of Biochemistry and Biophysics* 47(2): 117–120.

Website
Memorial Sloan-Kettering Cancer Center. www.mskcc.org.

Astragalus Root 🌱

Scientifically known as *Astragalus membranaceus,* the Chinese have con-sidered astragalus root to be a treatment for colds, respiratory infections, and the flu for at least 2,000 years. The Chinese, who believe that astraga-lus root stimulates the immune system, use astragalus root to prepare a hot water extract known as decoction.

However, astragalus root is also thought to have many more health bene-fits. It has been reported to be useful for diabetes, arthritis, asthma, nervous and liver conditions, blood pressure, breast and lung cancer, hepatitis, and cardiovascular problems. Astragalus root is even believed to be helpful for those dealing with overall weakness and fibromyalgia. Is astragalus really as effective as some people contend? Is there any serious scientific proof for these seemingly limitless claims? It is important to review what the re-searchers, who generally live and work in China, have learned.

Cardiovascular Disease

In a study published in 2009 in *Chinese Medicine,* researchers from China investigated the use of astragaloside IV, one of the main active ingredi-ents in astragalus root, on cardiovascular parameters in rats with long-term heart failure. Most of the rats, which were divided into several groups, re-ceived varying amounts of astragaloside IV. But, one group was placed on quinapril, a medication used to treat high blood pressure and heart failure and another group was given normal saline (salt water). All aspects of the trial took five weeks to complete.

The researchers found that astragaloside IV and quinapril improved car-diovascular parameters in the rats. For example, both the herb and the med-ication "suppressed the incidence of apoptotic myocytes [death of muscle cells, such as the muscle cells in the heart]."[1] This is an important finding. It means that this widely available herb may be useful for treating rats, and possibly people, with chronic heart failure, a difficult condition to manage.

Inhibits the Growth of Cancer Cells

In a study published in 2007 in *Carcinogenesis,* researchers from China and the United Kingdom combined human colon cancer cells with astragalus root saponins. (Saponins are phytochemicals that are found in most vegetables, beans, and herbs.) The researchers observed that the astragalus root inhibited cell proliferation and promoted apoptosis or cell death. When they studied the use of astragalus against colon cancer cells in mice, they found it to be comparable to a conventional chemotherapeutic medication. This was accomplished without the side effects, such as weight loss, that commonly occur with conventional chemotherapy. The researchers concluded that astragalus saponins "could be an effective chemotherapeutic agent in colon cancer treatment . . . [and] might also be used as an adjuvant in combination with other orthodox chemotherapeutic drugs to reduce the side effects of the latter compounds."[2]

In a study published in 2009 in *Phytomedicine: International Journal of Phytotherapy and Phytopharmacology*, researchers from China described the research they conducted on the ability of swainsonine, an extract from astragalus root, to kill C6 glioma cells. (A glioma is a primary brain tumor that begins in the brain or spinal cord.) In their in vitro testing, they treated C6 glioma cells with swainsonine; they observed that swainsonine inhibited the growth of cancer cells. In their in vivo testing, the researchers gave rats with glioma varying doses of swainsonine; they found that the weight of the tumor decreased. The researchers wrote that "swainsonine could inhibit the proliferation of C6 glioma cells *in vitro* and the growth of C6 glioma *in vivo*."[3]

Peripheral Nerve Regeneration

In a study published in 2010 in the *Journal of Trauma: Injury, Infection, and Critical Care,* researchers from Taiwan completed in vitro and in vivo investigations of the effect of astragalus on the regrowth of peripheral nerves. In both the cell studies and the trials with rats, there appeared to be a strong association between astragalus root and the regeneration of peripheral nerves. As a result, the researchers noted that astragalus root extract "can be a potential nerve growth-promoting factor." Nevertheless, the researchers cautioned that "further studies must be performed to delineate the mechanisms of *AM* [*Astragalus membranaceus*], to determine which components may contribute to the acceleration of the growth of nerves."[4]

Wound Healing

In a study published in 2009 in *Methods & Findings in Experimental & Clinical Pharmacology,* researchers from Seoul, Korea created wounds on the backs of anesthetized rats. Then, they evaluated the ability of astragalus root to help the wounds heal. When compared to the controls, the researchers observed that the astragalus root "significantly accelerated cutaneous [skin] healing by suppressing inflammation and stimulating basal cell growth."[5]

Lower Sugar Levels in Insulin Resistance and Type 2 Diabetes

In a study published in 2009 in *Phytomedicine: International Journal of Phytotherapy and Phytopharmacology*, researchers from China and Oklahoma City, Oklahoma, attempted to determine if astragalus polysaccharide (APS), a component of astragalus root, could lower levels of blood sugar both in a cell model and in mice with diet-induced insulin resistance. Following eight weeks, the researchers found that APS did indeed lower levels of blood sugar in both the cell model and the mice. The researchers concluded that their findings demonstrated that "APS has beneficial effects on insulin resistance and hyperglycemia [high levels of sugar in the blood]."[6]

In another study published in 2010 in the *Journal of Ethnopharmacology,* researchers from China treated 12-week-old diabetic and nondiabetic mice with APS. The trial continued for 8 weeks. The mice treated with APS had lower levels of hyperglycermia (elevated sugar) and insulin resistance. At the same time, APS did not have any effect on the nondiabetic mice. The researchers concluded that APS could become a component of the treatment for type 2 diabetes.[7]

Seasonal Allergic Rhinitis

In a double-blind, placebo-controlled clinical trial published in 2010 in *Phytotherapy Research,* researchers from Zagreb, Croatia investigated the efficiency and safety of using Lectranal, an herbal and mineral complex (HMC) with astragalus root as an active component, for seasonal allergic rhinitis

(SAR). The trial, which continued for 6 weeks, included 48 adults with moderate to severe SAR. When compared to the placebo, Lectranal "significantly decreased the intensity of rhinorrhea [runny nose] while for other primary efficacy variables the treatment groups did not differ." On the other hand, the researchers noted that "investigators and patients equally judged the treatment with HMC as more efficacious." Moreover, "the analysis of changes from baseline inside the groups for TSS [the symptom score], QoL [quality of life] and four main symptoms of SAR were strikingly in favor of active treatment." To bring more clarity to these results, the researchers recommended that their trial be followed by larger, multicenter trials.[8]

Is Astragalus Root Beneficial?

Astragalus root certainly seems to have a number of benefits.

Still, there have been reports of side effects, such as dehydration, belly bloating, and loose stools. Since some contend that astragalus root may interfere with blood clotting, it should not be used before surgery or by people who take aspirin or blood-thinning medications.

But, there are other people who should use astragalus root with even greater caution. Because astragalus may lower blood pressure, people on blood pressure medications who take astragalus root need to be monitored carefully. And, because it may lower blood sugar, people with type 2 diabetes who take astragalus should watch their sugar levels very closely.[9] If you are taking astragalus root, be sure to tell your medical provider.

There are some people who should simply avoid this herb. Astragalus root should not be used by people with autoimmune disorders, such as celiac disease, Crohn's disease, multiple sclerosis, rheumatoid arthritis, lupus, and psoriasis. Furthermore, unless a medical provider feels an exception is warranted, people on medications to suppress the immune system, such as corticosteroids, should not take astragalus root.

Notes

1. Zhao, Zhuanyou, Weiting Wang, Fang Wang, et al. April 2009. "Effects of Astragaloside IV on Heart Failure in Rats." *Chinese Medicine* 4(6): 6+.
2. Tin, Mandy M. Y., Chi-Hin Cho, Kelvin Chan, et al. 2007. "*Astragalus* Saponins Induce Growth Inhibition and Apoptosis in Human Colon Cancer Cells and Tumor Xenograft." *Carcinogenesis* 28(6): 1347–1355.
3. Sun, Ji-Yuan, Hao Yang, Shan Miao, et al. November 2009. "Suppressive Effects of Swainsonine on C6 Glioma Cell *In Vitro* and *In Vivo*." *Phytomedicine: International Journal of Phytotherapy and Phytopharmacology* 16(11): 1070–1074.

4. Lu, Ming-Chin, Chun-Hsu Yao, Ssu-Hung Wang, et al. February 2010. "Effect of *Astragalus membranaceus* in Rats on Peripheral Nerve Regeneration: In Vitro and In Vivo Studies." *Journal of Trauma: Injury, Infection, and Critical Care* 68(2): 434–440.

5. Han, D. O., H. J. Lee, and D. H. Hahm. March 2009. "Wound-Healing Activity of Astragali Radix in Rats." *Methods & Findings in Experimental & Clinical Pharmacology* 31(2): 95–100.

6. Mao, Xian-qing, Feng Yu, Nian Wang, et al. May 2009. "Hypoglycemia Effect of Polysaccharide Enriched Extract of *Astragalus membranaceus* in Diet Induced Insulin Resistant C57BL/6J Mice and Its Potential Mechanism." *Phytomedicine: International Journal of Phytotherapy and Phytopharmacology* 16(5): 416–425.

7. Liu, M., K. Wu, X. Mao, et al. January 2010. "Astragalus Polysaccharide Improves Insulin Sensitivity in KKAy Mice: Regulation of PKB/GLUT4 Signaling in Skeletal Muscle." *Journal of Ethnopharmacology* 127(1): 32–37.

8. Matkovic, Zinka, Visnja Zivkovic, Mirna Korica, et al. February 2010. "Efficacy and Safety of *Astragalus membranaceus* in the Treatment of Patients with Seasonal Allergic Rhinitis." *Phytotherapy Research* 24(2): 175–181.

9. American Cancer Society Website. www.cancer.org.

References and Resources

Magazines, Journals, and Newspapers

Han, D. O., H. J. Lee, and D. H. Hahm. March 2009. "Wound Activity of Astragali Radix in Rats." *Methods & Findings in Experimental & Clinical Pharmacology* 31(2): 95–100.

Jiang, Jun-Bing, Jian-Dong Qiu, Li-Hua Yang, et al. October 2010. "Therapeutic Effects of Astragalus Polysaccharides on Inflammation and Synovial Apoptosis in Rats with Adjuvant-Induced Arthritis." *International Journal of Rheumatic Diseases* 13(4): 396–405.

Liu, M., K. Wu, X. Mao, et al. January 2010. "Astragalus Polysaccharide Improves Insulin Sensitivity in KKAy Mice: Regulation of PKB/GLUT4 Signaling in Skeletal Muscle." *Journal of Ethnopharmacology* 127(1): 32–37.

Lu, Ming-Chin, Chun-Hsu Yao, Ssu-Hung Wang, et al. February 2010. "Effect of *Astragalus membranaceus* in Rats on Peripheral Nerve Regeneration: In Vitro and In Vivo Studies." *Journal of Trauma: Injury, Infection, and Critical Care* 68(2): 434–440.

Mao, Xian-qing, Feng Yu, Nian Wang, et al. May 2009. "Hypoglycemic Effect of Polysaccharide Enriched Extract of *Astragalus membranaceus* in Diet Induced Insulin Resistant C57BL/6J Mice and Its Potential Mechanism." *Phytomedicine: International Journal of Phytotherapy and Phytopharmacology* 16(5): 416–425.

Matkovic, Zinka, Visnja Zivkovic, Mirna Korica, et al. February 2010. "Efficacy and Safety of *Astragalus membranaceus* in the Treatment of Patients with Seasonal Allergic Rhinitis." *Phytotherapy Research* 24(2): 175–181.

Sun, Ji-Yuan, Hao Yang, Shan Miao, et al. November 2009. "Suppressive Effects of Swainsonine on C6 Glioma Cell *In Vitro* and *In Vivo.*" *Phytomedicine: International Journal of Phytotherapy and Phytopharmacology* 16(11): 1070–1074.

Tin, Mandy M. Y., Chi-Hin Cho, Kelvin Chan, et al. 2007. "*Astragalus* Saponins Induce Growth Inhibition and Apoptosis in Human Colon Cancer Cells and Tumor Xenograft." *Carcinogenesis* 28(6): 1347–1355.

Tyler, Varro E. January 2001. "Move Over, Echinacea!" *Prevention* 53(1): 95.

Zhao, Zhuanyou, Weiting Wang, Fang Wang, et al. April 2009. "Effects of Astragaloside IV on Heart Failure in Rats." *Chinese Medicine* 4(6): 6+.

Website

American Cancer Society. www.cancer.org.

B

Bacopa 🌿

Scientifically known as *Bacopa monnieri,* bacopa has been used for centuries in Ayurveda medicine, a holistic system of medicine that was founded in India. In fact, it is known that bacopa was referenced in a number of different ancient Ayurveda documents.

Bacopa is thought to be useful for a wide variety of medical problems. It is probably best known as an herb that may improve memory and the ability to concentrate. But, bacopa is also believed to be effective for anxiety, depression, and gastrointestinal upset.[1] It is important to review what researchers have learned.

Improves Cognitive Skills

In a randomized, placebo-controlled, double-blind trial published in 2010 in *The Journal of Alternative & Complementary Medicine,* researchers from Australia investigated the ability of bacopa to improve memory in older men and women. Initially, the cohort consisted of 98 healthy subjects between the ages of 55 and 86. For 12 weeks, they took either 300 mg bacopa per day or a placebo. Eighty-one subjects completed the trial. The researchers found that bacopa "significantly improved verbal learning, memory acquisition, and delayed recall." However, the researchers noted that bacopa "caused gastrointestinal side-effects of increased stool frequency, abdominal cramps, and nausea."[2]

In a study published in 2010 in the *Journal of Ethnopharmacology,* researchers from Thailand examined the effect of the administration of different doses of bacopa on rats before they are treated with a compound (ethylcholine aziridinium ion; AF64A) that causes symptoms seen in

Alzheimer's disease. The researchers found that the rats on bacopa had better spatial memory and an improved ability to navigate a maze. Apparently, the cholinergic neurons in the rats on bacopa produced more acetylcholine, a neurotransmitter in the brain that is chronically in short supply in people with Alzheimer's disease. The researchers commented that bacopa "could mitigate the memory impairment and the degeneration of neurons in hippocampus in animal models of Alzheimer's disease induced by AF46A." As a result, "this plant is a valuable candidate for cognitive enhances and neuroprotective agent in Alzheimer's disease."[3]

In an open-label, nonrandomized, prospective, uncontrolled trial published in 2011 in the *International Journal of Collaborative Research on Internal Medicine & Public Health,* researchers from India and Michigan (United States) evaluated the ability of bacopa to be useful for people with Alzheimer's disease. The cohort consisted of people who were newly diagnosed with Alzheimer's disease. Everyone took 300 mg of bacopa twice a day for six months. Thirty-nine people completed the trial; their mean age was 65.23. The researchers found that there was a significant improvement in a number of different components, such as "orientation of time, place and person," and in skills, such as reading, writing, and comprehension. They observed that the bacopa treatment resulted in "improvement in some aspects of cognitive function in geriatric patients suffering from Alzheimer's disease."[4]

In a randomized, double-blind, placebo-controlled trial published in 2008 in *Phytotherapy Research,* researchers from Australia and the United Kingdom examined the cognitive-enhancing effects of bacopa. Although the trial initially included 107 healthy subjects, 62 people actually completed the study. Of these, 33 were in the treatment group (9 males and 24 females, mean age of 41.6) and 29 were in the placebo group (12 males and 17 females, mean age of 44.3). After 90 days, the researchers found that bacopa did indeed have a cognitive-enhancing effect.[5]

Useful for Pain from Rheumatoid Arthritis

In a study published in 2010 in *Phytotherapy Research,* researchers from India wanted to learn if bacopa is useful for the pain associated with rheumatoid arthritis. They began by inducing rheumatoid arthritis in rats. That "significantly increased paw swelling compared to normal rats." After 14 days, the researchers treated some of the rats with bacopa. At the end of 60 days, the researchers learned that the administration of bacopa "significantly decreased the clinical signs of this disease, improved the arthritic index compared with arthritis control rats, [thus] indicating its protective effect." The researchers concluded that bacopa "possesses remarkable antiarthritic activity."[6]

Treatment for Anxiety and Depression

In a study published in 2010 in the *Indian Journal of Experimental Biology,* researchers from India assessed the use of bacopa and American Ginseng in mice that were given tasks that result in anxiety and depression. The researchers found that both herbs—bacopa at a dose of 80 mg/kg and American Ginseng at a dose of 100 mg/kg—"were effective as an anti-anxiety as well as anti-depressant activity." And, this goal was accomplished "without impairing the neuromuscular tone." The researchers concluded that "these extracts can be used as a potent therapeutic agent in treating mixed anxiety-depressive disorder."[7]

Protective Against Medical Problems Associated with Strokes

In a study published in 2010 in *Pharmacology, Biochemistry and Behavior,* researchers from India and Galveston, Texas wanted to learn if bacopa provided protection against strokes in Wistar rats. The researchers began by dividing rats into various groups; then, strokes were induced in the rats in all but one of the groups. Before a number of behavioral tests were conducted, the rats were fed different doses of bacopa for several days. The researchers learned that the bacopa reduced the infarct size and it improved neurological scores. According to the researchers, their findings "clearly suggest a protective effect" of bacopa. The researchers concluded that bacopa "attenuates the ischemia induced memory and other neurological deficits including infarct size by exerting antioxidant effects."[8]

Useful for Morphine-Induced Toxicity of the Liver and Kidneys

In a study published in 2009 in *Phytomedicine: International Journal of Phytotherapy and Phytopharmacology,* researchers from India investigated the ability of bacopa to provide a level of protection to the livers and kidneys of rats that are chronically exposed to morphine. The researchers began by dividing the rats into four groups. The rats in the first group were untreated. So, they served as controls. The rats in the other three groups were treated with morphine, or morphine and bacopa, or only bacopa. After

21 days, the rats were sacrificed. The researchers then learned that the bacopa "exerted a protection against morphine-induced liver and kidney toxicity."[9]

Protective against Nicotine-Induced Toxicity

In a study published in 2007 in *Phytotherapy Research,* researchers from India wanted to determine if bacopa could help reduce the toxicity caused by nicotine in mice. The researchers divided their mice into three groups. The mice in the first group, which served as the control, were treated with saline; the mice in the second group were treated with nicotine; and the mice in the third group were treated with bacopa and nicotine. The researchers found that bacopa "exerted protective effects by modulating the extent of lipid peroxidation and enhancing the antioxidant status."[10]

Is Bacopa Beneficial?

While bacopa is probably most useful as an herb that improves cognition, from a review of the literature, it is apparent that it may well assist with other health problems. Still, in at least one study, some of the subjects experienced bacopa-related gastrointestinal problems.

Notes

1. Gohil, Kashmira and Jagruti Patel. January–March 2010. "A Review on *Bacopa monniera*: Current Research and Future Prospects." *International Journal of Green Pharmacy* 4(1): 1–9.
2. Morgan, A. and J. Stevens. July 2010. "Does *Bacopa monnieri* Improve Memory Performance in Older Persons? Results of a Randomized, Placebo-Controlled, Double-Blind Trial." *The Journal of Alternative & Complementary Medicine* 16(7): 753–759.
3. Uabundit, N., S. Wattanathorn, S. Mucimapura, and K. Ingkaninan. January 2010. "Cognitive Enhancement and Neuroprotective Effects of *Bacopa monnieri* in Alzheimer's Disease Model." *Journal of Ethnopharmacology* 127(1): 26–31.
4. Goswami, Shiashir, Anand Saoji, Navneet Kumar, et al. March 2011. "Effect of *Bacopa monnieri* on Cognitive Functions in Alzheimer's Disease Patients." *International Journal of Collaborative Research on Internal Medicine & Public Health* 3(3): 179.
5. Stough, Con, Luke A. Downey, Jenny Lloyd, et al. 2008. "Examining the Nootropic Effects of a Special Extract of *Bacopa monniera* on Human Cognitive

Functioning: 90 Day Double-Blind Placebo-Controlled Randomized Trial." *Phytotherapy Research* 22: 1629–1634.

6. Vijayan, V., S. K. Kavitha, and A. Helen. September 2010. "*Bacopa monnieri* (L.) Wettst Inhibits Type II Collagen-Induced Arthritis in Rats." *Phytotherapy Research* 24(9): 1377–1383.

7. Chatterjee, M., P. Verma, and G. Palit. March 2010. "Comparative Evaluation of *Bacopa monniera* and *Panax quniquefolium* in Experimental Anxiety and Depressive Models in Mice." *Indian Journal of Experimental Biology* 48(3): 306–313.

8. Saraf, Manish Kumar, Sudesh Prabhakar, and Akshay Anand. 2010. "Neuroprotective Effect of *Bacopa monniera* on Ischemia Induced Brain Injury." *Pharmacology, Biochemistry and Behavior* 97: 192–197.

9. Sumathi, T. and S. Niranjali Devaraj. 2009. "Effect of *Bacopa monniera* on Liver and Kidney Toxicity in Chronic Use of Opioids." *Phytomedicine: International Journal of Phytotherapy and Phytopharmacology* 16: 897–903.

10. Vijayan, Viji and A. Helen. April 2007. "Protective Activity of *Bacopa monniera* Linn. on Nicotine-Induced Toxicity in Mice." *Phytotherapy Research* 21: 378–381.

References and Resources

Magazines, Journals, and Newspapers

Chatterjee, M., P. Verma, and G. Palit. March 2010. "Comparative Evaluation of *Bacopa monniera* and *Panax quniquefolium* in Experimental Anxiety and Depressive Models in Mice." *Indian Journal of Experimental Biology* 48(3): 306–313.

Erikson, Kim. May 2009. "Bacopa: Brains & Beauty: Known as One of the Best Herbs for Better Mental Function, Bacopa Also Offers Beauty Benefits." *Better Nutrition* 71(5): 30.

Gohil, Kashmira and Jagruti Patel. January–March 2010. "A Review on *Bacopa monniera*: Current Research and Future Prospects." *International Journal of Green Pharmacy* 4(1): 1–9.

Goswami, Shiashir, Anand Saoji, Navneet Kumar, et al. March 2011. "Effect of *Bacopa monnieri* on Cognitive Functions in Alzheimer's Disease Patients." *International Journal of Collaborative Research on Internal Medicine & Public Health* 3(3): 179.

Morgan, A. and J. Stevens. July 2010. "Does *Bacopa monnieri* Improve Memory Performance in Older Persons? Results of a Randomized, Placebo-Controlled, Double-Blind trial." *The Journal of Alternative & Complementary Medicine* 16(7): 753–759.

Saraf, Manish Kumar, Sudesh Prabhakar, and Akshay Anand. 2010. "Neuroprotective Effects of *Bacopa monniera* on Ischemia Induced Brain Injury." *Pharmacology, Biochemistry and Behavior* 97: 192–197.

Stough, Con, Luke A. Downey, Jenny Lloyd, et al. 2008. "Examining the Nootropic Effects of a Special Extract of *Bacopa monniera* on Human Cognitive Functioning 90 Day Double-Blind Placebo-Controlled Randomized Trial."
Phytotherapy Research 22: 1629–1634.

Sumathi, T. and S. Niranjali Devaraj. 2009. "Effect of *Bacopa monniera* on Liver
and Kidney Toxicity in Chronic Use of Opioids." *Phytomedicine: International
Journal of Phytotherapy and Phytopharmacology* 16: 897–903.

Uabundit, N., J. Wattanathorn, S. Mucimapura, and K. Ingkaninan. January 2010.
"Cognitive Enhancement and Neuroprotective Effects of *Bacopa monnieri* in
Alzheimer's Disease Model." *Journal of Ethnopharmacology* 127(1): 26–31.

Vijayan, V. and A. Helen. April 2007. "Protective Activity of *Bacopa monniera*
Linn. on Nicotine-Induced Toxicity in Mice." *Phytotherapy Research* 21:
378–381.

Vijayan, V., S.K. Kavitha, and A. Helen. September 2010. "*Bacopa monniera*
(L.) Wettst Inhibits Type II Collagen-Induced Arthritis in Rats." *Phytotherapy
Research* 24(9): 1377–1383.

Website
American Botanical Council. www.abc.herbalgram.org.

Boswellia 👻

Scientifically known as *Boswellia serrata,* Boswellia, a truly ancient herb
that grows in India and Africa, has traditionally been used to treat arthritis,
ulcerative colitis, coughs, sores, snakebites, and asthma.[1] A 2009 article in
the *Journal of Pharmacy and Pharmacology* observed that Boswellia resin
(known as frankincense or olibanum) has medicinal properties, "mainly
in the treatment of inflammatory conditions, as well as in some cancerous
diseases, wound healing and for its antimicrobial activity." But, it may well
be useful for other health problems, such as depression.[2] It is important to
review what researchers have learned.

Anti-Aging Properties

In a randomized, double-blind, split-face study published in 2010 in *Planta
Medica,* researchers from Italy examined the "efficacy, tolerability, and
safety" of the use of a base cream containing 0.5% Boswellic acid on
photoaging facial skin. The cohort consisted of 15 female volunteers. For

30 days, the women applied the cream containing Boswellic acid to one side of their face; they applied the same cream without the Boswellic acid to the other side of their face. After 30 days, the researchers noted that they observed "a significant improvement of tactile roughness and fine lines" in the sections of the faces treated with Boswellic acid. In addition, the treated areas had demonstrated improvements in skin sebum and elasticity. After 60 days, during follow-up appointments, the improvements were still evident. The researchers concluded that their findings "seem to indicate that the topical application of BAs [Boswellic acids] may represent a suitable treatment option for selected features of skin photoaging."[3]

Osteoarthritis

In a 90-day, randomized, double-blind, placebo-controlled single-center trial published in 2008 in *Arthritis Research & Therapy,* researchers from India evaluated the safety and efficacy of 5-Loxin, a Boswellia extract supplement for people with osteoarthritis. The initial cohort consisted of 75 people with osteoarthritis. The participants received either a 100-mg or 250-mg dose of 5-Loxin or a placebo. Seventy people completed the trial. The researchers found that the 250-mg dose "significantly improved joint function and exhibited better therapeutic efficacy" than the 100-mg dose. However, as early as one week after beginning treatment, relief was obtained from both doses. The researchers also learned that 5-Loxin "is safe for human consumption, even long term."[4]

Meanwhile, in a randomized, double-blind, placebo-controlled study published in 2010 in the *International Journal of Medical Sciences,* researchers from India and California compared the ability of 5-Loxin, Aflapin (another supplement with Boswellia), and a placebo to offer relief from osteoarthritis. The initial cohort consisted of 60 people with osteoarthritis. For 90 days, the subjects took either 100 mg of 5-Loxin, 100 mg of Aflapin, or a placebo. Fifty-seven subjects completed the trial. The researchers noted that by the end of the study "both 5-Loxin® and Aflapin® conferred clinically and statistically significant improvements in pain scores and physical function scores in OA [osteoarthritis] subjects."[5]

Treatment for Collagenous Colitis

A randomized, double-blind, placebo-controlled study on treating collagenous colitis (a type of colitis that tends to occur in middle-aged women) with Boswellia extract was summarized in an article in a 2008 issue of *Phytomedicine: International Journal of Phytotherapy & Phytopharmacology.* For six weeks, researchers from Germany provided 26 patients who had chronic diarrhea and histologically proven collagenous colitis with either 400 mg of oral Boswellia extract or a placebo—three times each day. The researchers found that by the end of the trial "the proportion of patients in clinical remission was higher in the BSE [Boswellia extract] than in the placebo group." The researchers concluded that Boswellia extract "might be clinically effective in patients with collagenous colitis."[6]

Improved Memory

In a 180-day study published in 2010 in *Archives of Pharmacal Research,* researchers from Iran investigated the effects of olibanum on adult rats with memory deficits caused by hypothyroidism (insufficient levels of thyroid hormone). The researchers began by dividing male rats into four groups. The rats in the first group received tap drinking water; the rats in the second group received drinking water containing 0.03% methimazol—to induce hypothyroidism. The rats in the third and fourth groups had drinking water containing 0.03% methimazole and, respectively, 100 and 500 mg/kg olibanum. The rats were then tested in a Morris water maze. The researchers found that "the swimming speed was significantly lower and the distance and time latency were higher in group 2 compared with group 1." Moreover, "in groups 3 and 4 the swimming speed was significantly higher while the length of the swim path and time latency were significantly lower in comparison with group 2." The researchers concluded that olibanum is able to prevent the learning and memory problems rats experienced from methimazole-induced hypothyroidism.[7]

Psychiatric Benefits

In a study published in 2008 in the *FASEB Journal,* researchers from Israel and several locations in the United States administered incensole acetate, a Boswellia resin constituent, to mice. The researchers found that incensole acetate significantly affected the areas of the brain that are involved with emotions as well as the nerve circuits that respond to drugs for anxiety and depression. Apparently, the incensole acetate activated a protein known as transient receptor potential vanilloid ($TRPV_3$), which is known to be

Notes

1. Memorial Sloan-Kettering Cancer Center Website. www.mskcc.org.
2. Moussaieff, A. and R. Mechoulam. October 2009. "Boswellia Resin: From Religious Ceremonies to Medical Uses; a Review of In-Vitro, In-Vivo and Clinical Trials." *Journal of Pharmacy and Pharmacology* 61(10): 1281–1293.
3. Pedretti, A., R. Capezzera, C. Zane, et al. April 2010. "Effects of Topical Boswellic Acid on Photo and Age-Damaged Skin: Clinical, Biophysical, and Echographic Evaluations in a Double-Blind, Randomized, Split-Face Study." *Planta Medica* 76(6): 555–560.
4. Sengupta, Krishanu, Alluri V. Krishnaraju, Andey Rama Satish, et al. July 2008. "A Double Blind, Randomized, Placebo Controlled Study of the Efficacy and Safety of 5-Loxin® for Treatment of Osteoarthritis of the Knee." *Arthritis Research & Therapy* 10: R85.
5. Sengupta, Krishanu, Alluri V. Krishnaraju, Amar A. Vishal, et al. 2010. "Comparative Efficacy and Tolerability of 5-Loxin® and Aflapin® Against Osteoarthritis of the Knee: A Double Blind, Randomized, Placebo Controlled Clinical Study." *International Journal of Medical Sciences* 7: 366–377.
6. Madisch, A., S. Miehlke, O. Eichele, et al. June 2008. "*Boswellia serrata* Extract for the Treatment of Collagenous Colitis: A Double-Blind Randomized, Placebo-Controlled, Multicenter Trial." *Phytomedicine: International Journal of Phytotherapy & Phytopharmacology* 15(6–7): 543.
7. Hosseini, Mahmoud, Mosa Al-Reza Hadjzadeh, Mohammad Derakhshan, et al. March 2010. "The Beneficial Effects of Olibanum on Memory Deficit Induced by Hypothyroidism in Adult Rats Tested in Morris Water Maze." *Archives of Pharmacal Research* 33(3): 463–468.
8. Moussaieff, Arieh, Neta Rimmerman, Tatiana Bregman, et al. 2008. "Incensole Acetate, an Incense Component, Elicits Psychoactivity by Activating $TRPV_3$ Channels in the Brain." *FASEB Journal* 22: 3024–3034.
9. Houssen, M.E., A. Ragab, A. Mesbah, et al. July 2010. "Natural Anti-Inflammatory Products and Leukotriene Inhibitors as Complementary Therapy for Bronchial Asthma." *Clinical Biochemistry* 43(10–11): 887–890.
10. Kirste, S., M. Treier, S.J. Wehrle, et al. 2011. "*Boswellia serrata* Acts on Cerebral Edema in Patients Irradiated for Brain Tumors: A Prospective, Randomized, Placebo-Controlled, Double-Blind Pilot Trial." *Cancer* 117(16): 3788–3795.

References and Resources

Magazines, Journals, and Newspapers

Hosseini, Mahmoud, Mosa Al-Reza Hadjzadeh, Mohammad Derakhshan, et al. March 2010. "The Beneficial Effects of Olibanum on Memory Deficit Induced by Hypothyroidism in Adults Rates Tested in Morris Water Maze." *Archives of Pharmacal Research* 33(3): 463–468.

present in mammalian brains. Interestingly, when mice were bred to not have the protein $TRPV_3$, incensole acetate had no effect on their brains.[8]

Controls Bronchial Asthma

In a study published in 2010 in *Clinical Biochemistry,* researchers from Egypt assessed the ability of an oral capsule containing Boswellia, licorice root, and turmeric root to aid people dealing with the symptoms of asthma. The cohort consisted of 63 people, between the ages of 18 and 60, who had at least a 1 year history of chronic bronchial asthma. The cohort was divided into two groups. One received capsules containing the herbs; they were told to take the capsules three times a day for four weeks. The other groups received placebos. The findings were rather notable. The researchers wrote that "there was a high statistically significant decrease in the number of asthma exacerbations, nocturnal awakening symptoms, daytime symptoms, and need for rescue medication per week in [the] target therapy group versus placebo group, while there were no statistically significant differences in the placebo group before and after taking [the] therapy." The researchers concluded that the herb combination was "effective in reducing asthma symptoms and the frequency of attacks with a gradual control of asthma."[9]

Reduces Cerebral Edema

In a prospective, randomized, placebo-controlled, double-blind pilot trial published in 2011 in *Cancer,* researchers from Egypt examined the ability of Boswellia to lower the cerebral edema associated with radiation treatments for brain tumors. (The current treatment, dexamethasone, is a steroid with side effects.) The researchers assigned 44 patients with primary or secondary malignant brain tumors to 4,200 mg/day Boswellia or a placebo. According to the researchers, "Compared with baseline and if measured immediately after the end of radiotherapy and BS [Boswellia] treatment, a reduction of cerebral edema of >75% was found in 60% of patients receiving BS and in 26% if patients receiving a placebo." The researchers concluded that "BS could potentially be steroid-sparing for patient receiving brain irradiation."[10]

Is Boswellia Beneficial?

It would be useful if there were more studies on this herb. But, it does appear to be beneficial and may well be helpful for many people.

Houssen, M. E., A. Ragab, A. Mesbah, et al. July 2010. "Natural Anti-Inflammatory Products and Leukotriene Inhibitors as Complementary Therapy for Bronchial Asthma." *Clinical Biochemistry* 43(10–11): 887–890.

Kirste, S., M. Treier, S. J. Wehrle, et al. 2011. "*Boswellia serrata* Acts on Cerebral Edema in Patients Irradiated for Brain Tumors: A Prospective, Randomized, Placebo-Controlled, Double-Blind Pilot Trial." *Cancer* 117(16): 3788–3795.

Madisch, A., S. Miehlke, O. Eichele, et al. June 2008. "*Boswellia serrata* Extract for the Treatment of Collagenous Colitis: A Double-Blind Randomized, Placebo-Controlled Multicenter Trial." *Phytomedicine: International Journal of Phytotherapy & Phytopharmacology* 15(6–7): 543.

Moussaieff, A. and R. Mechoulam. October 2009. "Boswellia Resin: From Religious Ceremonies to Medical Uses; a Review of In-Vitro, In-Vivo and Clinical Trials." *Journal of Pharmacy and Pharmacology* 61(10): 1281–1293.

Moussaieff, Arieh, Neta Rimmerman, Tatiana Bregman, et al. 2008. "Incensole Acetate, an Incense Component, Elicits Psychoactivity by Activating $TRPV_3$ Channels in the Brain." *FASEB Journal* 22: 3024–3034.

Pedretti, A., R. Capezzera, C. Zane, et al. April 2010. "Effects of Topical Boswellic Acid on Photo and Age-Damaged Skin: Clinical, Biophysical, and Echographic Evaluations in a Double-Blind, Randomized, Split-Face Study." *Planta Medica* 76(6): 555–560.

Sengupta, Krishanu, Alluri V. Krishnaraju, Andey Rama Satish, et al. July 2008. "A Double-Blind, Randomized, Placebo Controlled Study of the Efficacy and Safety of 5-Loxin® for Treatment of Osteoarthritis of the Knee." *Arthritis Research & Therapy* 10: R85.

Sengupta, Krishanu, Alluri V. Krishnaraju, Amar A. Vishal, et al. 2010. "Comparative Efficacy and Tolerability of 5-Loxin® and Aflapin® Against Osteoarthritis of the Knee: A Double Blind, Randomized, Placebo Controlled Clinical Study." *International Journal of Medical Sciences* 7: 366–377.

Website
Memorial Sloan-Kettering Cancer Center. www.mskcc.org.

C

Cayenne Pepper

Scientifically known as *Capsicum annuum,* cayenne pepper has very high concentrations of a substance called capsaicin, which is believed to add heat and spice to foods. It is also thought to reduce pain, support cardiovascular health, and drain congested nasal passages. Also known as chili pepper, cayenne pepper has excellent amounts of vitamin A and good amounts of vitamins B, C, and K, manganese, and dietary fiber.[1] But, it is important to review what the researchers have learned.

Pain Management
In a single-center, randomized, double-blind, placebo-controlled trial published in 2008 in *Anesthesia & Analgesia,* researchers from the United States, Belgium, and Denmark investigated the ability of capsaicin to help manage postoperative pain. The cohort consisted of 41 adult male patients who had groin hernia repair surgery. During the surgery, half of the men received 1,000 μg of ultra purified capsaicin injected directly into the wound; the other half received a placebo. Other than the injection, both groups of patients received the same amount of pain medication, with equal amounts of acetaminophen and ibuprofen. The findings are notable. When compared with patients who received the placebo, the patients who received the capsaicin injection had significantly lower pain scores during the first few days after surgery. The researchers wrote that the "instillation of purified capsaicin resulted in superior analgesia to placebo with regards to average pain during the first 3 to 4 postoperative days after inguinal herniotomy."[2]

Heart Protection

In a study published in 2009 in *Circulation,* researchers from Cincinnati, Ohio, applied capsaicin to certain locations on the skin of mice that were undergoing induced heart attacks. The researchers found that this caused sensory nerves in the skin to trigger signals in the nervous system. Amazingly, these signals activated certain protective pathways, thereby protecting the heart from injury. In fact, the application of capsaicin resulted in an 85% reduction in cardiac cell death. But, the testing was conducted on mice. Would it work the same way in humans? It is not known. Still, the researchers emphasized that "topical capsaicin has no known serious adverse effects, and could be easily applied in an ambulance or emergency room setting."[3]

Lower Blood Pressure

In a study published in 2010 in *Cell Metabolism,* researchers from China, Germany, and Chapel Hill, North Carolina, tested the ability of capsaicin to lower the blood pressure of rats bred to have high blood pressure (hypertension). For seven months, researchers fed capsaicin to hypertensive rats. They found that the capsaicin activated the transient receptor potential vanilloid 1 (TRPV1) channel in the lining of the rats' blood vessels. This increased the production of nitric oxide, a gas molecule known for protecting blood vessels from inflammation and dysfunction. The researchers concluded that "TRPV1 activation through chronic dietary capsaicin may represent a promising intervention of lifestyle in high-risk populations with hypertension and related vascular disorders."[4]

Weight Loss

In a study published in 2011 in *Physiology & Behavior,* researchers from Purdue University in Indiana tested the ability of dried ground cayenne red pepper to control appetite. The cohort consisted of 25 people who were not overweight. Thirteen of the people liked spicy food; 12 did not. At various times, the subjects ate food containing 1 g of dried cayenne red pepper, the equivalent of half a teaspoon. Interestingly, the researchers found that the subjects who were not regular consumers of cayenne red peppers experienced a decrease in hunger, especially for fatty, salty, and sweet foods. But, the researchers speculated that this effect may diminish if people begin to eat this food more frequently.[5]

In a randomized, double-blind, placebo-controlled study published in 2009 in *The American Journal of Clinical Nutrition,* researchers from Japan and several locations in the United States examined "the safety and efficacy" of taking 6 mg/day of capsinoids from capsaicin "for weight loss, fat loss, and change in metabolism." Forty men and 40 women, who were all overweight or obese, were assigned to take capsinoid or placebo. At the end of 12 weeks, the researchers found that the ingestion of capsinoid appeared to be safe and well tolerated and was "associated with a loss of abdominal fat." Additionally, capsinoid ingestion was related to an increase in the oxidation of fat that was "nearly significant."[6]

In randomized, double-blind, placebo-controlled trial published in *The American Journal of Clinical Nutrition* in 2010, researchers from Baton Rouge, Louisiana, examined the acute and chronic effect of dihydrocapsiate (a capsinoid similar to capsaicin, which is found in chili peppers) on the resting metabolic rate in humans. The researchers began by assigning 78 healthy men to one of three groups. For 28 days, the members of one group took 3 mg dihydrocapsiate per day; the members of the second group took 9 mg dihydrocapsiate per day; and the members of the third group took placebos. The researchers wrote that they "observed no significant increase in metabolic rate after acute consumption of dihydrocapsiate." It was only after they combined the results from the two dihydrocapsiate-consuming groups that a modest increase in metabolic rate could be seen. The researchers noted that "a small but consistent increase in energy expenditure will help individuals maintain body weight, if not lose weight."[7]

Treatment for Irritable Bowel Syndrome

In a randomized, double-blind study published in 2011 in *Digestive Diseases and Sciences,* researchers from Italy wanted to learn if red pepper powder could help the millions of people dealing with irritable bowel syndrome. The researchers began with 50 men and women, between the ages of 18 and 65, with irritable bowel syndrome. After a two-week washout period, 23 people took four pills per day that contained 150 mg of red pepper powder (0.50 mg of capsaicin). The pills had a special coating that enabled them to remain intact until they reached the colon, thus avoiding the possibility of absorption in the small intestine. Twenty-seven people were given placebos. For the next six weeks, the participants recorded daily scores of their levels of abdominal pain and bloating.

During the course of the trial, eight people dropped out; six were taking the red pepper and two were on placebos. Additionally, because of abdominal pain, eight people reduced their dosage to two pills per day. Still, by the end of the study, the "red pepper group scored significantly better than placebo." The researchers commented that their results found "that the chronic administration of red pepper powder in IBS patients with enteric-coated pills was significantly more effective than placebo in decreasing the intensity of abdominal pain and bloating and was considered by patients more effective than placebo."[8]

Kills Pancreatic Cancer Cells

In a study published in 2008 in *Apoptosis,* researchers from Pittsburgh, Pennsylvania, and Amarillo, Texas, conducted in vitro and in vivo research on the ability of capsaicin to kill pancreatic cancer cells. In their in vitro studies, the researchers treated human pancreatic cancer cells with capsaicin. They found that the capsaicin triggered apoptosis or cell death, without having any negative impact on the normal pancreatic cells. Similar results were obtained from their in vivo studies in which mice with pancreatic cancer xenografts were orally treated with capsaicin. According to the researchers, the "oral administration of capsaicin significantly suppressed the growth of pancreatic tumor xenograft by inducing apoptosis of the tumor cells" in a manner similar to what their observed in their in vitro studies. The researchers concluded that their findings "provide a rational for the development of capsaicin as [a] chemotherapeutic agent against pancreatic cancer in the clinical setting."[9]

Is Cayenne Pepper Beneficial?

Cayenne pepper may well have a number of benefits. For those who enjoy spicier foods, cayenne pepper may be a wonderful addition to the diet. At the very least, capsaicin appears to be useful for pain. And, products containing capsaicin are readily available in over-the-counter topical creams, gels, and patches.

Notes

1. The George Mateljan Foundation Website. www.whfoods.com.
2. Asavang, E. K., J. B. Hansen, J. Malmstrøm, et al. July 2008. "The Effect of Wound Instillation of a Novel Purified Capsaicin Formulation on Postherni-

otomy Pain: A Double-Blind, Randomized, Placebo-Controlled Study." *Anesthesia & Analgesia* 107(1): 282–291.

3. Jones, W. Keith, Guo-Chang Fan, Siyun Liao, et al. 2009. "Peripheral Nociception Associated with Surgical Incision Elicits Remote Nonischemic Cardioprotection via Neurogenic Activation of Protein Kinase C Signaling." *Circulation* 120: S1–S9.

4. Yang, Dachun, Zhidan Luo, Shauangtao Ma, et al. August 2010. "Activation of TRPV1 by Dietary Capsaicin Improves Endothelium-Dependent Vasorelaxation and Prevents Hypertension." *Cell Metabolism* 12(2): 130–141.

5. Ludy, Mary-Jon and Richard D. Mattes. March 2011. "The Effects of Hedonically Acceptable Red Pepper Doses on Thermogenesis and Appetite." *Physiology & Behavior* 102(3–4): 251–258.

6. Snitker, S., Y. Fujishima, H. Shen, et al. January 2009. "Effects of Novel Capsinoid Treatment on Fatness and Energy Metabolism in Humans: Possible Pharmacogenetic Implications." *The American Journal of Clinical Nutrition* 89(1): 45–50.

7. Galgani, Jose E. and Eric Ravussin. November 2010. "Effect of Dihydrocapsiate on Resting Metabolic Rate in Humans." *The American Journal of Clinical Nutrition* 92(5): 1089–1093.

8. Bortolotti, M. and S. Porta. 2011. "Effect of Red Pepper on Symptoms of Irritable Bowel Syndrome: Preliminary Study." *Digestive Diseases and Sciences* 56(11): 3288–3295.

9. Zhang, R., I. Humphreys, R. P. Sahu, et al. December 2008. "In Vitro and In Vivo Induction of Apoptosis by Capsaicin in Pancreatic Cancer Cell is Mediated Through ROS Generation and Mitochondrial Death Pathway." *Apoptosis* 13(12): 1465–1478.

References and Resources

Magazines, Journals, and Newspapers

Aasvang, E. K., J. B. Hansen, J. Malmstrøm, et al. July 2008. "The Effect of Wound Instillation of a Novel Purified Capsaicin Formulation on Postherniotomy Pain: A Double-Blind, Randomized, Placebo-Controlled Study." *Anesthesia & Analgesia* 107(1): 282–291.

Bortolotti, M. and S. Porta. 2011. "Effect of Red Pepper on Symptoms of Irritable Bowel Syndrome: Preliminary Study." *Digestive Diseases and Sciences* 56(11): 3288–3295.

Galgani, Jose E. and Eric Ravussin. November 2010. "Effect of Dihydrocapsiate on Resting Metabolic Rate in Humans." *The American Journal of Clinical Nutrition* 92(5): 1089–1093.

Jones, W. Keith, Guo-Chang Fan, Siyun Liao, et al. 2009. "Peripheral Nociception Associated with Surgical Incision Elicits Remote Nonischemic Cardioprotection via Neurogenic Activation of Protein Kinase C Signaling." *Circulation* 120: S1–S9.

Ludy, Mary-Jon and Richard D. Mattes. March 2011. "The Effects of Hedonically Acceptable Red Pepper Doses on Thermogenesis and Appetite." *Physiology & Behavior* 102(3–4): 251–258.

Snitker, S., Y. Fujishima, H. Shen, et al. January 2009. "Effects of Novel Capsinoid Treatment on Fatness and Energy Metabolism in Humans: Possible Pharmaco-genetic Implications." *The American Journal of Clinical Nutrition* 89(1): 45–50.

Yang, Dachun, Zhidan Luo, Shauangtao Ma, et al. August 2010. "Activation of TRPV1 by Dietary Capsaicin Improves Endothelium-Dependent Vasorelax-ation and Prevents Hypertension." *Cell Metabolism* 12(2): 130–141.

Zhang, R., I. Humphreys, R.P. Sahu, et al. December 2008. "In Vitro and In Vivo Induction of Apoptosis by Capsaicin in Pancreatic Cancer Cells Is Medi-ated through ROS Generation and Mitochondrial Death Pathway." *Apoptosis* 13(12): 1465–1478.

Website
The George Mateljan Foundation. www.whfoods.com.

Chamomile 🌿

There are two types of chamomile that are used for health conditions— German chamomile and Roman chamomile. While they are both believed to have similar effects on the body, German chamomile is the form generally available in the United States. So, this review will present only the research on German chamomile.

Chamomile has ancient roots. Historically, chamomile has been used for digestive upset, inflammation, healing wounds, and insomnia.[1] Today, chamomile is believed to help relieve anxiety, digestive disorders, skin problems, and inflammatory conditions.[2] A 2010 article in *Molecular Medicine Reports* noted that chamomile is also effective for hay fever, menstrual disorders, muscle spasms, rheumatic pain, and hemorrhoids.[3] But, it is important to review what researchers have learned.

Generalized Anxiety Disorder
In a randomized, double-blind, placebo-controlled, eight-week trial published in 2009 in the *Journal of Clinical Psychopharmacology,* researchers based at the University of Pennsylvania Medical Center investigated the use of chamomile extract to treat mild to moderate generalized anxiety

disorder in 57 patients with a mean age of 46. The patients received either a placebo ($n = 29$) or a pharmaceutical grade of German chamomile extract ($n = 28$). In the end, one patient in each treatment group discontinued therapy. Chamomile treatment began at 220 mg and progressed, if tolerated, to 1,100 mg. The researchers found that the patients taking chamomile had significant improvements in their symptoms. They noted that their "results suggest that chamomile may have modest anxiolytic activity in patients with mild to moderate GAD [generalized anxiety disorder]."[4]

Psychological Benefits

In a study published in 2008 in *Homeopathy,* researchers from Brazil investigated whether chamomile could benefit mice subjected to two different types of experimental stress. In the first trial, mice that received daily treatment with chamomile had roommates with growing tumors. Other mice served as the controls. The researchers found that the "mice who cohabitated with a sick cage-mate showed a decrease in their general activity, but those treated with Chamomile . . . were less severely affected." In the second study, mice pretreated with chamomile were subjected to forced swimming. There were also control mice. The researchers found that chamomile helped the mice recover from the stressful swimming and return to their previous behavior.[5]

Wound Healing

In a study published in 2009 in *Phytotherapy Research,* researchers from Brazil compared the ability of chamomile, two different corticosteroids, and a control to heal wounds in both in vitro and in vivo (rat) trials. During the trials, the researchers consistently found that chamomile had the best wound-healing ability. They concluded that "chamomile is a phytotherapic drug able to significantly improve wound healing by speeding the lesions recovery in comparison to the treatment with corticosteroids."[6] (Steroids tend to delay wound healing.)

A year later, in a study published in 2010 in *Natural Product Research,* researchers from Iran made 3-cm linear incisions on the skin of the backs of 30 male Wistar rats. The rats were then randomly divided into one of three experimental groups. The rats in the first group became the controls. They received no treatment for their wounds. Olive oil was applied daily to the wounds of the rats in the second group. And, chamomile extract dissolved in olive oil was applied daily to the rats in the third groups. The wounds were evaluated several times over 20 days. During most of the evaluations, the researchers found that chamomile accelerated the healing process. They concluded that chamomile extract "administered topically has wound healing potential in linear incisional wound model in rats."[7]

Useful for People with Diabetes

In a study published in 2008 in the *Journal of Agricultural and Food Chemistry,* researchers from Japan and the United Kingdom wanted to determine if chamomile was useful for symptoms of diabetes, such as hyperglycemia or elevated levels of sugar in the blood. In their in vitro studies, the researchers learned that chamomile hot water extract inhibited the activity of enzymes that contributed to hyperglycemia. Meanwhile, in their in vivo trials in rats with streptozotocin-induced diabetes, the administration of chamomile hot water extract decreased blood glucose levels. Then, in a final in vitro study, the researchers found that active components of chamomile inhibited the accumulation of sorbitol, a type of sugar, in red blood cells, which is associated with the diabetic complications of cataracts and neuropathy. The researchers concluded that their findings "suggested that daily consumption of chamomile tea with meals could contribute to the prevention of the progress of hyperglycemia and diabetic complications."[8]

Attention-Deficit Hyperactivity Disorder

In a small observational study published in 2009 in *Phytomedicine: International Journal of Phytotherapy and Phytopharmacology,* a researcher from Germany attempted to learn if chamomile would be useful for two 14- to 16-year-old teens who had been dealing with the symptoms of attention-deficit hyperactivity disorder (ADHD) for more than six years. After a seven-day washout period, one teen was placed on chamomile three times per day and the other teen took a placebo. After four weeks, the teens switched treatments for an additional four-week period. The researcher reported that while the teens took chamomile, there were improvements in a number of measurements of ADHD. For example, the teens experienced reductions in levels of inattention and hyperactivity or impulsivity. Meanwhile, when taking the placebo, their scores were similar to what they were before the study began. Chamomile appeared to have no serious side effects. Though limited conclusions may be drawn from a study that contains only two people, the author noted that further studies may determine if chamomile is a useful component of ADHD treatment. Additionally, it is possible that by adding chamomile to ADHD treatment, clinicians may be able to lower levels of ADHD medication.[9]

Antibacterial Activity against *Helicobacter pylori*

In a study published in 2008 in *Phytotherapy Research,* researchers from Russia evaluated the antibacterial properties of chamomile oil extract against *Helicobacter pylori,* the bacteria that causes stomach ulcers. The researchers determined that chamomile inhibited the activity of this bacterium. And, they concluded that chamomile oil extract "may be useful as [an] additional remedy in the complex treatment of stomach ulcers and duodenal intestinal diseases, especially for patients with allergic responses to antibacterial drugs." Moreover, "this oil extract may be useful in cases of antibiotic resistant strains of *H. pylori.*"[10]

Is Chamomile Beneficial?

There are numbers of people who swear that chamomile relieves anxiety and eases them into a restful sleep. And, there is no doubt that chamomile has some wound-healing properties. But, the research literature on chamomile also contains some caveats. For example, a 2008 article in the *International Journal of Food Microbiology* noted that some people use chamomile to treat infants suffering from colic. But, chamomile may contain botulism spores. The authors noted that botulism spores are much more likely to be found in unwrapped chamomile that is sold by weight. A far safer offering is chamomile sold in tea bags.[11] A 2005 article in *Drugs of Today* suggested that people should not apply chamomile in or around the eye. This action has the potential to cause "severe conjunctivitis."[12] In fact, when chamomile is applied to the skin, it is not uncommon for skin reactions to occur. When this happens, the application of chamomile should be discontinued.

Notes

1. Craig, Winston J. January–February 2011. "Chamomile: You Know Chamomile Makes a Nice Cup of Tea, But What Else Do you Know About It?" *Vibrant Life* 27(1): 19.
2. National Center for Complementary and Alternative Medicine Website. Nccam.nih.gov.

3. Srivastava, Janmejai K., Eswar Shankar, and Sanjay Gupta. November–December 2010. "Chamomile: A Herbal Medicine of the Past with Bright Future." *Molecular Medicine Reports* 3(6): 895–901.
4. Amsterdam, J.D., Y. Li, I. Soeller, et al. August 2009. "A Randomized, Double-Blind, Placebo-Controlled Trial of Oral *Matricaria recutita* (Chamomile) Extract Therapy for Generalized Anxiety Disorder." *Journal of Clinical Psychopharmacology* 29(4): 378–382.
5. Pinto, Sandra Augusta Gordinho, Elisabeth Bohland, Cideli de Paula Coelho, et al. July 2008. "An Animal Model for the Study of *Chamomilla* in Stress and Depression: Pilot Study." *Homeopathy* 97(3): 141–144.
6. Martins, M.D., M.M. Marques, S.K. Bussadori, et al. February 2009. "Comparative Analysis between *Chamomilla recutita* and Corticosteroids on Wound Healing: An In Vitro and In Vivo Study." *Phytotherapy Research* 23(2): 274–278.
7. Jarrahi, M., A.A. Vafaei, A.A. Taherian, et al. May 2010. "Evaluation of Topical *Matricaria chamomilla* Extract Activity on Linear Incisional Wound Healing in Albino Rats." *Natural Product Research* 24(8): 697–702.
8. Kato, Atsushi, Yuka Minoshima, Jo Yamamoto, et al. 2008. "Protective Effects of Dietary Chamomile Tea on Diabetic Complications." *Journal of Agricultural and Food Chemistry* 56(17): 8206–8211.
9. Niederhofer, H. April 2009. "Observational Study: *Matricaria chamomilla* may Improve Some Symptoms of Attention-Deficit Hyperactivity Disorder." *Phytomedicine: International Journal of Phytotherapy and Phytopharmacology* 16(4): 284–286.
10. Shikov, Alexander N., Olga N. Pozharitskaya, Valery G. Makarov, and Asya S. Kvetnaya. February 2008. "Antibacterial Activity of *Chamomilla recutita* Oil Extract against *Helicobacter pylori*." *Phytotherapy Research* 22(2): 252–253.
11. Bianco, Maria I., Carolina Luquez, Laura I.T. de Jong, and Rafael A. Fernandez. February 2008. "Presence of *Clostridium botulinum* Spores in *Matricaria chamomilla* (Chamomile) and Its Relationship with Infant Botulism." *International Journal of Food Microbiology* 121(3): 357–360.
12. Fraunfelder, F.W. August 2005. "Ocular Side Effects Associated with Dietary Supplements and Herbal Medicines." *Drugs of Today* 41(8): 537–545.

References and Resources

Magazines, Journals, and Newspapers

Amsterdam, J.D., Y. Li, I. Soeller, et al. August 2009. "A Randomized, Double-Blind, Placebo-Controlled Trial of Oral *Matricaria Recutita* (Chamomile) Extract Therapy for Generalized Anxiety Disorder." *Journal of Clinical Psychopharmacology* 29(4): 378–382.
Bianco, Maria I., Carolina Luquez, Laura I.T. de Jong, and Rafael A. Fernandez. February 2008. "Presence of *Clostridium botulinum* Spores in *Matricaria chamomilla* (Chamomile) and Its Relationship with Infant Botulism." *International Journal of Food Microbiology* 121(3): 357–360.

Craig, Winston J. January–February 2011. "Chamomile: You Know Chamomile Makes a Nice Cup of Tea, but What Else Do You Know About It?" *Vibrant Life* 27(1): 19.

Finney-Brown, Tessa. Spring 2009. "ADHD and Chamomile." *Australian Journal of Medical Herbalism* 21(1): 19–20.

Fraunfelder, F. W. August 2005. "Ocular Side Effects Associated with Dietary Supplements and Herbal Medicine." *Drugs of Today* 41(8): 537–545.

Jarrahi, M., A. A. Vafaei, A. A. Taherian, et al. May 2010. "Evaluation of Topical *Matricaria chamomilla* Extract Activity on Linear Incisional Wound Healing in Albino Rats." *Natural Product Research* 24(8): 697–702.

Kato, Atsushi, Yuka Minoshima, Jo Yamamoto, et al. 2008. "Protective Effects of Dietary Chamomile Tea on Diabetic Complications." *Journal of Agricultural and Food Chemistry* 56(17): 8206–8211.

Martins, M. D., M. M. Marques, S. K. Bussadori, et al. February 2009. "Comparative Analysis between *Chamomilla recutita* and Corticosteroids on Wound Healing: An In Vitro and In Vivo Study." *Phytotherapy Research* 23(2): 274–278.

Niederhofer, H. April 2009. "Observational Study: *Matricaria chamomilla* may Improve Some Symptoms of Attention-Deficit Hyperactivity Disorder." *Phytomedicine: International Journal of Phytotherapy and Phytopharmacology* 16(4): 284–286.

Pinto, Sandra Augusta Gordinho, Elisabeth Bohland, Cideli de Paula Coelho, et al. July 2008. "An Animal Model for the Study of *Chamomilla* in Stress and Depression: Pilot Study." *Homeopathy* 97(3): 141–144.

Shikov, Alexander N., Olga N. Pozharitskaya, Valery G. Makarov, and Asya S. Kvetnaya. February 2008. "Antibacterial Activity of *Chamomilla recutita* Oil Extract against *Helicobacter pylori*." *Phytotherapy Research* 22(2): 252–253.

Srivastava, Janmejai K., Eswar Shankar, and Sanjay Gupta. November–December 2010. "Chamomile: A Herbal Medicine of the Past with Bright Future." *Molecular Medicine Reports* 3(6): 895–901.

Website
National Center for Complementary and Alternative Medicine. nccam.nih.gov.

Cinnamon 🌿

Cinnamon, which has long been used both to enhance the flavor of various foods and as a medicine, is sold in a dried tubular form known as quill or as a ground powder. The two varieties of cinnamon, Chinese (*Cinnamomum aromaticum*) and Ceylonese (*Cinnamonum verum*), are similar, though the Ceylonese cinnamon is slightly sweeter and more refined. Cinnamon contains excellent amounts of manganese and very good amounts of dietary fiber, iron, and calcium.[1] But, what have the researchers learned?

Overall Health of People with Type 2 Diabetes

In a study published in 2003 in *Diabetes Care,* Pakistani researchers assisted by one researcher from the United States wanted to determine if cinnamon could improve the blood glucose, triglyceride, total cholesterol, high-density lipoprotein (HDL; good) cholesterol, and low-density lipoprotein (LDL; bad) cholesterol levels of people with type 2 diabetes. The cohort consisted of 60 people with type 2 diabetes. The 30 men and 30 women were randomly divided into 6 groups of 10. Groups 1, 2, and 3 consumed 1, 3, and 6 g of cinnamon daily, respectively; groups 4, 5, 6 were given placebos. After 40 days on the cinnamon or placebos, there was a 20-day washout period.

The researchers determined that all three levels of cinnamon reduced the mean fasting serum glucose, triglyceride, LDL cholesterol, and total cholesterol levels. There were no significant changes in the HDL levels or in the people who took placebos. The researchers suggested that people with and without type 2 diabetes may want to consider including cinnamon in the diet. "Because cinnamon would not contribute to caloric intake, those who have type 2 diabetes or those who have elevated glucose, triglyceride, LS cholesterol or total cholesterol levels may benefit from the regular inclusion of cinnamon in their daily diet. In addition, cinnamon may be beneficial for the remainder of the population to prevent and control elevated and blood lipid levels."[2]

A few years later, in a study published in 2006 in the *Journal of the American College of Nutrition,* researchers from Washington, DC, and Maryland investigated the effects of dietary cinnamon on systolic blood pressure and "various glucose- and insulin-related parameters" in rats that were bred to have high blood pressure. In a series of three trials, rats with high blood pressure that had diets with or without sucrose were given various amounts of cinnamon, cinnamon extract, or chromium. The trials continued for three to four weeks. The researchers found that the rats that had diets high in sucrose were more likely to have metabolic syndrome and elevated blood pressure levels. When cinnamon was added to the diets, the blood pressure of the rats that ate sucrose was lowered to "virtually the same levels" as the rats that ate no sucrose. Moreover, the cinnamon also lowered the blood pressure of the rats that did not consume sucrose. While the cinnamon did not decrease the levels of blood glucose, it did lower "circulating insulin concentrations." Aqueous extracts of cinnamon also reduced blood pressure. The researchers noted that cinnamon may play a role in blood pressure regulation and glucose metabolism. "Therefore, BP [blood pressure] regulation may not only be influenced favorably by limiting the amounts of dietary substances that have negative effects on BP and insulin function but also by the additional of beneficial ones, such as cinnamon, that have positive effects."[3]

In a placebo-controlled, double-blind study published in 2006 in the *European Journal of Clinical Investigation,* German researchers evaluated the use of water-soluble cinnamon extract for glycemic control and cardiovascular risk factors in people with type 2 diabetes. The cohort consisted of 79 people who were being treated for their diabetes with oral medication or diet therapy. The subjects were randomly assigned to take either a cinnamon extract or placebo capsule three times daily for four months. The cinnamon capsule contained the equivalent of 1 g of cinnamon powder. When compared to the placebo group, the group taking cinnamon had a significant reduction in fasting plasma glucose levels. There were some indications that those people with higher glucose levels obtained greater benefits from the cinnamon. The researchers wrote that the cinnamon extract had "a moderate effect in reducing fasting plasma glucose concentrations in diabetic patients with poor glycemic control."[4]

In a placebo-controlled, double-blind study published in 2009 in the *Journal of the American College of Nutrition,* researchers from the United States and France examined the effects of dried aqueous extract of cinnamon on the antioxidant status of people who were overweight or obese and had impaired fasting glucose. The cohort consisted of 22 people who had body mass indexes between 25 and 45. For 12 weeks, two times each day, subjects took either 250 mg of aqueous extract of cinnamon or a placebo. The researchers found that the cinnamon improved several antioxidant variables by as much as 13 to 23%. Furthermore, including water soluble compounds in the diet has the potential to "reduce risk factors associated with diabetes and cardiovascular disease."[5]

On the other hand, there are studies that find cinnamon having no effect. For example, in a prospective, double-blind, placebo-controlled study published in 2007 in *Diabetes Care,* researchers from the Dartmouth-Hitchcock Medical Center in New Hampshire attempted to learn the effect of cinnamon on glycemic control in adolescents with type 1 diabetes. For 90 days, 72 adolescents with type 1 diabetes were treated in an outpatient setting with 1 g of cinnamon per day or a placebo. The cinnamon was found not to be effective in improving glycemic control among these adolescents.[6]

In a study published in 2007 in *Diabetes Care,* researchers from Oklahoma City, Oklahoma, randomly divided 60 men and women with type 2 diabetes into two groups. One group took two capsules daily of 500 mg cinnamon; the other group took placebos. At the end of three months, 43 subjects completed the study. The researchers found no significant differences between the two groups, and, as a result, they noted that "cinnamon cannot be generally recommended for treatment of type 2 diabetes in an American population."[7]

In a truly striking piece of research published in 2008 in *Diabetes Care,* researchers from the University of Connecticut and Hartford Hospital conducted a meta-analysis of five randomized placebo-controlled trials that included a total of 282 subjects. Following their evaluation, the researchers were unable to find an association between improvements in problems faced by people with type 1 or type 2 diabetes, such as elevated levels of blood sugar, and intake of cinnamon.[8]

Cervical Cancer

In a study published in 2010 in *BMC Cancer,* researchers from India reported that they used aqueous cinnamon extract (ACE-c) from the bark of *Cinnamomum cassia* (SiHa) to kill human cervical cancer cells. How is this done? According to the researchers, "Cinnamon alters the growth kinetics of SiHa cells in a dose-dependent manner. Cells treated with ACE-c exhibited reduced number of colonies compared to the control cells." The researchers concluded that "cinnamon extract could be proposed to be a potent anticancer drug candidate in cervical cancer."[9]

Is Cinnamon Beneficial?

The results of the research on cinnamon are clearly inconclusive. Obviously, people should not expect cinnamon to cure their metabolic syndrome and type 2 diabetes. Far more impressive results may be obtained from dietary changes and exercise. As for treating cervical cancer, more research is needed. Still, for those dealing with these health problems, supplementing with cinnamon for a few months is probably worth a try.

However, before beginning such supplementation, it is a good idea to check with a health care provider.

Notes

1. The George Mateljan Foundation Website. www.whfoods.com.
2. Khan, Alam, Mahpara Safdar, Mohammad Muzaffar, et al. December 2003. "Cinnamon Improves Glucose and Lipids of People with Type 2 Diabetes." *Diabetes Care* 26(12): 3215–3218.
3. Preuss, Harry G., Bobby Echard, Marilyn M. Polansky, and Richard Anderson. 2006. "Whole Cinnamon and Aqueous Extracts Ameliorate Sucrose-Induced Blood Pressure Elevations in Spontaneously Hypertensive Rats." *Journal of the American College of Nutrition* 25(2): 144–150.
4. Mang, B., M. Wolters, B. Schmitt, et al. May 2006. "Effects of a Cinnamon Extract on Plasma Glucose, HbA1c, and Serum Lipids in Diabetes Mellitus Type 2." *European Journal of Clinical Investigation* 36(5): 340–344.
5. Roussel, Anne-Marie, Isabelle Hininger, Rachida Benaraba, et al. 2009. "Antioxidant Effects of a Cinnamon Extract in People with Impaired Fasting Glucose That Are Overweight or Obese." *Journal of the American College of Nutrition* 28(1): 16–21.
6. Altschuler, Justin A., Samuel J. Casella, Todd A. MacKenzie, and Kevin M. Curtis. April 2007. "The Effect of Cinnamon on A1C among Adolescents with Type 1 Diabetes." *Diabetes Care* 30(4): 813–816.
7. Blevins, Steve M., Misti J. Leyva, Joshua Brown, et al. September 2007. "Effect of Cinnamon on Glucose and Lipid Levels in Non-Insulin-Dependent Type 2 Diabetes." *Diabetes Care* 30(9): 2236–2237.
8. Baker, William L., Gabriela Gutierrez-Williams, C. Michael White, et al. January 2008. "Effect of Cinnamon on Glucose Control and Lipid Parameters." *Diabetes Care* 31(1): 41–43.
9. Koppikar, Soumya J., Amit S. Choudhari, Snehal A. Suryavanshi, et al. May 2010. "Aqueous Cinnamon Extract (ACE-c) from the Bark of *Cinnamomum cassia* Causes Apoptosis in Human Cervical Cancer Cell Line (SiHa) through Loss of Mitochondrial Membrane Potential." *BMC Cancer* 10: 210.

References and Resources

Magazines, Journals, and Newspapers

Altschuler, Justin, Samuel J. Casella, Todd A. MacKenzie, and Kevin M. Curtis. April 2007. "The Effect of Cinnamon on A1C among Adolescents with Type 1 Diabetes." *Diabetes Care* 30(4): 813–816.

Baker, William L., Gabriela Gutierrez-Williams, C. Michael White, et al. January 2008. "Effect of Cinnamon on Glucose Control and Lipid Parameters." *Diabetes Care* 31(1): 41–43.

Blevins, Steve M., Misti J. Leyva, Joshua Brown, et al. September 2007. "Effects of Cinnamon on Glucose and Lipid Levels in Non-Insulin-Dependent Type 2 Diabetes." *Diabetes Care* 30(9): 2236–2237.

Khan, Alam, Mahpara Safdar, Mohammad Muzaffar, et al. December 2003. "Cinnamon Improves Glucose and Lipids of People with Type 2 Diabetes." *Diabetes Care* 26(12): 3215–3218.

Koppikar, Soumya J., Amit S. Choudhari, Snehal A. Suryavanshi, et al. May 2010. "Aqueous Cinnamon Extract (ACE-c) from the Bark of *Cinnamomum cassia* Cause Apoptosis in Human Cervical Cancer Cell Line (SiHa) through Loss of Mitochondrial Membrane Potential." *BMC Cancer* 10: 210.

Mang, B., M. Wolters, B. Schmitt, et al. May 2006. "Effects of a Cinnamon Extract on Plasma Glucose, HbA1c, and Serum Lipids in Diabetes Mellitus Type 2." *European Journal of Clinical Investigation* 36(5): 340–344.

Preuss, Harry G., Bobby Echard, Marilyn M. Polansky, and Richard Anderson. 2006. "Whole Cinnamon and Aqueous Extracts Ameliorate Sucrose-Induced Blood Pressure Elevations in Spontaneously Hypertensive Rats." *Journal of the American College of Nutrition* 25(2): 144–150.

Roussel, Anne-Marie, Isabelle Hininger, Rachida Benaraba, et al. 2009. "Antioxidant Effects of a Cinnamon Extract in People with Impaired Fasting Glucose That Are Overweight or Obese." *Journal of the American College of Nutrition* 28(1): 16–21.

Websites

American Diabetes Association. www.diabetes.org.

The George Mateljan Foundation. www.whfoods.com.

Cloves 🌰

Known for their warm, sweet, and aromatic taste, cloves are the unopened pink flower buds of the evergreen clove tree. Picked when they are still pink, the buds, which are about a half inch long and one quarter inch in diameter, are dried until they turn brown. At that point, they look like nails. (It is interesting to note that their English name is derived from the Latin word for nail—*clavus*.) While cloves are hard on the outside, their flesh contains eugenol, an oily compound that has antibacterial and anti-inflammatory properties.[1]

Scientifically known as *Eugenia caryophyllus,* cloves have been consumed in Asia for about 2,000 years. Around the fourth century, Arab traders brought them to Europe. By the Middle Ages, they were widely used.

Today, cloves are grown in Zanzibar (eastern Africa), Sri Lanka (Asia), Madagascar (in the Indian Ocean off the southeast coast of Africa), India, Brazil, and the West Indies.[2]

Cloves contain a number of different vitamins and nutrients. They have excellent amounts of manganese and very good amounts of omega 3 fatty acids, dietary fiber, and vitamins C and K. Cloves also have good amounts of magnesium and calcium. In addition to its anti-inflammatory properties, cloves are said to fight bacteria and reduce dental pain.[3] But, what have the researchers learned?

Improving Food Safety

In a study published in 2010 in the *Journal of Food Safety,* researchers from Tunisia noted that the bacterium *Listeria monocytogenes* has been known to survive and grow on foods, such as milk, cheese, beef, pork, chicken, fish, fruits, and vegetables, even when these items are refrigerated. According to the researchers, human listeriosis, the illness caused by *L. monocytogenes,* may have severe symptoms, and it has the potential to be deadly. As a result, this bacterium has become a "public health concern."

So, these researchers decided to investigate whether 1% or 2% concentrations of essential oil of clove could inhibit the growth of Listeria. They inoculated fresh cut salmon with three strains of this bacterium. For two weeks, some of the salmon was stored at 4°C and other salmon was stored at 25°C. The salmon pieces that were inoculated with the bacterium but received no essential oil of clove served as controls.

The researchers found that the clove oil did indeed inhibit the growth of *L. monocytogenes* in the salmon. Moreover, they found that "the effect was more pronounced with 2% of clove oil compared with 1%." Furthermore, the clove oil decreased more growth at the 25°C temperature than the lower temperature. Still, the clove oil did not completely stop the growth of the bacterium. The researchers concluded that "clove oil has a good potential as an antilisterial substance in food preservation as it may be more acceptable to consumers and the regulatory agencies in comparison with chemical compounds."[4]

In another study published in 2009 in the *Journal of Food Science,* U.S. Department of Agriculture (USDA) researchers tested the ability of the essential oil of clove buds, cinnamon, and allspice to protect apple puree from bacteria. While all three oils were effective against bacteria, the researchers determined that relatively low concentrations of clove buds and allspice oils suppressed the growth of *L. monocytogenes*. This occurred during both direct contact with the bacteria and indirect contact via vapors.[5]

In a study published in 2007 in the *Journal of Food Safety,* researchers from Spain evaluated the antifungal properties of cloves, oregano, and thyme on two types of mold—*Aspergillus niger* and *Aspergillus flavus*— "two of the more important molds of foodborne diseases and/or food spoilage." While oregano demonstrated the highest inhibition of mold growth, clove was second. Clove essential oil inhibited more *A. niger* than *A. flavus.* The researchers noted that consumers are comfortable with essential oils, and they do not harm the environment as some other types of antifungal agents may. Moreover, there is a "very low risk that pathogens will develop resistance to the mixture of components that make up the oils with their apparent diversity of antifungal mechanisms."[6]

Overall Health

In a study published in 2010 in the *Flavour and Fragrance Journal,* Spanish researchers determined the antioxidant activity of five herbs and spices—clove, thyme, rosemary, oregano, and sage—that are commonly used in the Mediterranean diet.

Of the herbs and spices tested, cloves had the highest levels of antioxidants. So, they have the highest ability to fight damaging free radicals.[7]

Useful for Diabetes and Supportive of Healthy Aging

In a similar study published in 2008 in the *Journal of Medicinal Food,* researchers from the University of Georgia in Athens, Georgia, tested extracts from 24 well-known herbs and spices, such as cloves. They learned that cloves had very high amounts of antioxidant-rich compounds known as phenols. Moreover, the researchers found a direct correlation between phenol content and the ability to stop the formation of compounds (advanced glycation end products or AGE) that support the damage and inflammation caused by aging and diabetes. The researchers noted that "the most potent inhibitors included extracts of cloves, ground Jamaican allspice, and cinnamon."[8]

Prevention of Lung Cancer

In a study published in 2006 in *Carcinogenesis,* researchers from India injected mice with benzopyrene, a cancer-causing agent in tobacco.

Then, they divided the mice into two groups. In one group, the mice received an oral clove infusion made from soaking cloves in distilled water; in the other group, the mice were given only distilled water. When compared to the mice that had only water, the mice treated with cloves had fewer abnormal cells in their lungs. Additionally, cloves reduced the abnormal crowding of cells in certain sections of lung tissue and stopped the growth of premalignant cells by more than 85%. And, cloves increased the levels of some proteins that triggered cell death and helped to stop the creation of a protein that fuels abnormal cells growth. As if that were not enough, cloves inhibited the action of an enzyme that fosters inflammation and the growth of cancer cells. The researchers commented that "the most notable implication of our work is that the oral infusion of clove could result in a significant inhibition in the progression of cancer in the animal model that emulates human disease."[9]

Topical Dental Anesthetic

In a single-blind study published in 2006 in the *Journal of Dentistry,* researchers from Kuwait investigated whether cloves could replace benzocaine as a tropical anesthetic. So, they recruited 73 volunteers, who were healthy medical, dental, or pharmacy students. Five minutes before receiving two needle sticks to the same section of the mouth, one of the following topical agents was applied—homemade clove gel, benzocaine 20% gel, a placebo that resembled clove, and a placebo that resembled benzocaine. The researchers found that when compared with the placebos, both the clove and benzocaine gels significantly reduced pain from the needle sticks. Since there was no significant difference in pain reduction between the clove and benzocaine gels, it is possible that cloves could be substituted for benzocaine. Why is this important? The researchers noted that "topical anesthetics are drugs with toxicity and side effects." There is also the concern that benzocaine may be absorbed into the system. On the other hand, the researchers commented that the eugenol in cloves may result in "tissue irritation." Four of the volunteers developed small ulcers. Nevertheless, the researchers concluded that "clove might replace the widely used topical anesthetic benzocaine, thereby reducing the dose of drugs the patient absorbs, lowering the cost on the dentist and allowing more patients throughout the world to benefit from a cheap and largely available topical anesthetic."[10]

Are Cloves Beneficial?

They certainly appear to have a number of beneficial characteristics. Hopefully, further research on cloves will yield more definitive information.

Notes

1. The George Mateljan Foundation Website. www.whfoods.com.
2. The George Mateljan Foundation Website. www.whfoods.com.
3. The George Mateljan Foundation Website. www.whfoods.com.
4. Miladi, Hanene, Kamel Chaieb, Emna Ammar, and Amina Bakhrouf. May 2010. "Inhibitory Effect of Clove Oil (*Syzium aromaticum*) against *Listeria monocytegenes* Cells Incubated in Fresh-Cut Salmon." *Journal of Food Safety* 30(2): 432–442.
5. Du, W.-X., C. W. Olsen, R. J. Avena-Bustillos, et al. September 2009. "Effects of Allspice, Cinnamon, and Clove Bud Essential Oils in Edible Apple Films on Physical Properties and Antimicrobial Activities." *Journal of Food Science* 74(7): M372–M378.
6. Viuda-Martos, M., Y. Ruiz-Navajas, J. Fernández-López, and J. A. Pérez-Álvarez. February 2007. "Antifungal Activities of Thyme, Clove and Oregano Essential Oils." *Journal of Food Safety* 27(1): 91–101.
7. Viuda-Martos, Manuel, Yolanda Ruiz Navajas, Elena Sánchez Zapata, et al. January–February 2010. "Antioxidant Activity of Essential Oils of Five Spice Plants Widely Used in a Mediterranean Diet." *Flavour and Fragrance Journal* 25(1): 13–19.
8. Dearlove, Rebecca P., Phillip Greenspan, Diane K. Hartle, et al. June 2008. "Inhibition of Protein Glycation by Extracts of Culinary Herbs and Spices." *Journal of Medicinal Food* 11(2): 275–281.
9. Banerjee, Sarmistha, Chinmay Kr. Panda, and Sukta Das. 2006. "Clove (*Syzygium aromaticum* L.), a Potential Chemopreventive Agent for Lung Cancer." *Carcinogenesis* 27(8): 1645–1654.
10. Alqareer, Athbi, Asma Alyahya, and Lars Andersson. November 2006. "The Effect of Clove and Benzocaine versus Placebo as Topical Anesthetics." *Journal of Dentistry* 34(10): 747–750.

References and Resources

Magazines, Journals, and Newspapers

Alqareer, Athbi, Asma Alyahya, and Lars Andersson. November 2006. "The Effect of Clove and Benzocaine versus Placebo as Topical Anesthetics." *Journal of Dentistry* 34(10): 747–750.

Banerjee, Sarmistha, Chinmay Kr. Panda, and Sukta Das. 2006. "Clove (*Syzygium aromaticum* L.), a Potential Chemopreventive Agent for Lung Cancer." *Carcinogenesis* 27(8): 1645–1654.

Dearlove, Rebecca P., Phillip Greenspan, Diane K. Hartle, et al. June 2008. "Inhibition of Protein Glycation by Extracts of Culinary Herbs and Spices." *Journal of Medicinal Food* 11(2): 275–281.

Du, W.-X., C.W. Olsen, R.J. Avena-Bustillos, et al. September 2009. "Effects of Allspice, Cinnamon, and Clove Bud Essential Oils in Edible Apple Films on Physical Properties and Antimicrobial Activities." *Journal of Food Science* 74(7): M372–M378.

Miladi, Hanene, Kamel Chaieb, Emna Ammar, and Amina Bakhrouf. May 2010. "Inhibitory Effect of Clove Oil (*Syzium aromaticum*) against *Listeria monocytogenes* Cells Incubated in Fresh-Cut Salmon." *Journal of Food Safety* 30(2): 432–442.

Viuda-Martos, M., Y. Ruiz-Navajas, J. Fernández-López, and J. A. Pérez-Álvarez. February 2007. "Antifungal Activities of Thyme, Clove and Oregano Essential Oils." *Journal of Food Safety* 27(1): 91–101.

Viuda-Martos, Manuel, Yolanda Ruiz Navajas, Elena Sánchez Zapata, et al. January–February 2010. "Antioxidant Activity of Essential Oils of Five Spice Plants Widely Used in a Mediterranean Diet." *Flavour and Fragrance Journal* 25(1): 13–19.

Website
The George Mateljan Foundation. www.whfoods.com.

Coriander/Cilantro 🌿

Coriander refers to the seeds of the coriander plant and cilantro refers to the leaves. In actuality, at least in the United States, coriander and cilantro tend to be used interchangeably to describe an herb that belongs in the parsley family and may be traced to ancient times.

Scientifically known as *Coriandrum sativum,* coriander is one of the world's oldest herbs. It is even mentioned in the Old Testament. The ancient Chinese were known to have considered coriander as both food and medicine. Hippocrates, and other ancient Greek physicians, used it as a medicine. And, ancient Romans seasoned their food with coriander and introduced the herb to the English. Of course, it was the English who brought coriander to the New World. It has been said that coriander is useful for people with diabetes and/or cardiovascular problems. Coriander is also said to help with gastrointestinal concerns, food poisoning, and inflammation. But, what have the researchers learned?

Cardiovascular Health

In a study published in 2008 in the *Journal of Environmental Biology,* researchers from India fed two groups of female albino rats a diet high in fat and cholesterol. The diet of the experimental group of rats also contained coriander seeds; the other group became the control. After more than two months, the animals were sacrificed, and the researchers conducted a number of studies. The researchers found that the rats whose diet included coriander seed had "a significant decrease in cholesterol and triglyceride level." So, the researchers concluded that "the administration of coriander seeds had a profound influence on the metabolism of lipids in animals fed on cholesterol containing diet."[1]

A similar study on coriander seed oil was conducted by Egyptian researchers and published in 2008 in *European Food Research and Technology.* In this study, 24 male albino rats were placed on a cholesterol-rich diet. The researchers then added coriander seed oil to the diets of some of the rats; they added a blend of soybean oil, sunflower oil, and coriander oil (blended oil) to the diets of other rats. By the end of the 60-day study, the researchers found that both the coriander seed oil and the blended oil lowered levels of total cholesterol and low-density lipoprotein (LDL; bad) cholesterol. In addition, both groupings of oils raised high-density lipoprotein (HDL; good) cholesterol. They noted that "the results demonstrated that COR [coriander seed oil], and to a relatively lesser degree Blend, have hypocholesterolemic [cholesterol lowering] properties in rats fed a cholesterol-rich diet."[2]

In a study published in 2008 in the *Journal of Ethnopharmacology,* Moroccan researchers compared the diuretic ability of coriander to furosemide, a standard diuretic. During the investigation, anesthetized Wistar rats received intravenous infusions of aqueous extract of coriander seeds. Though the researchers found that forosemide "was more potent as a diuretic and saluretic [drug that promotes the excretion of salt in the urine]," coriander seed "possesses diuretic and saluretic activity."[3]

Overall Health and Well-Being

In a study published in 2009 in *Journal of Ethnopharamcology,* researchers from Pakistan used mice, rats, and guinea pigs to examine the usefulness of coriander crude extract for dyspepsia (painful, difficult, or disturbed digestion), vomiting, diarrhea, abdominal colic, and hypertension. The researchers found that coriander had both stimulating and inhibiting effects on digestion. Since it also demonstrated diuretic properties, it is useful for those with hypertension.[4]

In a study published in 2010 in *Plant Foods for Human Nutrition,* researchers from Cork, Ireland, determined the amount of bioactive phytochemicals, such as carotenoids, in eight different herbs. After these amounts were learned, they used a simulated human in vitro digestion model to assess carotenoid bioaccessibility from these herbs. They wanted to determine "the amount of carotenoids transferred to micelles after digestion when compared with the original amount present in the food." The researchers found that coriander was the second best source of carotenoids. (Basil was the first.) And, they concluded that "of the herbs analyzed, basil and coriander were superior in carotenoid content and bioaccessibility."[5]

Possible Help in Preventing Foodborne Infectious Agents

In a study published in 2004 in the *Journal of Agricultural and Food Chemistry,* researchers from the University of California, Berkley, determined that dodecenal, a chemical in coriander, may well be useful in the fight against salmonella, a potentially deadly food-borne disease. These researchers observed that dodecenal was two times as potent as gentamicin, the allopathic medicine normally used to treat salmonella.[6]

In an in vitro study, published in 2010 in *Bioscience, Biotechnology, and Biochemistry,* researchers from Thailand investigated the antimicrobial effectiveness of 12 essential oils, including coriander oil, against *Campylobacter jejuni,* a common food-borne bacteria. In this instance, the bacteria were placed on raw chicken and raw beef at 4°C and 32°C. Of the 12 tested oils, the researchers found that coriander oil "exhibited the strongest antimicrobial activity against all tested strains." The antimicrobial activity of the oil, which reduced bacteria in a dose-dependent manner, was not affected by the type of meat or the temperature of the meat. The researchers noted that coriander has the potential "to serve as a natural antimicrobial agent against *C. jejuni.*" They added that "Its availability, low cost, and effectiveness at a wide range of temperatures contribute to its advantages as a food preservative and prospective alternative to currently used chemical-based inhibitors."[7]

On the other hand, in a study published in 2005 in the *World Journal of Gastroenterology,* researchers from the United Kingdom examined the ability of 25 different plants, including coriander, to destroy *Helicobacter pylori,* a type of bacteria associated with the vast majority of stomach ulcers. Of the plants tested, eight were found to have no ability to kill *H. pylori.* Those eight included coriander.[8]

Skin Protection

In a randomized, placebo-controlled, double-blind study published in 2008 in the *Journal der Deutschen Dermatologischen Gesellschaft (Journal of the German Society of Dermatology),* researchers from Freiburg, Germany attempted to determine if a lotion containing coriander oil could have anti-inflammatory properties. During the study, test areas on the backs of 40 volunteers were placed under ultraviolet radiation. Then, some of the test areas were treated for two days with lotions containing 0.5% or 1.0% of coriander oil; other test areas were treated with either hydrocortisone or betamethasone valerate, creams known for treating inflammation, itching, and swelling. Test areas were treated with a lotion that had no additional additives, and some irradiated areas were untreated. The researchers found that untreated areas that received radiation were red. The 0.5% coriander oil lotion significantly reduced redness, but it was not as effective as the 1% hydrocortisone. Interestingly, the 1.0% coriander oil was not as effective as the 0.5%. The researchers noted that the lotion containing 0.5% coriander showed "moderate anti-inflammatory effects," and because coriander oil has "anti-inflammatory and antimicrobial properties," the lotion "might be useful in the concomitant treatment of inflammatory skin disease such as atopic dermatitis."[9]

Is Coriander Beneficial?

From this brief review, coriander appears to have a number of useful qualities. And, since it is so readily available and reasonably priced, it may well be a good idea to add a little to the diet.

Notes

1. Dhanapakiam, P., J. Mini Joseph, V. K. Ramaswamy, et al. January 2008. "The Cholesterol Lowering Property of Coriander Seeds (*Coriandrum sativum*): Mechanism of Action." *Journal of Environmental Biology* 29(1): 53–56.

2. Ramadan, Mohamed Fawzy, Mohamed Mostafa Afify Amer, and Ahmed El-Said Awad. 2008. "Coriander (*Coriandrum sativum* L.) Seed Oil Improves Plasma Lipid Profile in Rats Fed a Diet Containing Cholesterol." *European Food Research and Technology* 227(4): 1173–1182.

3. Aissaoui, A., J. El-Hilaly, Z. H. Israili, and B. Lyoussi. January 2008. "Acute Diuretic Effect of Continuous Intravenous Infusion of an Aqueous Extract of *Coriandrum sativum* L. in Anesthetized Rats." *Journal of Ethnopharmacology* 115(1): 89–95.

4. Jabeen Q., S. Bashir, B. Lyoussi, and A. H. Gilani. February 2009. "Coriander Fruit Exhibits Gut Modulatory, Blood Pressure Lowering, and Diuretic Activities." *Journal of Ethnopharmacology* 122(1): 123–130.

5. Daly, Trevor, Marvin A. Jiwan, Nora M. O'Brien, and S. Aisling Aherne. June 2010. "Carotenoid Content of Commonly Consumed Herbs and Assessment of Their Bioaccessibility Using an *In Vitro* Digestion Model." *Plant Foods for Human Nutrition* 65(2): 164–169.

6. Kubo, I., K. Fujita, A. Kubo, et al. 2004. "Antibacterial Activity of Coriander Volatile Compounds against *Salmonella choleraesuis*." *Journal of Agricultural and Food Chemistry* 52(11): 3329–3332.

7. Rattanachaikunsopon, P. and P. Phumkhachorn. 2010. "Potential of Coriander (*Coriandrum sativam*) Oil as a Natural Antimicrobial Compound in Controlling *Campylobacter jejuni* in Raw Meat." *Bioscience, Biotechnology, and Biochemistry* 74(1): 31–35.

8. O'Mahony, R., H. Al-Khtheeri, D. Weerasekera, et al. December 2005. "Bactericidal and Anti-Adhesive Properties of Culinary and Medicinal Plants against *Helicobacter pylori*." *World Journal of Gastroenterology* 11(47): 7499–7507.

9. Reuter, J., C. Huyke, F. Casetti, et al. October 2008. "AntiInflammatory Potential of a Lipolotion Containing Coriander Oil in the Ultraviolet Erythema Test." *Journal der Deutschen Dermatologischen Gesellschaft* [*Journal of the German Society of Dermatology*] 6(10): 847–851.

References and Resources

Magazines, Journals, and Newspapers

Aissaoui, A, J. El-Hilaly, Z. H. Israili, and B. Lyoussi. January 2008. "Acute Diuretic Effect of Continuous Intravenous Infusion of an Aqueous Extract of *Coriandrum sativum* L. in Anesthetized Rats." *Journal of Ethnopharmacology* 115(1): 89–95.

Daly, Trevor, Marvin A. Jiwan, Nora M. O'Brien, and S. Aisling Aherne. June 2010. "Carotenoid Content of Commonly Consumed Herbs and Assessment of Their Bioaccessibility Using an *In Vitro* Digestion Model." *Plant Foods for Human Nutrition* 65(2): 164–169.

Dhanapakiam, P., J. Mini Joseph, V. K. Ramaswamy, et al. January 2008. "The Cholesterol Lowering Property of Coriander Seeds (*Coriandrum sativum*): Mechanism of Action." *Journal of Environmental Biology* 29(1): 53–56.

Jabeen, Q., S. Bashir, B. Lyoussi, and A. H. Gilani. February 2009. "Coriander Fruits Exhibits Gut Modulatory, Blood Pressure Lowering, and Diuretic Activities." *Journal of Ethnopharmacology* 122(1): 123–130.

Kubo, I., K. Fujita, A. Kubo, et al. June 2004. "Antibacterial Activity of Coriander Volatile Compounds against *Salmonella choleraesuis*." *Journal of Agricultural and Food Chemistry* 52(11): 3329–3332.

O'Mahony, R., H. Al-Khtheeri, D. Weerasekera, et al. December 2005. "Bacterial and Anti-Adhesive Properties of Culinary and Medicinal Plants against *Helicobacter pylori*." *World Journal of Gastroenterology* 11(47): 7499–7507.

Ramadan, Mohamed Fawzy, Mohamed Mostafa Afify Amer, and Ahmed El-Said Awad. 2008. "Coriander (*Coriandrum sativum* L.) Seed Oil Improves Plasma Lipid Profile in Rats Fed a Diet Containing Cholesterol." *European Food Research and Technology* 227(4): 1173–1182.

Rattanachaikunsopon, P. and P. Phumkhachorn. 2010. "Potential of Coriander (*Coriandrum sativum*) Oil as a Natural Antimicrobial Compound in Controlling *Campylobacter jejuni* in Raw Meat." *Bioscience, Biotechnology, and Biochemistry* 74(1): 31–35.

Reuter, J., C. Huyke, F. Casetti, et al. October 2008. "Anti-Inflammatory Potential of a Lipolotion Containing Coriander Oil in the Ultraviolet Erythema Test." *Journal der Deutschen Dermatologischen Gesellschaft* [*Journal of the German Society of Dermatology*] 6(10): 847–851.

Website

The George Mateljan Foundation. www.whfoods.com.

D

Dandelion ❦

While many people think dandelions are useless weeds, dandelions have historically been considered medicinal herbs. Scientifically known as *Taraxacum officinale,* dandelions have traditionally been used to treat liver and kidney problems as well as swelling, skin disorders, heartburn, and gastrointestinal distress. Today, dandelions are frequently viewed to be a diuretic, appetite stimulant, and digestive aid. Moreover, they are thought to improve the functioning of the liver and the gallbladder. Nutritional analyses of dandelions have found that they contain rich amounts of vitamins and minerals.[1] But, what have the researchers learned?

Diuretic

In a study published in 2009 in *The Journal of Alternative and Complementary Medicine,* researchers from Maryland, Massachusetts, and North Carolina wondered if the ingestion of high-quality ethanolic extract of fresh leaf dandelion would cause volunteers to have increased output and frequency of urination. Initially, 28 female subjects were enrolled. They were told to monitor fluid intake for four consecutive days and record urine output for three consecutive days—one day before taking the extract (control), the day the extract is consumed, and, a third, the day after taking the extract. On the day the volunteers took the extract, they consumed 8-mL doses at 8 A.M., 1 P.M., and 6 P.M.

Unfortunately, 11 of the 28 volunteers had difficulty collecting and/or measuring the fluids. So, they were eliminated. Nevertheless, the researchers found that there was a significant increase in urination in the five-hour period after the first dose. There was also a significant increase in the excretion ratio in the five-hour period after the second dose. Following the third dose, there were no changes in the measured parameters. The researchers concluded that dandelion ethanolic extract "shows promise as a diuretic in humans."[2]

Cardiovascular Health

In a study published in 2010 in the *International Journal of Molecular Sciences,* researchers from Korea examined some of the cardiovascular benefits of dandelion when fed to rabbits on a high-cholesterol diet. The researchers randomly divided 28 male rabbits into four equal groups. For one week, all the rabbits were fed a normal diet. The rabbits in one group remained on the regular diet. The three other groups of rabbits were switched to a high-cholesterol diet. One of these groups was also placed on dandelion leaf supplement; another group took dandelion root supplement; and the third group ate only the high-cholesterol diet. The researchers found that the dandelion had a number of cardiovascular benefits, such as reducing total cholesterol and low-density lipoprotein (LDL; bad cholesterol) and raising high-density lipoprotein (HDL; good cholesterol).[3]

Kills Human Leukemia Cells

In a study published in 2011 in the *Journal of Ethnopharmacology,* researchers from Ontario, Canada, investigated the ability of dandelion root extract to kill human leukemia cells. In their in vitro studies, the researchers exposed human leukemia cells to increasing concentrations of dandelion root extract. They found that dandelion root extract "effectively induces apoptosis [cell death] in human leukemia cell lines in a dose and time dependent manner." At the same time, the dandelion root extract did not harm any of the noncancerous cells.[4]

Kills Breast and Prostate Cancer Cells

In an in vitro study published in 2008 in the *International Journal of Oncology,* researchers from New Mexico tested the ability of dandelion leaves, roots, and flowers to destroy breast and prostate cancer cells. The researchers found that dandelion leaf extract slowed the growth of breast cancer cells and stopped the spread of prostate cancer cells. However, neither dandelion flower extract nor dandelion root extract had any effect on either type of cancer cell. Still, the researchers concluded that dandelion "extracts or individual components present in the extracts may be of value as novel anti-cancer agents."[5]

Kills Melanoma Cells

In a study published in 2011 in *Evidence-Based Complementary and Alternative Medicine,* researchers from Ontario, Canada, tested the ability of dandelion root extract to destroy melanoma (the most serious type of skin cancer) cells. Melanoma that has spread tends to be resistant to conventional therapies. The researchers found that dandelion root extract did indeed kill melanoma cells, and it did so without harming healthy cells. Additionally, "melanoma cells retain the signals to commit suicide long after DRE [dandelion root extract] has been removed from the system."[6]

Liver Protection

In a study published in 2010 in *Food and Chemical Toxicology,* researchers from Korea examined the ability of dandelion to help heal liver cells impaired by alcohol. In their in vitro studies, the researchers damaged liver cells with alcohol. Yet, when they added dandelion root to the mix, they could not observe any cell damage. Similar results were seen in the researchers' studies on mice. Again, dandelion protected the liver cells. One of the ways that it accomplished this goal was to increase the antioxidant activity within the liver. The researchers wrote that their findings "suggest that the aqueous extract of *T. officinale root* has protective action against alcohol-induced toxicity in the liver."[7]

In a study published in 2010 in the *Journal of Ethnopharmacology,* researchers from Croatia investigated the use of dandelion root water-ethanol extract (DWE) to treat mice with livers that have been harmed by carbon tetrachloride. After sufficiently damaging the livers of the mice, the researchers treated the mice with once daily doses of DWE. There were also two groups of control mice. The researchers observed that "the DWE treatment . . . promoted the complete regression of fibrosis and the enhancement of hepatic [liver] regenerative capabilities." Moreover, "the results obtained from this study strongly suggest the therapeutic potential of DWE in patients with liver fibrosis."[8]

Weight Loss

In a study published in 2008 in *Nutrition Research and Practice,* researchers from Alabama and Korea noted that the medication Orlistat inhibits pancreatic lipase, a key enzyme for the digestion of fat. In so doing, it prevents some fats from being absorbed into the body. "However, gastrointestinal side effects caused by Orlistat may limit its use." So, the researchers decided to examine the ability of dandelion to have in vitro and in vivo pancreatic lipase–inhibiting properties. The researchers found that in both their in vitro and in vivo studies dandelion had "inhibitory activities against pancreatic lipase."[9]

Is Dandelion Beneficial?

Though dandelion appears to have some benefits, there are insufficient studies to make a definitive determination. Of even more importance are the references in research literature of medical problems associated with the intake of dandelion. For example, a letter to the editor of the *International Journal of Cardiology,* published in 2006, describes a 39-year-old obese woman who arrived at the hospital with palpitations and fainting spells. For approximately three weeks, she had been hoping to lose weight with the assistance of a supplement containing three herbs, including dandelion.[10] In another example, published in 2010 in *The American Journal of Emergency Medicine,* physicians in Turkey reported on a 58-year-old woman with type 2 diabetes who came to the hospital with palpitations, nausea, anxiety, and excessive sweating. About two weeks earlier, she started eating dandelion with her salads. Physicians diagnosed her with hypoglycemia—low blood sugar—and she was told to stop eating dandelion. Once she eliminated dandelion from her diet, the woman did not have a recurrence of the symptoms.[11]

Notes

1. University of Maryland Medical Center Website. www.umm.edu.
2. Clare, B. A., R. S. Conroy, and K. Spelman. August 2009. "The Diuretic Effect in Human Subjects of an Extract of *Taraxaxum officinale* Folium over a Single Day." *The Journal of Alternative and Complementary Medicine* 15(8): 929–934.
3. Choi, U. K., O. H. Lee, J. H. Yim, et al. January 2010. "Hypolipidemic and Antioxidant Effects of Dandelion (*Taraxacum officinale*) Root and Leaf on Cholesterol-Fed Rabbits." *International Journal of Molecular Sciences* 11(1): 67–78.
4. Ovadje, P., S. Chatterjee, C. Griffin, et al. January 2011. "Selective Induction of Apoptosis through Activation of Caspase-8 in Human Leukemia Cells (Jurkat) by Dandelion Root Extract." *Journal of Ethnopharmacology* 133(1): 86–91.

5. Sigstedt, S.C., C.J. Hooten, M.C. Callewaert, et al. May 2008. "Evaluation of Aqueous Extracts of *Taraxacum officinale* on Growth and Invasion of Breast and Prostate Cancer Cells." *International Journal of Oncology* 32(5): 1085–1090.

6. Chatterjee, S.J., P. Ovadje, M. Mousa, et al. 2011. "The Efficacy of Dandelion Root Extract in Inducing Apoptosis in Drug-Resistant Human Melanoma Cells." *Evidence-Based Complementary and Alternative Medicine* Epub December 20, 2010.

7. You, Yanghee, Soonam Yoo, Ho-Geun Yoon, et al. June 2010. "In Vitro and In Vivo Hepatoprotective Effects of the Aqueous Extract from *Taraxacum officinale* (Dandelion) Root against Alcohol-Induced Oxidative Stress." *Food and Chemical Toxicology* 48(6): 1632–1637.

8. Domitrović, R., H. Jakovac, Z. Romić, et al. August 2010. "Antifibrotic Activity of *Taraxacum officinale* Root in Carbon Tetrachloride-Induced Liver Damage in Mice." *Journal of Ethnopharmacology* 130(3): 569–577.

9. Zhang, J., M.J. Kang, M.J. Kim, et al. Winter 2008. "Pancreatic Lipase Inhibitory Activity of *Taraxacum officinale* In Vitro and In Vivo." *Nutrition Research and Practice* 2(4): 200–203.

10. Agarwal, S.C., J.R. Crook, and C.B. Pepper. 2006. "Herbal Remedies—How Safe Are They? A Case Report of Polymorphic Ventricular Tachycardia/Ventricular Fibrillation Induced by Herbal Medication Used for Obesity." *International Journal of Cardiology* 106: 260–261.

11. Goksu, Erkan, Cenker Eken, Ozgur Karadeniz, and Oguz Kucukyilmaz. January 2010. "First Report of Hypoglycemia Secondary to Dandelion (*Taraxacum officinale*) Ingestion." *The American Journal of Emergency Medicine* 28(1): 111.e1–111.e2.

References and Resources

Magazines, Journals, and Newspapers

Agarwal, S.C., J.R. Crook, and C.B. Pepper. January 2006. "Herbal Remedies—How Safe Are They? A Case Report of Polymorphic Ventricular Tachycardia/Ventricular Fibrillation Induced by Herbal Medication Used for Obesity?" *International Journal of Cardiology* 106: 260–261.

Chatterjee, S.J., P. Ovadje, M. Mousa, et al. 2011. "The Efficacy of Dandelion Root Extract in Inducing Apoptosis in Drug-Resistant Human Melanoma Cells." *Evidence-Based Complementary and Alternative Medicine* Epub December 30, 2010.

Choi, U.K., O.H. Lee, J.H. Yim, et al. January 2010. "Hypolipidemic and Antioxidant Effects of Dandelion (*Taraxacum officinale*) Root and Leaf on Cholesterol-Fed Rabbits." *International Journal of Molecular Sciences* 11(1): 67–78.

Clare, B.A., R.S. Conroy, and K. Spelman. August 2009. "The Diuretic Effect in Human Subjects of an Extract of *Taraxacum officinale* Folium over a Single Day." *The Journal of Alternative and Complementary Medicine* 15(8): 929–934.

Domitrović, R., H. Jakovac, Z. Romić, et al. August 2010. "Antifibrotic Activity of *Taraxacum officinale* Root in Carbon Tetrachloride-Induced Liver Damage in Mice." *Journal of Ethnopharmacology* 130(3): 569–577.

Goksu, Erkan, Cenker Eken, Ozgur Karadeniz, and Oguz Kucukyilmaz. January 2010. "First Report of Hypoglycemia Secondary to Dandelion (*Taraxacum officinale*) Ingestion." *The American Journal of Emergency Medicine* 28(1): 111.e1–111.e2.

Ovadje, P., S. Chatterjee, C. Griffin, et al. January 2011. "Selective Induction of Apoptosis through Activation of Caspase-8 in Human Leukemia Cells (Jurkat) by Dandelion Root Extract." *Journal of Ethnopharmacology* 133(1): 86–91.

Sigstedt, S.C., C.J. Hooten, M.C. Callewaert, et al. May 2008. "Evaluation of Aqueous Extracts of *Taraxacum officinale* on Growth and Invasion of Breast and Prostate Cancer Cells." *International Journal of Oncology* 32(5): 1085–1090.

You, Yanghee, Soonam Yoo, Ho-Geun Yoon, et al. June 2010. "In Vitro and In Vivo Hepatoprotective Effects of the Aqueous Extract from *Taraxacum officinale* (Dandelion) Root against Alcohol-Induced Oxidative Stress." *Food and Chemical Toxicology* 48(6): 1632–1637.

Zhang, J., M.J. Kang, M.J. Kim, et al. Winter 2008. "Pancreatic Lipase Inhibitory Activity of *Taraxacum officinale* In Vitro and In Vivo." *Nutrition Research and Practice* 2(4): 200–203.

Websites

MedlinePlus. www.medlineplus.gov.

University of Maryland Medical Center Website. www.umm.edu.

E

Elderberry

Elderberry has roots that date back thousands of years. The ancient Greeks and Romans used it to treat a wide variety of medical problems including arthritis and asthma. By the Middle Ages, it was considered useful for influenza and other types of infections.[1]

In the early 1990s, elderberry took a huge step forward when Hadassah researchers in Jerusalem used elderberry to treat an influenza outbreak at an Israeli kibbutz. While those who took elderberry, which was processed into a syrup, recovered in three days, those who did not take the herb required twice the time—six days.[2]

But, elderberry is also believed to be useful for additional medical problems. It is important to examine what the researchers have learned.

Influenza

One of the most well-known trials on the role that elderberry may play in the treatment of influenza was published in 2004 in *The Journal of International Medical Research.* Researchers from Israel, Norway, and Sweden investigated the efficacy and safety of using oral elderberry syrup for treating influenza A and B infections. This randomized, double-blind, placebo-controlled study enrolled 60 people between the ages of 18 and 54 who had experienced influenza-like symptoms for 48 hours or less. For five days, the participants took either 15 mL of elderberry or placebo four times a day. The people taking elderberry had symptom relief "an average of four days earlier" than those on placebos; they also took significantly less medication for their influenza symptoms. The researchers noted that "elderberry extract offers an efficient, safe and cost-effective supplement to the present . . . medications for the prophylaxis and treatment of influenza." Nevertheless, they cautioned that their trial "involved only adult influenza patients who were otherwise healthy and did not include any high-risk patients."[3]

Another well-known in vitro study on the use of elderberry for influenza was published in 2009 in *Phytochemistry*. Researchers from Florida and Singapore determined that elderberry extract directly bound to the H1N1 (a type of influenza) virus and blocked its ability to enter cells, thereby providing protection against the virus. In fact, elderberry compared favorably with oseltamivir and amantadine, prescription drugs used to treat influenza.[4] Still, it is important to add that laboratory results do not necessarily translate into clinical efficacy. However, as has been noted, there is some evidence that elderberry is effective when used by people during the early stages of influenza infection.

Antibacterial Activity

In a study published in 2010 in the *Journal of Medicinal Plants Research,* researchers from Northern Ireland noted that the World Health Organization and other health authorities have acknowledged that antimicrobial resistance "is a major emerging problem of public health importance." Many pathogens have become resistant to antibiotics. So, the researchers wondered whether herbs, such as elderberry, may play a role in fighting pathogens. From their studies, they learned that elderberry does indeed have antimicrobial activity. The researchers commented that "the constituents identified in elder flower or berry (*S. nigra* L.) were toxic to all noscomial pathogens [infections acquired in a hospital] tested particularly, *S. aureus* (MRSA)."[5]

Anti-Inflammatory Activity

In a study published in 2006 in the *Journal of Periodontology,* researchers from Louisiana and New York examined the ability of elderberry to reduce the inflammation of periodontitis, a chronic inflammatory disease of the gums and bone around the teeth. In their in vitro studies, these researchers found that "the elder flower [elderberry] was found to potently inhibit all proinflammatory activities tested." They concluded that "the elder flower extract displays useful anti-inflammatory properties that could be exploited therapeutically for the control of inflammation in human periodontitis."[6]

Constipation

Writing in *BMC Complementary and Alternative Medicine* in 2010, researchers from Porto Alegre, Brazil noted that a compound containing elderberry, sweet fennel, anise, and senna is often used in Brazil for chronic constipation. However, no clinical trials have been conducted to determine whether this combination of herbs is actually effective.

In a randomized, crossover, placebo-controlled, single-blind trial, the researchers selected 20 people with chronic constipation. Half of the subjects received the compound for five days; during that time, the other subjects took a placebo. After a nine-day washout period, the subjects received the reverse treatment for five days. When the subjects were taking the compound, they had more evacuations per day; they also thought that their bowel function had improved. The researchers concluded that the compound "assessed has laxative efficacy and is a safe alternative option for the treatment of constipation."[7]

Weight Loss

In a study published in 2008 in *Phytotherapy Research,* researchers from Germany and Australia wanted to learn if a short-term elderberry- and asparagus-based low-calorie diet could be an effective and safe way to begin to make lifestyle changes that would result in weight loss. The researchers found that after two weeks on this diet, measures of body mass index, blood pressure, well-being, and quality of life had improved "to some extent." Most of the people who completed the study rated the "effectiveness and tolerability of the regimen . . . as very good or good." The researchers noted that their findings indicated "that the popular elder- and asparagus-based hypocaloric [very low calorie] diet may well serve as a starter for lifestyle change."[8]

Cardiovascular Health

In a study published in 2006 in the *Journal of Applied Physiology,* researchers from the Indiana University School of Medicine examined the cardiovascular effects of three extracts—elderberry, bilberry, and chokeberry—which are all rich in anthocyanins (antioxidant flavonoids that are protective of many body systems). The researchers determined that all three extracts had a number of positive cardiovascular benefits, and they noted that "these results suggest that such extracts could have significant beneficial effects in vascular disease."[9]

In a parallel-designed, randomized, placebo-controlled study published in 2009 in *The Journal of Nutrition*, researchers from the United Kingdom examined the cardiovascular effects of ingesting 500 mg elderberry per day for a total of 12 weeks. The cohort consisted of 52 healthy postmenopausal women; 26 took elderberry and 26 took a placebo. By the end of the trial, the researchers found "no significant change in biomarkers of CVD [cardiovascular disease]." The researchers concluded that the daily consumption of 500 mg elderberry "is apparently safe," but it fails to alter "biomarkers of CVD in healthy postmenopausal women."[10]

Anticancer Properties

In a study published in 2006 in the *Journal of Medicinal Food*, Illinois researchers examined the anticancer properties of both European elderberry (*Sambucus nigra*) and American elderberry (*Sambucus canadensis*). They noted that European elderberry is known to contain antioxidants such as "anthocyanins, flavonoids and other polyphenolics." However, they noted that less is known about American elderberry. After testing the berries, the researchers commented that both types "demonstrated significant chemopreventive potential."[11]

Is Elderberry Beneficial?

It is not uncommon to meet people who maintain that they have dramatically reduced their battles with viral infections by taking elderberry at the first sign of a cold or influenza. And, the limited scientific evidence that is available is compelling. It is hoped that future research will reveal even more uses for this herb.

Still, people on certain medications should not use elderberry without first discussing the issue with their medical providers. The drugs of particular concern are chemotherapies, laxatives, theophylline (respiratory problems), immunosuppressants, and medications for diabetes.

Notes

1. Castleman, Michael. November 2006. "Elder Statesman: The Venerable Elderberry Has Been Successfully Fighting Flu for Centuries." *Natural Health* 36(10): 96.
2. Castleman, Michael. November 2006. "Elder Statesman: The Venerable Elderberry Has Been Successfully Fighting Flu for Centuries." *Natural Health* 36(10): 96.

3. Zakay-Rones, Z., E. Thom, T. Wollan, and J. Wadstein. March–April 2004. "Randomized Study of the Efficacy and Safety of Oral Elderberry Extract in the Treatment of Influenza A and B Virus Infection." *The Journal of International Medical Research* 32(2): 132–140.

4. Roschek Jr., Bill, Ryan C. Fink, Matthew D. McMichael, et al. July 2009. "Elderberry Flavonoids Bind to and Prevent H1N1 Infection *In Vitro.*" *Phytochemistry* 70(10): 1255–1261.

5. Hearst, Caroline, Graham McCollum, David Nelson, et al. September 2010. "Antibacterial Activity of Elder (*Sambucus nigra* L.) Flower or Berry against Hospital Pathogens." *Journal of Medicinal Plants Research* 4(7): 1805–1809.

6. Harokopakis, E., M. H. Albzreh, E. M. Haase, et al. February 2006. "Inhibition of Proinflammatory Activities of Major Periondontal Pathogens by Aqueous Extracts from Elder Flower (*Sambucus nigra*)." *Journal of Periodontology* 77(2): 271–279.

7. Picon, P. D., R. V. Picon, A. F. Costa, et al. April 2010. "Randomized Clinical Trial of a Phytotherapic Compound Containing *Pimpinella anisum, Foeniculum vulgare, Sambucus nigra,* and *Cassia augustifolia* for Chronic Constipation." *BMC Complementary and Alternative Medicine* 10: 17.

8. Chrubasik, C., T. Maier, C. Dawid, et al. July 2008. "An Observational Study and Quantification of the Actives in a Supplement with *Sambucus nigra* and *Asparagus officinalis* Used for Weight Reduction." *Phytotherapy Research* 22(7): 913–918.

9. Bell, D. R. and K. Gochenaur. April 2006. "Direct Vasoactive and Vasoprotective Properties of Anthocyanin-Rich Extracts." *Journal of Applied Physiology* 100(4): 1164–1170.

10. Curtis, Peter J., Paul A. Kroon, Wendy J. Hollands, et al. December 2009. "Cardiovascular Disease Risk Biomarkers and Liver and Kidney Function Are Not Altered in Postmenopausal Women after Ingesting an Elderberry Extract Rich in Anthocyanins for 12 Weeks." *The Journal of Nutrition* 139(12): 2266–2271.

11. Thole, J. M., T. F. Kraft, L. A. Sueiro, et al. Winter 2006. "A Comparative Evaluation of the Anticancer Properties of European and American Elderberry Fruits." *Journal of Medicinal Food* 9(4): 498–504.

References and Resources

Magazines, Journals, and Newspapers

Bell, D. R. and K. Gochenaur. April 2006. "Direct Vasoactive and Vasoprotective Properties of Anthocyanin-Rich Extracts." *Journal of Applied Physiology* 100(4): 1164–1170.

Castleman, Michael. November 2006. "Elder Statesman: The Venerable Elderberry Has Been Successfully Fighting Flu for Centuries." *Natural Health* 36(10): 96.

Chrubasik, C., T. Maier, C. Dawid, et al. July 2008. "An Observational Study and Quantification of the Actives of a Supplement with *Sambucus nigra* and *Asparagus officinalis* Used for Weight Reduction." *Phytotherapy Research* 22(7): 913–918.

Curtis, Peter J., Paul A. Kroon, Wendy J. Hollands, et al. December 2009. "Cardiovascular Disease Risk Biomarkers and Liver and Kidney Function Are Not Altered in Postmenopausal Women after Ingesting an Elderberry Extract Rich in Anthocyanins for 12 Weeks." *The Journal of Nutrition* 139(12): 2266–2271.

Harokopakis, E., M. H. Albzreh, E. M. Haase, et al. February 2006. "Inhibition of Proinflammatory Activities of Major Periodontal Pathogens by Aqueous Extracts from Elder Flower (*Sambucus nigra*)." *Journal of Periodontology* 77(2): 271–279.

Hearst, Caroline, Graham McCollum, David Nelson, et al. September 2010. "Antibacterial Activity of Elder (*Sambucus nigra* L.) Flower or Berry against Hospital Pathogens." *Journal of Medicinal Plants Research* 4(17): 1805–1809.

Picon, P. D., R. V. Picon, A. F. Costa, et al. April 2010. "Randomized Clinical Trial of a Phytotherapic Compound Containing *Pimpinella anisum, Foeniculum vulgare, Sambucus nigra,* and *Cassia augustifolia* for Chronic Constipation." *BMC Complementary and Alternative Medicine* 10: 17.

Roschek Jr., Bill, Ryan C. Fink, Matthew D. McMichael, et al. July 2009. "Elderberry Flavonoids Bind to and Prevent H1N1 Infection *In Vitro.*" *Phytochemistry* 70(10): 1255–1261.

Thole, J. M., T. F. Kraft, L. A. Sueiro, et al. Winter 2006. "A Comparative Evaluation of Anticancer Properties of European and American Elderberry Fruits." *Journal of Medicinal Food* 9(4): 498–504.

Zakay-Rones, Z., E. Thom, T. Wollan, and J. Wadstein. March–April 2004. "Randomized Study of the Efficacy and Safety of Oral Elderberry Extract in the Treatment of Influenza A and B Virus Infection." *The Journal of International Medical Research* 32(2): 132–140.

Website
University of Maryland Medical Center. www.umm.edu.

Evening Primrose Oil 🌱

Scientifically known as *Oenothera biennis,* evening primrose is a wildflower that grows throughout the United States. The oil, which is located in the seeds, is filled with omega-6 essential fatty acids, such as linoleic acid and gamma-linolenic acid (GLA). Evening primrose is thought to be useful for a number of different health problems, including breast pain, premenstrual symptoms, menopausal symptoms, atopic dermatitis, arthritis, and diabetic neuropathy.[1] It is important to review what researchers have learned.

Breast Pain (Mastalgia)

In a study published in 2010 in *The Internet Journal of Surgery,* researchers from India wanted to determine if evening primrose oil (EPO) was useful for mastalgia (breast pain). The cohort consisted of 89 women, between the ages of 17 and 40, with mild to severe breast pain. All the women were given 500-mg capsules of evening primrose and instructed to take them twice daily for six months. In addition, each woman was given a breast pain chart and told to record a daily pain assessment. The researchers completed follow-ups with the women at three months and, again, at six months. Seventy-eight women completed the trial. Of these, 58 were found to have cyclical mastalgia and 20 had noncyclical mastalgia.

At the end of six months, the researchers determined that 42 women in the cyclical group had either an excellent or substantial response to their breast pain, while 16 had a poor or no response. Among the noncyclical women, after six months, 16 had an excellent or substantial response and 4 had a poor or no response. Thus, while substantial numbers of women were helped, many were not as fortunate. The researchers concluded that EPO may "be used as [a] first line of treatment in mild to moderate mastalgia; however, its efficacy for moderate to severe mastalgia remains doubtful."[2]

In a double-blind, randomized, placebo-controlled trial published in 2010 in the *Alternative Medicine Review,* researchers from the Mayo Clinic in Minnesota evaluated the use of EPO, vitamin E, and the combination of EPO and vitamin E to control pain in women with cyclical mastalgia. The cohort consisted of 85 women who had premenstrual cyclical breast discomfort; they ranged in age from 19 to 56, with a mean age of 40.4.

For six months, the women were placed on one of four different regimens—3,000 mg/day EPO, 1,200 IU/day vitamin E, 3,000 mg/day EPO, and 1,200 IU/day vitamin E, or placebo. Unfortunately, only 41 women completed the study. Nevertheless, the researchers noted that their findings "suggest that EPO, vitamin E, and EPO in combination with vitamin E may improve cyclical mastalgia." They added that "it is reasonable in a clinical setting to offer premenopausal women with severe cyclical mastalgia a short-term duration trial with either vitamin E at a daily dose of 1,200 IU, EPO at a daily dose of 3,000 mg, or the combination of vitamin E and EPO in the same dosages."[3]

Treatment for Atopic Dermatitis

In a study published in 2008 in the *Indian Journal of Dermatology, Venereology and Leprology,* researchers from India tested the efficacy and safety of EPO for atopic dermatitis, a chronic itchy skin disease that often starts in childhood.

Researchers assigned patients with atopic dermatitis to one of two groups. One group of 29 people received tablets containing 500 mg EPO, while another group of 36 people received placebo tablets that looked identical in appearance but contained 300 mg of sunflower oil. Treatment continued for five months. Twenty-six people in the EPO group and 27 people in the control group completed the study. The results were significant. By the end of the five months, a stunning 96% of the EPO group and 32% of the placebo group showed improvement. The researchers concluded that "evening primrose oil is a safe and effective medicine in management of AD."[4]

Anticoagulant Properties

In a study published in 2009 in the *Pakistan Journal of Pharmaceutical Sciences,* researchers from Pakistan assessed the anticoagulant properties of EPO in five different groups of white rabbits. One group of rabbits was fed warfarin, a blood-thinning medication, and another group, which served as the control, was fed water. The rabbits in three groups were fed normal, moderate, or high doses of EPO. The researchers found that EPO had "anticoagulant properties and its anticoagulant activity is supported by its anti-inflammatory effect." Why is this important? According to the researchers, "These effects along with antiplatelet activity suggest that EPO may be of value in cardiovascular diseases."[5]

Reduce the Need for Births by Cesarean Section

In a randomized, double-blind, placebo-controlled clinical trial published in 2006 in the *American Journal of Obstetrics & Gynecology,* a researcher from Manila, Philippines, examined the use of EPO in 71 Filipino women who were nearing the end of their pregnancies. For one week, 38 women were assigned to take one EPO capsule three times per day. Thirty-three women took placebos. The researcher found that the mean Bishop score (a measure used to determine whether a woman is likely to have a successful vaginal delivery and whether labor should be induced) was significantly better in the EPO group than in the placebo group. Moreover, the mean cervical length decreased significantly more in the EPO group than in the placebo group. But, the final finding was probably the most important. While 51% of the placebo group delivered vaginally, 70% of those in the EPO delivered vaginally. Still, there was no significant difference between the birth weights of the newborns in both groups. The researcher concluded that the use of EPO "as a cervical priming agent to enhance success rate for vaginal delivery may be considered for healthy term gravidas awaiting onset of labor."[6]

On the other hand, in an article published in 2008 in the *Journal of Pediatrics,* two physicians from Cincinnati Children's Hospital Medical Center in Cincinnati, Ohio, reported on a female newborn who developed petechiae (pinpoint, round spots that appear on the skin as a result of bleeding under the skin) shortly after birth. Apparently, to improve childbirth, the mother's health care provider had recommended that she take EPO and raspberry leaf tea. The physicians noted that the EPO probably "inhibited platelet function" in the newborn. The physicians wrote that "although it is reasonable to optimize the process of childbirth, this case raises concerns regarding the safety of primrose oil in this clinical setting."[7]

Lessens Symptoms of Dyslexia

In an open pilot study published in 2007 in the *Journal of Medicinal Food,* researchers from Sweden investigated the effect that a supplement containing EPO and high-docosahexaenoic acid (DHA) fish oil could help 20 Swedish children and adolescents, with an average age of 12, diagnosed with dyslexia. Dyslexia is an inherited condition in which people with normal intelligence have difficulties with reading, writing, and spelling in their native language. The children took eight capsules per day of the combination supplements for a total of five months. Subjective assessments by the parents and children were made at 6, 12, and 20 weeks. For the millions of people throughout the world who deal with this challenging disorder, the results were notable. These subjective assessments "showed increasing numbers of positive responders over time in reading speed, general schoolwork, and overall perceived benefit." Additionally, "significant improvements were observed in reading speed and motor-perceptual velocity." When objective tests were conducted, the researchers found an average of 23% improvement in word recognition and a 60% improvement in reading speed. The researchers commented that the supplementation "provided positive and clear beneficial effect on variables usually impaired by dyslexia."[8]

Is Evening Primrose Beneficial?

While it is evident that evening primrose may well be useful for some medical problems, it is also apparent that it may not be as effective as some claim. Likewise, it has the potential to cause problems, as it did with the previously described newborn. Before using evening primrose, it should be discussed with a medical provider.

Notes

1. Bayles, Bryan, and Richard Usatine. December 2009. "Evening Primrose Oil." *American Family Physician* 80(12): 1405–1408.
2. Thakur, Natasha, Babar Rashid Zargar Zargar, Nadeem U. I. Nazeer, et al. July 2010. "Mastalgia—Use of Evening Primrose Oil in Treatment of Mastalgia." *The Internet Journal of Surgery* 24(2): NA.
3. Pruthi, S., D. L. Wahner-Roedler, C. J. Torkelson, et al. April 2010. "Vitamin E and Evening Primrose Oil for Management of Cyclical Mastalgia: A Randomized Pilot Study." *Alternative Medicine Review* 15(1): 59–67.
4. Senapati, S., S. Banerjee, D. N. Gangopadhyay. September–October 2008. "Evening Primrose Oil Is Effective in Atopic Dermatitis: A Randomized Placebo-Controlled Trial." *Indian Journal of Dermatology, Venereology and Leprology* 74(5): 447–452.
5. Riaz, A., R. A. Khan, and S. P. Ahmed. October 2009. "Assessment of Anticoagulant Effect of Evening Primrose Oil." *Pakistan Journal of Pharmaceutical Sciences* 22(4): 355–359.
6. Ty-Torredes, Karen Alessandra. 2006. "The Effect of Oral Evening Primrose Oil on Bishop Score and Cervical Length among Term Gravidas." *American Journal of Obstetrics & Gynecology* 195(6) Supplement: S30.
7. Wedig, Kathy E., and Jeffrey A. Whitsett. January 2008. "Down the Primrose Path: Petechiae in a Neonate Exposed to Herbal Remedy for Parturition." *Journal of Pediatrics* 152: 140–141.
8. Lindmark, L., and P. Clough. December 2007. "A Five-Month Open Study with Long-Chain Polyunsaturated Fatty Acids in Dyslexia." *The Journal of Medicinal Food* 10(4): 662–666.

References and Resources

Magazines, Journals, and Newspapers

Bayles, Bryan and Richard Usatine. December 2009. "Evening Primrose Oil." *American Family Physician* 80(12): 1405–1408.

Lindmark, L. and P. Clough. December 2007. "A Five-Month Open Study with Long-Chain Polyunsaturated Fatty Acids in Dyslexia." *The Journal of Medicinal Food* 10(4): 662–666.

Pruthi, S., D.L. Wahner-Roedler, C.J. Torkelson, et al. April 2010. "Vitamin E and Evening Primrose Oil for Management of Cyclical Mastalgia: A Randomized Pilot Study." *Alternative Medicine Review* 15(1): 59–67.

Riaz, A., R.A. Khan, S.P. Ahmed. October 2009. "Assessment of Anticoagulant Effect of Evening Primrose Oil." *Pakistan Journal of Pharmaceutical Sciences* 22(4): 355–359.

Senapati, S., S. Banerjee, and D.N. Gangopadhyay. September–October 2008. "Evening Primrose Oil Is Effective in Atopic Dermatitis: A Randomized Placebo-Controlled Trial." *Indian Journal of Dermatology, Venereology and Leprology* 74(5): 447–452.

Thakur, Natasha, Babar Rashid Zargar Zargar, Nadeem U.I. Nazeer, et al. July 2010. "Mastalgia—Use of Evening Primrose Oil in Treatment of Mastalgia." *The Internet Journal of Surgery* 24(2): 1.

Ty-Torredes, Karen Alessandra. 2006. "The Effect of Oral Evening Primrose Oil on Bishop Score and Cervical Length among Term Gravidas." *American Journal of Obstetrics and Gynecology* 195(6) Supplement: S30.

Website
University of Maryland Medical Center. www.umm.edu.

F

Fennel 🌿

Fennel may be traced back to the ancient Greeks and Romans. Since then, it has been valued for both its medicinal and culinary properties. Today, fennel is grown mainly in the United States, France, India, and Russia.[1]

Fennel, which is scientifically known as *Foeniculum vulgare,* is rich in a number of vitamins and nutrients. It has excellent amounts of vitamin C and very good amounts of dietary fiber, potassium, manganese, folate, and molybdenum. Fennel also has good amounts of phosphorus, calcium, magnesium, iron, copper, and vitamin B3.[2] But, what have the researchers learned?

Painful Menstruation

In a study published in 2006 in the *Eastern Mediterranean Health Journal,* researchers from Iran compared the effectiveness of fennel and mefenamic acid (a nonsteroidal anti-inflammatory pain medication) for treating menstrual pain. The researchers divided girls, with a mean age of 13, into two groups. All the girls had a history of painful menstruation. For two months, one group of 55 girls took fennel and the other group of 55 took mefenamic acid. The researchers found that 80% of the girls who took fennel and 73% of the girls who took mefenamic acid "showed complete pain relief or pain decrease." Moreover, "80% of the fennel group and 62% of the mefenamic acid group no longer needed to rest." The researches concluded that "there was no significant difference between the two groups in the level of pain relief."[3] Still, it is important to know that fennel may relieve such a common problem.

Cardiovascular Health

In a study published in 2007 in *Pharmacological Research,* researchers from Parma, Italy, tested anethole, the main component in fennel essential oil, for elements that support cardiovascular health in guinea pigs, rats, and mice. They found that anethole relaxed blood vessels, and it had antiplatelet properties. Moreover, fennel demonstrated antithrombotic activity—it worked to prevent the formation of clots, which may be life-threatening. The researchers concluded that fennel essential oil and anethole had "safe antithrombotic activity that seems due to their broad spectrum antiplatelet activity, clot destabilizing effect and vasorelaxant action."[4]

Treatment for Infantile Colic

In a prospective, randomized study published in 2008 in the *Journal of Clinical Nursing,* Turkish researchers evaluated the effectiveness of four different treatments for infantile colic (persistent unexplained crying in a healthy baby)—massage, sucrose solution, fennel tea, and hydrolyzed formula (a pediatric formula in which the proteins are broken down into smaller, easier to digest, parts). A total of 175 infants were included in the study.

Parents and their infants were randomly assigned to one of the four treatment groups or a control group. The researchers found "a significant reduction in crying hours per day in all intervention groups." The infants switched to the hydrolyzed formula experienced the most improvement; the infants in the massage group experienced the least. So, the infants on fennel tea were in the middle.[5]

In a randomized, placebo-controlled trial published in 2003 in *Alternative Therapies in Health and Medicine,* Russian researchers noted that the only known effective pharmaceutical treatment for colic is dicyclomine hydrochloride. However, 5% of infants treated with this medication "develop serious side effects, including death." (It is no longer advised to give this medicine to infants under the age of six months.) So, these researchers wanted to learn if an herb, in this case fennel, could be an effective treatment for colic.

The cohort consisted of 125 infants, between the ages of 2 and 12 weeks, who had colic. Some of the infants were treated with fennel seed oil emulsion; other infants received no intervention. Sixty-five percent of the infants receiving fennel were significantly improved; only 23.7% of the infants in the control group were significantly better. There were no reports of side effects in either group. The researchers concluded that "fennel seed oil emulsion is superior to placebo in decreasing intensity of infantile colic."[6]

Reducing the Risk for Diabetic Complications

When pressure builds inside the eye or nerve cells of people with diabetes, it may trigger a host of different medical concerns such as problems with eyesight and with nerve damage. To understand how this occurs, one must briefly discuss aldose reductase, an enzyme that is normally found in the eyes and other parts of the body. Aldose reductase helps convert glucose in the body to a sugar alcohol known as sorbital. If aldose reductase converts too much glucose to sorbital, there may be excess amounts of damage inducing sorbital in the eyes and nerve cells. So, researchers search for aldose reductase inhibitors.

In a study published in 2008 in the *Asian Pacific Journal of Clinical Nutrition,* researchers from India investigated the aldose reductase inhibiting potential of 22 different plant-derived aqueous extracts. They found that 10 of the extracts had "considerable inhibitory potential." Fennel was among these. The researchers concluded that including herbs and certain other foods in the diet may help people with diabetes with "the management of diabetic complications."[7]

In a study published in 2008 in the *Indian Journal of Physiology and Pharmacology,* researchers from India evaluated the response of a single drop of fennel aqueous extract on rabbits' eyes that had normal and excess amounts of fluid. The researchers found that the fennel reduced fluid in both the normal eyes and the eyes with excess fluid. In fact, fennel was found to be comparable to timolol, a medication used to reduce fluid pressure within the eye.[8]

Antibacterial Activity

In a study published in 2009 in the *Pakistan Journal of Biological Sciences,* researchers from Iran evaluated the ability of fennel essential oil to destroy isolates of *Acinetobacter baumannii,* a bacterium that is naturally resistant to a number of antibiotics. The researchers tested fennel essential oil on 48 isolates collected from burn wards of hospitals in Tehran. They learned that fennel essential oil possessed antibacterial effect against all *A. baumannii* isolates. As a result, the researchers noted, fennel has the potential to be used for *A. baumannii* infections. "However, more adequate studies must be carried out to verify the possibility of using it for fighting bacterial infections in humans."[9]

Possible Concerns about Fennel

In an article published in a 2008 issue of the *Journal of Pediatric Surgery,* members of the Department of Pediatric Surgery at Gazi University in Ankara, Turkey noted that thelarche, the development of breast in a young girl with no other signs of puberty, has been associated with the long-term use of herbs, such as fennel, for gastrointestinal problems in children. Thus, the authors advise that the use of such herbs be "limited."[10]

The website of *American Family Physician* (FamilyDoctor.org) notes that intake of fennel has been associated with galactorrhea, a condition in which one or both breasts make milk. Though the condition is more common in women, it may occur in men. This production of milk takes place in people who are not nursing babies.[11]

And, the website of the American Society for Reproductive Medicine (www.asrm.org) includes information on a medical problem known as hyperprolactinemia, the production of excess prolactin by the body. Prolactin plays a role in the development of breast and the production of milk by a nursing mother. With hyperprolactinemia, women who are not pregnant have too much prolactin in their bodies. However, it also occurs in men. According to the society, one of the causes of this disorder is the consumption of herbs such as fennel.[12]

Is Fennel Beneficial?

Though some have expressed concerns, in all probability modest amounts of fennel are a good addition to the diet. And, parents who are dealing with a baby with colic, a very stressful and exhausting problem, may wish to discuss fennel with their child's health care provider.

Notes

1. The George Mateljan Foundation Website. www.whfoods.com.
2. The George Mateljan Foundation Website. www.whfoods.com.
3. Modaress Nejad, V., and M. Asadipour. May–July 2006. "Comparison of the Effectiveness of Fennel and Mefenamic Acid on Pain Intensity in Dysmenorrhoea." *Eastern Mediterranean Health Journal* 12(3–4): 423–427.

4. Tognolini, Massimiliano, Vigilio Ballabeni, Simona Bertoni, et al. September 2007. "Protective Effect of *Foeniculum vulgare* Essential Oil and Anethole in an Experimental Model of Thrombosis." *Pharmacological Research* 56(3): 254–260.

5. Arikan, Duygu, Handan Alp, Gözüm Sebahat, et al. July 2008. "Effectiveness of Massage, Sucrose Solution, Herbal Tea or Hydrolysed Formula in the Treatment of Infantile Colic." *Journal of Clinical Nursing* 17(13): 1754–1761.

6. Alexandrovich, I., O. Rakovitskaya, E. Kolmo, et al. July–August 2003. "The Effect of Fennel (*Foeniculum vulgare*) Seed Oil Emulsion in Infantile Colic: A Randomized, Placebo-Controlled Study." *Alternative Therapies in Health and Medicine* 9(4): 58–61.

7. Saraswat, M., P. Muthenna, P. Suryanarayana, et al. 2008. "Dietary Sources of Aldose Reductase Inhibitors: Prospects for Alleviating Diabetic Complications." *Asian Pacific Journal of Clinical Nutrition* 17(4): 558–565.

8. Agarwal, R., S. K. Gupta, S. S. Agrawal, et al. January–March 2008. "Oculohypotensive Effects of *Foeniculum vulgare* in Experimental Models of Glaucoma." *Indian Journal of Physiology and Pharmacology* 52(1): 77–83.

9. Janzani, N. H., M. Zartoshti, H. Babazadeh, et al. May 2009. "Antibacterial Effects of Iranian Fennel Essential Oil on Isolates of *Acinetobacter baumannii*." *Pakistan Journal of Biological Sciences* 12(9): 738–741.

10. Türkyilmaz, Z., R. Karabulut, K. Sönmez, and A. Can Başaklar. November 2008. "A Striking and Frequent Cause of Premature Thelarche in Children: *Foeniculum vulgare*." *Journal of Pediatric Surgery* 43(11): 2109–2111.

11. American Family Physician Website. www.FamilyDoctor.org.

12. American Society for Reproductive Medicine Website. www.asrm.org.

References and Resources

Magazines, Journals, and Newspapers

Agarwal, R., S. K. Gupta, S. S. Agrawal, et al. January–March 2008. "Oculohypotensive Effects of *Foeniculum vulgare* in Experimental Models of Glaucoma." *Indian Journal of Physiology and Pharmacology* 52(1): 77–83.

Alexandrovich, I., O. Rakovitskaya, E. Kolmo, et al. July–August 2003. "The Effect of Fennel (*Foeniculum vulgare*) Seed Oil Emulsion in Infantile Colic: A Randomized, Placebo-Controlled Study." *Alternative Therapies in Health and Medicine* 9(4): 58–61.

Arikan, Duygu, Handan Alp, Gözüm Sebahat, et al. July 2008. "Effectiveness of Massage, Sucrose Solution, Herbal Tea or Hydrolysed Formula in the Treatment of Infantile Colic." *Journal of Clinical Nursing* 17(13): 1754–1761.

Jazani, N. H., M. Zartoshti, H. Babazadeh, et al. May 2009. "Antibacterial Effects of Iranian Fennel Essential Oil on Isolates of *Acinetobacter baumannii*." *Pakistan Journal of Biological Sciences* 12(9): 738–741.

Modaress Nejad, V., and M. Asadipour. May–July 2006. "Comparison of the Effectiveness of Fennel and Mefenamic Acid on Pain Intensity in Dysmenorrhoea." *Eastern Mediterranean Health Journal* 12(3–4): 423–427.

Saraswat, M., P. Muthenna, P. Suryanarayana, et al. 2008. "Dietary Sources of Aldose Reductase Inhibitors: Prospects for Alleviating Diabetic Complications." *Asian Pacific Journal of Clinical Nutrition* 17(4): 558–565.

Tognolini, Massimiliano, Vigilio Ballabeni, Simona Bertoni, et al. September 2007. "Protective Effect of *Foeniculum vulgare* Essential Oil and Anethole in an Experimental Model of Thrombosis." *Pharmacological Research* 56(3): 254–260.

Türkyilmaz, Z., R. Karabulut, K. Sönmez, and A. Can Başaklar. November 2008. "A Striking and Frequent Cause of Premature Thelarche in Children: *Foeniculum vulgare.*" *Journal of Pediatric Surgery* 43(11): 2109–2111.

Websites

American Family Physician. www.FamilyDoctor.org.

American Society for Reproductive Medicine. www.asrm.org.

The George Mateljan Foundation. www.whfoods.com.

Fenugreek 🌿

Scientifically known as *Trigonella foenum-graecum,* fenugreek may be traced to ancient times. An Egyptian papyrus dated to 1500 BC described how fenugreek was commonly used in cooking.[1]

Historically, fenugreek, which is sometimes called fenugreek seed, was considered an effective treatment for a wide variety of medical concerns, such as inducing childbirth, digestive problems, and menopausal symptoms. Today, fenugreek is often cited as a means to stimulate milk production in breastfeeding moms as well as a treatment for type 2 diabetes and skin inflammation.[2] Additionally, fenugreek is believed to have properties that support cardiovascular health and fight cancer cells.[3] Is this funny-sounding herb really so valuable? It is important to review what researchers have learned.

Insulin Resistance and Type 2 Diabetes

In a double-blind, randomized study published in 2009 in the *Journal of Medicinal Food,* researchers from Louisiana developed a whole wheat bread containing fenugreek that was indistinguishable from their regular whole wheat bread. Then, they tested the bread on eight people who had diet-controlled diabetes. During one session, the participants were given two slices of the fenugreek-containing bread. After consumption, blood glucose insulin tests were taken over a four-hour time period. One week later, the researchers completed the same testing with the whole wheat bread. The researchers found that the bread with fenugreek did reduce insulin resistance. They concluded that "acceptable baked products can be prepared with added fenugreek, which will reduce insulin resistance and treat type 2 diabetes."[4] Still, it should be noted that the sample was probably too small to offer any definitive conclusions.

In a study published in 2009 in the *Indian Journal of Medical Research,* researchers from India investigated the effects of administering fenugreek, quercetin (plant-derived flavonoid found in fruits, vegetables, leaves, and grains), and metformin (prescription medication used to treat type 2 diabetes) in rats with insulin resistance. Researchers divided the rats into seven groups. The rats in the first group served as normal control. The rats in groups 2, 3, 4, and 5 were fed a high-fructose diet for 60 days, and, as a result, they developed insulin resistance. From day 16, the rats in the third group were also fed fenugreek seed polyphenolic extract; the rats in the fourth group were also fed quercetin; and the rats in the fifth group were also fed metformin. Rats in the sixth and seventh groups, respectively, served as the fenugreek and quercetin controls. The researchers determined that the fenugreek and quercetin separately "improved insulin signaling and sensitivity and thereby promoted the cellular actions of insulin." Moreover, their effects were similar to those obtained by metformin.[5] As a result, at least in this trial, fenugreek worked as well as prescription medication to control type 2 diabetes.

Anticancer Properties
In a study published in 2009 in *Cancer Biology & Therapy,* researchers from Baltimore, Maryland and Aurora, Colorado wanted to determine if fenugreek had anti-cancer properties. During the trial, the researchers examined the ability of fenugreek to kill in vitro breast, pancreatic, and prostate cancer cells. They found that "fenugreek seeds possess potent anti-cancer properties." At the same time, they do not harm normal cells.[6]

Diuretic Properties

In a study published in 2009 in *The Internet Journal of Alternative Medicine,* researchers from India evaluated the diuretic properties of fenugreek. The researchers began by dividing rats into seven groups. Prior to the experiment, the rats were deprived of food and water for 18 hours. The first group of rats, which served as the control, received normal saline. The second group received furosemide, a medicine used to reduce swelling and fluid retention in the body, in saline. The other groups received fenugreek extract doses of 150 mg/kg and 350 mg/kg injected into the cavity that holds the stomach and intestines. Immediately thereafter, the animals were placed in special cages designed to separate urine and feces. When compared to the control rats, the researchers found that the rats on either dose of fenugreek as well as furosemide had significant increases in the volume of urine. They concluded that their "work supports the traditional claim about the fenugreek seeds being used as diuretic."[7]

Weight Control

In a double-blind, randomized, placebo-controlled, three-period crossover trial published in 2009 in the *European Journal of Clinical Pharmacology,* researchers from France tested the ability of two different doses of fenugreek (588 and 1,176 mg) to control the consumption of fat in 12 healthy male volunteers between the ages of 19 and 26. The trial had three 14-day treatment periods that were separated by 14-day washout periods. The researchers found that when compared to the placebo the "daily fat consumption was significantly decreased by the higher dose of fenugreek seed extract." And, they concluded that "a 14-day treatment with a fenugreek seed extract reduces daily fat consumption in healthy, normal weight volunteers, with a tendency toward a decrease in total energy intake."[8]

The next year, in 2010, the *European Journal of Clinical Pharmacology* published another French study that examined the use of fenugreek seed extract for overweight subjects. This six-week, double-blind, randomized, placebo-controlled parallel trial included 39 healthy overweight male volunteers between the ages of 18 and 59. The researchers found that when compared to the subjects on the placebo, the subjects taking the fenugreek had significant reductions in daily consumption of fat.[9]

In a single-blind, randomized, crossover study published in 2009 in *Phytotherapy Research,* researchers from the University of Minnesota tested three different breakfasts—containing 0 g of fenugreek fiber, 4 g of fenu-greek fiber, or 8 g of fenugreek fiber—on 18 healthy obese subjects. For 3 ½ hours after the breakfasts, the subjects rated their feelings of hunger, satiety, and fullness every 30 minutes. After blood samples were taken, the subjects had an unlimited lunch buffet, and they recorded their food intake for the remainder of the day. The researchers found that "the 8 gram dose of fenugreek fiber significantly increased mean ratings of satiety and full-ness and reduced ratings of hunger and prospective food consumption."[10]

Heartburn Relief

In a study published in 2011 in *Phytotherapy Research,* researchers from Ohio and the Netherlands examined the use of fenugreek fiber in people who suffer from frequent heartburns. The cohort consisted of nonsmok-ing males and nonpregnant females who had heartburn after three to eight meals per week for at least a month. No participant could be taking pre-scription medication to treat heartburn symptoms. People were also elimi-nated who had any of the following characteristics: heavy use of alcohol, regular use of over-the-counter antacids, gastrointestinal diseases, and use of medications that may trigger heartburn such as low-dose aspirin. Not surprisingly, people with active cancer, gastric bypass surgery, or problems that limit food intake were also not allowed to participate.

After a week baseline period in which the subjects described their heart-burn symptoms, subjects were randomly assigned to one of three treat-ments for two weeks. The members of the first group took four placebo capsules twice each day; the members of the second group took 75 mg ran-tidine (Zantac 75, an over-the-counter heartburn medication) twice each day; and the members of the third group took fenugreek fiber, 500-mg cap-sules, four capsules twice each day. The subjects all kept a diary in which they rated the frequency and severity of their symptoms. While the people on fenugreek and Zantac both experienced similar levels of relief, they still had pain. The researchers wondered whether a trial that continues for a longer period of time may be more effective.[11]

Is Fenugreek Beneficial?

Fenugreek certainly appears to have a number of beneficial properties. You may wish to share some of the research on fenugreek with your medical provider. What about increasing the milk of nursing moms? While there are numerous anecdotal references and products marketed to nursing moms, at present, there is little scientific research on the topic.

Notes

1. National Center for Complementary and Alternative Medicine Website. www.nccam.nih.gov.
2. National Center for Complementary and Alternative Medicine Website. www.nccam.nih.gov.
3. Memorial Sloan-Kettering Cancer Center Website. www.mskcc.org.
4. Losso, Jack N., Darryl L. Holliday, John W. Finley, et al. October 2009. "Fenugreek Bread: A Treatment for Diabetes Mellitus." *Journal of Medicinal Food* 12(5): 1046–1049.
5. Kannappan, S., and C. V. Anuradha. April 2009. "Insulin Sensitizing Actions of Fenugreek Seed Polyphenols, Quercetin & Metformin in a Rat Model." *Indian Journal of Medical Research* 129(4): 401–408.
6. Shabbeer, Shabana, Michelle Sobolewski, Ravi Kumar Anchoori, et al. February 2009. "Fenugreek: A Naturally Occurring Edible Spice as an Anticancer Agent." *Cancer Biology & Therapy* 8(3): 272–278.
7. Rohini, R. M., Naira Nayeem, and Amit Kumar. 2009. "Diuretic Effect of *Trigonella foenum graecum* Seed Extracts." *The Internet Journal of Alternative Medicine* 6(2): NA.
8. Chevassus, Hugues, Nathalie Molinier, Françoise Costa, et al. 2009. "A Fenugreek Seed Extract Selectively Reduces Spontaneous Fat Consumption in Healthy Volunteers." *European Journal of Clinical Pharmacology* 65: 1175–1178.
9. Chevassus, Hugues, Jean-Baptiste Gaillard, Anne Farret, et al. 2010. "A Fenugreek Seed Extract Selectively Reduces Spontaneous Fat Intake in Overweight Subjects." *European Journal of Clinical Pharmacology* 66: 449–455.
10. Mathern, Jocelyn R., Susan K. Raatz, William Thomas, and Joanne L. Slavin. November 2009. "Effects of Fenugreek Fiber on Satiety, Blood Glucose and Insulin Response and Energy Intake in Obese Subjects." *Phytotherapy Research* 23(11): 1543–1548.
11. DiSilvestro, Robert A., Marian A. Verbruggen, and E. Jann Offutt. January 2011. "Anti-Heartburn Effects of a Fenugreek Fiber Product." *Phytotherapy Research* 25(1): 88–91.

References and Resources

Magazines, Journals, and Newspapers

Chevassus, Hugues, Jean-Baptist Gaillard, Anne Farret, et al. 2010. "A fenugreek Seed Extract Selectively Reduces Spontaneous Fat Intake in Overweight Subjects." *European Journal of Clinical Pharmacology* 66: 449–455.

Chevassus, Hugues, Nathalie Molinier, Françoise Costa, et al. 2009. "A Fenugreek Seed Extract Selectively Reduces Spontaneous Fat Consumption in Health Volunteers." *European Journal of Pharmacology* 65: 1175–1178.

DiSilvestro, Robert A., Marian A. Verbruggen, and E. Jann Offutt. January 2011. "Anti-Heartburn Effects of a Fenugreek Fiber Products." *Phytotherapy Research* 25(1): 88–91.

Kannappan, S., and C. V. Anuradha. April 2009. "Insulin Sensitizing Actions of Fenugreek Seed Polyphenols, Quercetin & Metformin in a Rat Model." *Indian Journal of Medical Research* 129(4): 401–408.

Losso, Jack N., Darryl L. Holliday, John W. Finley, et al. October 2009. "Fenugreek Bread: A Treatment for Diabetes Mellitus." *Journal of Medicinal Food* 12(5): 1046–1049.

Mathern, Jocelyn R., Susan K. Raatz, William Thomas, and Joanne L. Slavin. November 2009. "Effect of Fenugreek Fiber on Satiety, Blood Glucose and Insulin Response and Energy Intake in Obese Subjects." *Phytotherapy Research* 23(11): 1543–1548.

Rohini, R. M., Haira Nayeem, and Amit Kumar Das. 2009. "Diuretic Effects of *Trigonella foenum graecum* Seed Extracts." *The Internet Journal of Alternative Medicine* 6(2): NA.

Shabbeer, Shabana, Michelle Sobolewski, Ravi Kumar, et al. February 2009. "Fenugreek: A Naturally Occurring Edible Spice as an Anticancer Agent." *Cancer Biology & Therapy* 8(3): 272–278.

Websites
Memorial Sloan-Kettering Cancer Center. www.mskcc.org.

National Center for Complementary and Alternative Medicine. www.nccam. nih.gov.

Feverfew 🌿

Scientifically known as *Tanacetum parthenium,* feverfew has been used for centuries to treat a wide variety of medical problems. These include fevers, headaches, stomach aches, skin conditions, asthma, toothaches, infertility, insect bites, rheumatoid arthritis, menstruation, and labor pain.[1]

But, several decades ago, interest in feverfew grew exponentially. A 2007 article in *Townsend Letter: The Examiner of Alternative Medicine* described how the fascination with feverfew escalated in the 1970s after a Welsh lady, named Mrs. Anne Jenkins, reported that she took three fresh leaves of feverfew each day to stop debilitating recurrent migraines. At some point, Dr. Stewart Johnson, a London migraine specialist, heard about Mrs. Jenkins and her use of feverfew. So, he started to conduct his own research on the herb. Dr. Johnson found that an astonishing 72% of the people he surveyed who suffered from migraines obtained relief from feverfew. Since then, other researchers have examined the use of feverfew for migraines and a host of other concerns. It is important to review what they have learned.

Migraine Relief

In a randomized, double-blind, multicenter, placebo-controlled study published in 2005 in *Cephalalgia,* researchers from Germany reviewed the "efficacy and tolerability" of a carbon dioxide extract of feverfew (MIG-99) in patients with migraines. After a four-week baseline period, for 16 weeks, 80 patients took 6.25 mg of the extract, 3 times each day; 81 patients took placebos. At the beginning of the study, the participants experienced an average of 4.79 migraine attacks per month. By the end of the trial, the participants on feverfew had an average decrease of 1.9 attacks per month; the participants on placebos had an average reduction of 1.3 attacks. This difference was statistically significant.[2]

In a prospective, open-label study published in 2006 in *Clinical Drug Investigation,* French researchers attempted to determine if combining feverfew with white willow (*Salix alba*) would provide more protection from migraines than feverfew alone. The cohort initially consisted of 12 patients diagnosed with migraine without aura. Later, it was reduced to 10 patients. All the patients took 300-mg feverfew and 300-mg white willow twice each day. The researchers found that at the end of six weeks the frequency of migraine attacks was reduced by 57.2% in 9 of the 10 patients; at the end of 12 weeks, this reduction was 61.7%. In all 10 patients, the attack intensity was reduced by 38.7% at 6 weeks and by 62.6% at 12 weeks. All the patients experienced a decrease in attack duration of 67.2% at 6 weeks and 76.2% at 12 weeks. The researchers noted that "the remarkable efficacy of Mig-RL [the treatment] in not only reducing the frequency of migraine attacks but also their pain intensity and duration in this trial warrant further investigation."[3]

Kills Melanoma Cells

In an in vitro study published in 2010 in *Melanoma Research,* researchers from Lodz, Poland, examined the anticancer effects of parthenolide, a sesquiterpene lactone that is an active component of feverfew, on melanoma cells obtained "directly from a surgical excision." (A sesquiterpene lactone is a substance found in some plants that may have anti-inflammatory and anticancer effects. Melanoma is the most serious type of skin cancer.) The researchers found that parthenolide "reduced the number of viable adherent cells in melanoma cultures." They concluded that "the observed anticancer activity makes parthenolide an attractive drug candidate for further testing in melanoma therapy."[4]

Kills Glioblastoma Cells

In a study published in 2008 in the *Journal of Pharmacological Sciences,* researchers from Western Michigan University in Kalamazoo, Michigan, treated glioblastoma cells with varying doses of parthenolide. (Glioblastoma is a type of brain cancer.) The researchers then observed obvious glioblastoma cell death. According to the researchers, "glioblastomas are difficult to treat and frequently aggressive and fatal." As a result, "parthenolide or its derivatives may represent a new class of compounds that will be useful in the treatment of brain tumors."[5]

Kills Pancreatic Cancer Cells

In a study published in 2010 in the *Journal of Experimental & Clinical Cancer Research,* researchers from China examined the ability of parthenolide to destroy pancreatic cancer cells. During the trial, they treated human pancreatic cancer cells with different concentrations of parthenolide. The researchers learned that parthenolide "inhibited cell growth, migrations, and induced the apoptosis [cell death] in human pancreatic cancer." And, they added that their findings "may provide a novel approach for pancreatic cancer treatment."[6] The prognosis for people diagnosed with pancreatic cancer is often not very hopeful.

Kills Other Types of Cancer Cells

In a study published in 2006 in the *Journal of Medicinal Food,* researchers from Clemson University in Clemson, South Carolina, and China reviewed the ability of golden feverfew and components of golden feverfew, such as parthenolide camphor, luteolin, and apigenin, to kill cancer cells in two human breast cancer cell lines and one human cervical cancer cell line. The researchers learned that feverfew inhibited the growth of all three cancer cell lines. Among the tested components of feverfew, "parthenolide showed the highest inhibitory effect."[7]

In still another study published in 2007 in *Pharmacological Reports,* researchers from Lublin, Poland, tested the anticancer potential of parthenolide against three different types of human cancer cell lines—human lung cancer, human medulloblastoma (a type of brain cancer), and human colon adenocarcinoma (colorectal cancer). The researchers found that parthenolide "inhibited proliferation of all three types of cancer." Commenting on their results, the researchers wrote, "Based on our results and experiments performed by others, it may be suggested that parthenolide possesses antiproliferative properties and its use as an anticancer drug should be considered and carefully evaluated in clinical studies."[8]

Anti-Inflammatory Properties

In a study published in 2009 in *Inflammopharmacology,* researchers at the Johnson & Johnson Skin Research Center in Skillman, New Jersey, developed an extract of feverfew that contained no parthenolide. This enabled them to prevent the possibility of any allergic reactions. The researchers then conducted a variety of tests to determine the usefulness of the parthenolide-depleted extract of feverfew (PD-Feverfew) as an anti-inflammatory agent. (Inflammation in the body has been associated with a variety of chronic medical conditions, such as cardiovascular disease and cancer.) The researchers found that their PD-Feverfew had strong anti-inflammatory properties. In fact, "in some models of inflammation, PD-Feverfew was actually found to be more potent than whole Feverfew."[9]

Skin Protection

In a study published a year earlier, in 2008, in the *Archives of Dermatological Research,* researchers from the same Johnson & Johnson Skin Research Center noted that the skin "is under continual assault from a variety of damaging environmental factors such as ultraviolet irradiation and atmospheric pollutants." This results in "chronic inflammation and premature aging." The researchers maintained that feverfew, with its antioxidants, could "replenish the depleted cutaneous stores and perhaps forestall these degenerative changes." So, as in the previous notation, they developed parthenolide-depleted extract of feverfew (PD-Feverfew), which was free of any allergic potential. The researchers noted dramatic improvements in their in vitro and in vivo studies. "Through the ability to scavenge free radicals, preserve endogenous antioxidant levels, reduce depleted extract of Feverfew may protect skin from the numerous external aggressions encountered daily by the skin and reduce the damage to oxidatively challenged skin."[10]

Is Feverfew Beneficial?

It is very evident that feverfew appears to have a number of benefits. But, it is also obvious that there have been too few studies of this herb. Certainly, people who are dealing with debilitating migraines may wish to discuss feverfew with their medical providers. It is possible that feverfew may offer some relief.

Notes

1. National Center for Complementary and Alternative Medicine Website. www.nccam.nih.gov.
2. Diener, H. C., V. Pfaffenrath, J. Schnitker, et al. November 2005. "Efficacy and Safety of 6.25 mg t.i.d. Feverfew CO_2-Extract (MIG-99) in Migraine Prevention—a Randomized, Double-Blind, Multicentre, Placebo-Controlled Study." *Cephalalgia* 25(11): 1031–1041.
3. Shrivastava, J. C. Pechadra, and G. W. John. 2006. *"Tanacetum parthenium* and *Salix alba* (Mig-RL) Combination in Migraine Prophylaxis: A Prospective, Open-Label Study." *Clinical Drug Investigation* 26(5): 287–296.
4. Lesiak, K., K. Koprowska, I. Zalesna, et al. February 2010. "Parthenolide, a Sesquiterpene Lactone from the Medical Herb Feverfew, Shows Anticancer Activity against Human Melanoma Cells In Vitro." *Melanoma Research* 20(1): 21–34.
5. Anderson, K. N., and B. E. Bejcek. February 2008. "Parthenolide Induces Apoptosis in Glioblastomas without Affecting NF-kappaB." *Journal of Pharmacological Sciences* 106(2): 318–320.
6. Liu, J. W., M. X. Cai, Y. Xin, et al. August 2010. "Parthenolide Induces Proliferation Inhibition and Apoptosis of Pancreatic Cancer Cells In Vitro." *Journal of Experimental & Clinical Cancer Research* 29: 108.
7. Wu, C., F. Chen, J. W. Rushing, et al. Spring 2006. "Antiproliferative Activities of Parthenolide and Golden Feverfew Extract against Three Human Cancer Cell Lines." *Journal of Medicinal Food* 9(1): 55–61.
8. Parada-Turska, Jolanta, Roman Paduch, Maria Majdan, et al. March–April 2007. "Antiproliferative Activity of Parthenolide against Three Human Cancer Cell Lines and Human Umbilical Vein Endothelial Cells." *Pharmacological Reports* 59(2): 233–237.

9. Sur, R., K. Martin, F. Liebel, et al. February 2009. "Anti-Inflammatory Activity of Parthenolide-Depleted Feverfew (*Tanacetum parthenium*)." *Inflammopharmacology* 17(1): 42–49.

10. Martin, Katharine, Runa Sur, Frank Liebel, et al. February 2008. "Parthenolide-Depleted Feverfew (*Tanacetum parthenium*) Protects Skin from UV Irradiation and External Aggression." *Archives of Dermatological Research* 300(2): 69–80.

References and Resources

Magazines, Journals, and Newspapers

Anderson, K. N., and B. E. Bejcek. February 2008. "Parthenolide Induces Apoptosis in Glioblastomas without Affecting NF-kappaB." *Journal of Pharmacology Sciences* 106(2): 318–320.

Bone, Kerry. November 2007. "Feverfew and Migraine Headaches." *Townsend Letter: The Examiner of Alternative Medicine* 292: 61–65.

Diener, H. C., V. Pfaffenrath, J. Schnitker, et al. November 2005. "Efficacy and Safety of 6.25 t.i.d. Feverfew CO_2-Extract (MIG-99) in Migraine Prevention—a Randomized, Double-Blind, Multicentre, Placebo-Controlled Study." *Cephalalgia* 25(11): 1031–1041.

Lesiak, K., K. Koprowska, I. Zalesna, et al. February 2010. "Parthenolide, a Sesquiterpene Lactone from the Medical Herb Feverfew, Shows Anticancer Activity against Human Melanoma Cells in Vitro." *Melanoma Research* 20(1): 21–34.

Liu, J. W., M. X. Cai, Y. Xin, et al. August 2010. "Parthenolide Induces Proliferation Inhibition and Apoptosis of Pancreatic Cancer Cells In Vitro." *Journal of Experimental & Clinical Cancer Research* 29: 108.

Martin, Katharine, Runa Sur, Frank Liebel, et al. February 2008. "Parthenolide-Depleted Feverfew (*Tanacetum parthenium*) Protects Skin from UV Irradiation and External Aggression." *Archives of Dermatological Research* 300(2): 69–80.

Parada-Turska, Jolanta, Roman Raduch, Maria Majdan, et al. March–April 2007. "Antiproliferative Activity of Parthenolide against Three Human Cancer Cell Lines and Human Umbilical Vein Endothelial Cells." *Pharmacological Reports* 59(2): 233–237.

Shrivastava, R., J. C. Pechadre, and G. W. John. 2006. "*Tanacetum parthenium* and *Salix alba* (Mig-RL) Combination in Migraine Prophylaxis: A Prospective, Open-Label Study." *Clinical Drug Investigation* 26(5): 287–296.

Sur, R., K. Martin, F. Liebel, et al. February 2009. "Anti-Inflammatory Activity of Parthenolide-Depleted Feverfew (*Tanacetum parthenium*)." *Inflammopharmacology* 17(1): 42–49.

Wu, C., F. Chen, J. W. Rushing, et al. Spring 2006. "Antiproliferative Activities of Parthenolide and Golden Feverfew Extract against Three Human Cancer Cell Lines." *Journal of Medicinal Food* 9(1): 55–61.

Website
National Center for Complementary and Alternative Medicine. www.nccam .nih.gov.

G

Garlic 🌰

Scientifically known as *Allium sativum,* garlic has been used as a food and medicine for thousands of years. Today, garlic remains a very popular herb that is rich in free radical–destroying antioxidants. Garlic is thought to support cardiovascular health. Additionally, garlic has anti-inflammatory and anticancer properties. Garlic may even protect nerve cells.[1] But, it is important to review what researchers have learned.

Lowers Blood Pressure

In a randomized, double-blind, placebo-controlled trial published in 2010 in *Maturitas,* researchers from Australia wanted to determine if garlic could lower blood pressure levels in people with treated but uncontrolled high blood pressure. The trial began with 50 participants—25 were assigned to take four capsules of aged garlic per day (equivalent of 2.5 g of fresh garlic) and 25 took placebos. Systolic and diastolic blood pressure measurements were taken at baseline and at 4, 8, and 12 weeks. At the end of 12 weeks, the researchers noted that "aged garlic extract was superior to placebo in lowering systolic blood pressure in patients with treated, but uncontrolled, blood pressure." Moreover, "aged garlic extract was generally well-tolerated, and the level of blood pressure reduction achieved was comparable to that of common antihypertensive medication."[2]

In a study published in 2011 in *Clinical and Experimental Hypertension,* researchers from Serbia compared the ability of ethanol extracts of ginkgo, garlic, and onion to lower blood pressure levels and heart rates in anesthetized normotensive rats (rats with normal blood pressure). The researchers divided 18 rats into three groups of 6. The first group received the ginkgo; the second received the garlic; and the third received onion. The researchers found that when they administered the extracts intravenously, "the extract produced dose-dependent and reversible hypotensive and bradycardiac [slowing heart rate] effects." Of the three extracts, garlic was the most effective in reducing arterial blood pressure and heart rate. Still, the researchers added, that "there were statistically significant differences in bradycardiac and hypotensive effects of the garlic and ginkgo extracts."[3]

Improves Cardiovascular Health

In a randomized, double-blind, placebo-controlled trial published in 2010 in *Lipids in Health and Disease,* researchers from Russia investigated the ability of time-released garlic supplementation to help people dealing with coronary heart disease (CHD). Initially, the cohort consisted of 63 people between the ages of 40 and 65. For 12 months, the members of one group took one garlic powder tablet twice daily; the members of the second group took an identical placebo tablet twice daily. Fifty-one people completed the study. The treatment group consisted of 14 men and 12 women; the placebo group included 14 men and 11 women. The researchers found that the members of the garlic supplement group experienced significant reductions in total and low-density lipoprotein (LDL; bad) cholesterol. Their total cholesterol decreased by 12.4%, and their LDL decreased by 16.3%. The most significant results were observed in men. The researchers concluded that the 12-month supplementation of time-released garlic powder results "in the significant decrease of cardiovascular risk."[4]

In a study published in 2010 in the *Journal of Agriculture and Food Chemistry,* researchers from Taiwan noted that people with diabetes have at least twice the risk of developing heart disease as people who do not have diabetes. In addition, they are especially at risk for diabetic cardiomyopathy, a heart disease that inflames and weakens heart muscles and tissues. Could garlic oil help? The researchers divided 24 rats with laboratory induced diabetes into four groups. The rats in three groups were fed different amounts of garlic oil; the rats in the fourth group were fed corn oil. At the end of 16 days, when the rats were sacrificed, the researchers learned that the animals fed garlic oil experienced a number of different beneficial changes that are associated with protection against heart disease. The cardiovascular problems created by diabetes, such as a decrease in heart rate, lessened. "All these cardiac abnormalities induced by diabetes are improved by GO [garlic oil] treatment." The researchers noted that the changes appeared to be related to the potent antioxidant properties of garlic oil. The researchers concluded that "garlic oil possesses significant potential for protecting hearts from diabetes-induced cardiomyopathy."[5]

Controls Oral Pathogens

In an in vitro study published in 2011 in the *Journal of Medicinal Food,* researchers from Jerusalem, Israel tested the antimicrobial activity of the allicin contained in garlic against the oral pathogens that foster the development of dental cavities (caries) and periodontitis (inflammation and infection of ligaments and bones that support the teeth). (Allicin is not present in whole garlic. However, it is produced instantly when garlic is crushed or damaged.) The researchers found that "allicin was effective in inhibiting the growth of all tested bacteria." They noted that their findings "support the traditional medicinal use of garlic and suggest the use of allicin for alleviating dental disease." The researchers concluded that "allicin might be a useful candidate for *in vivo* testing as an agent for the prevention and treatment of dental diseases."[6]

Protects Lung Cells

In a study published in 2011 in *Phytotherapy Research,* researchers from Korea wanted to learn if garlic extracts could prevent cigarette smoke extract (CSE)–induced cell death in human bronchial smooth muscle cells. The researchers began by preparing garlic extract from fresh raw garlic, aged black garlic, and aged red garlic. Then, to induce cell death, they treated human bronchial smooth muscle cells with 10% cigarette smoke. The researchers found that of the three garlic extracts tested, treatment with aged red extract reduced cell death. Since the researchers noted that cigarette smokers may not eat a sufficient amount of aged red extract, smokers may require aged red extract supplementation. The researchers commented that "further studies will be needed to analyze the components in ARG [aged red garlic] extracts to identify the molecular mechanism by which antioxidative components are effective against CSE-induced cell death."[7]

Protects Gastric Cells

In a study published in 2010 in *Oncology Reports,* researchers from China explored the effects of allicin on gastric cancer cells. The researchers found that allicin reduced the cell viability in a dose-dependent manner. This was partially accomplished by triggering the induction of cell death in the gastric cancer cells. The researchers concluded that data from their study "demonstrated that allicin should be further investigated as a novel cancer preventive or therapeutic agent in control of gastric cancer, with potential uses in other tumor types."[8]

In a study published in 2010 in the *Chinese Journal of Cancer Research,* researchers from China examined the risk factors for precancerous gastric lesions primarily in rural China. Their cohort consisted of 1,179 subjects from Zhuanghe County. Because of smoking and drinking, all were considered at increased risk for precancerous gastric lesions. After the researchers controlled for gender, smoking, and alcohol, they found a significant correlation between deep-fried food consumption and gastric epithelial dysplasia. At the same, the researchers found that "garlic eating was shown to confer protection against the development of gastric ulcer."[9]

Is Garlic Beneficial?

The evidence is truly overwhelming. Eating garlic has a host of different benefits. Still, people who eat a good deal of garlic tend to release garlic odors from both their breath and body. And, it is well known that not everyone appreciates these smells. There are a few suggestions to help reduce garlic breath and body odor. Some people advise drinking whole milk and/or green tea or chewing parsley when eating garlic. There is also the belief that cooking garlic with button mushrooms may be useful. Do all these work? Probably not. But, for those who wish to eat garlic frequently, they are certainly worth trying.

Notes

1. University of Maryland Medical Center Website. www.umm.edu.
2. Ried, K., O. R. Frank, and N. P. Stocks. October 2010. "Aged Garlic Extract Lowers Blood Pressure in Patients with Treated by Uncontrolled Hypertension: A Randomised Controlled Trial." *Maturitas* 67(2): 144–150.
3. Brankovic, S., M. Radenkovic, and D. Kitic. 2011. "Comparison of the Hypotensive and Bradycardiac Activity of Ginkgo, Garlic, and Onion Extracts." *Clinical and Experimental Hypotension* 33(2): 95–99.
4. Sobenin, I. A., V. V. Pryanishnikov, L. M. Kunnova, et al. October 2010. "The Effects of Time-Released Garlic Powder Tablets on Multifunctional Cardiovascular Risk in Patients with Coronary Artery Disease." *Lipids in Health and Disease* 9: 119.

5. Ou, H.-C., B.-S. Tzang, M.-H. Chang, et al. October 2010. "Cardiac Contractile Dysfunction and Apoptosis in Streptozotocin-Induced Diabetic Rats Are Ameliorated by Garlic Oil Supplementation." *Journal of Agriculture and Food Chemistry* 58(19): 10347–10355.

6. Bachrach, G., A. Jamil, R. Naor, et al. November 2011. "Garlic Allicin as a Potential Agent for Controlling Oral Pathogens." *Journal of Medicinal Food* 14(11): 1338–1343.

7. Jeong, Y.Y., H.J. Park, Y.W. Cho, et al. 2011. "Aged Red Garlic Extract Reduces Cigarette Smoke Extract-Induced Cell Death in Human Bronchial Smooth Muscle Cells by Increasing Intracellular Glutathione Levels." *Phytotherapy Research.* dol:10.1002/ptr.3502.

8. Zhang, W., M. Ha, Y. Gong, et al. December 2010. "Allicin Induces Apoptosis in Gastric Cancer Cells through Activation of Both Extrinsic and Intrinsic Pathways." *Oncology Reports* 24(6): 1585–1592.

9. Liu, Jian, Li-Ping Sun, Yue-Hua Gong, and Yuan Yuan. December 2010. "Risk Factors of Precancerous Gastric Lesions in a Population at High Risk of Gastric Cancer." *Chinese Journal of Cancer Research* 22(4): 267–273.

References and Resources

Magazines, Journals, and Newspapers

Bachrach, G., A. Jamil, R. Naor, et al. November 2011. "Garlic Allicin as a Potential Agent for Controlling Oral Pathogens." *Journal of Medicinal Foods* 14(11): 1338–1343.

Brankovic, S., M. Radenkovic, and D. Kitic. 2011. "Comparison of the Hypotensive and Bradycardiac Activity of Ginkgo, Garlic, and Onion Extracts." *Clinical and Experimental Hypertension* 33(2): 95–99.

Jeong, Y.Y., H.J. Park, Y.W. Cho, et al. 2011. "Aged Red Garlic Extract Reduces Cigarette Smoke Extract-Induced Cell Death in Human Bronchial Smooth Muscle Cells by Increasing Intracellular Glutathione Levels." *Phytotherapy Research.* dol:10.1002/ptr.3502.

Liu, Jian, Li-Ping Sun, Yue-Hua Gong, and Yuan Yuan. December 2010. "Risk Factors of Precancerous Gastric Lesions in a Population at High Risk of Gastric Cancer." *Chinese Journal of Cancer Research* 22(4): 267–273.

Ou, H.-C., B.-S. Tzang, M.-H. Chang, et al. October 2010. "Cardiac Contractile Dysfunction and Apoptosis in Streptozotocin-Induced Diabetic Rats Are Ameliorated by Garlic Oil Supplementation." *Journal of Agriculture and Food Chemistry* 58(19): 10347–10355.

Ried, K., O.R. Frank, and N.P. Stocks. October 2010. "Aged Garlic Extract Lowers Blood Pressure in Patients with Treated but Uncontrolled Hypertension: A Randomised, Controlled Trial." *Maturitas* 67(2): 144–150.

Sobenin, I.A., V.V. Pryanishnikov, L.M. Kunnova, et al. October 2010. "The Effects of Time-Released Garlic Powder Tablets on Multifunctional

Cardiovascular Risk in Patients with Coronary Artery Disease." *Lipids in Health and Disease* 9: 119.

Zhang, W., M. Ha, Y. Gong, et al. December 2010. "Allicin Induces Apoptosis in Gastric Cancer Cells through Activation of Both Extrinsic and Intrinsic Pathways." *Oncology Reports* 24(6): 1585–1592.

Website
University of Maryland Medical Center. www.umm.edu.

Ginger ❦

Scientifically known as *Zingiber officinale,* ginger has historically been considered an excellent remedy for gastrointestinal distress. It was thought to soothe the intestinal tract and aid in the elimination of internal gas. Today, ginger is also believed to have antioxidant effects and inhibit inflammation in the body. In fact, it has been determined that ginger contains good amounts of potassium, magnesium, copper, manganese, and vitamin B6 (pyridoxine).[1] But, it is important to review what researchers have learned.

Antioxidant and Antimicrobial Properties
In a study published in 2010 in *Phytotherapy Research,* researchers from Taiwan tested the ability of four compounds found in ginger to destroy *Acinetobacter baumannii* (exceedingly drug-resistant *Acinetobacter baumannii,* XDRAB), a bacterium that is "a growing and serious nosocomial [hospital acquired] infection worldwide." The researchers found that "all these compounds showed antibacterial effects against XDRAB." And, the compounds lowered the drug resistance properties of XDRAB. Moreover, when tetracycline (an antibiotic) was used in conjunction with these compounds, there was an even better antibacterial effect. The researchers concluded that "ginger compounds have antioxidant effects that partially contribute to their antimicrobial activity and are candidates for use in the treatment of infections with XDRAB."[2] Given the serious nature of hospital-acquired infections, the importance of this finding should not be ignored.

Helps Prevent Oxidative Damage of Kidneys

In a study published in 2011 in the *Journal of Renal Nutrition,* researchers from India, Taiwan, and New Jersey investigated the protective ability of ginger against chronic alcohol-induced oxidative stress and tissue damage in rat kidneys. The researchers divided 24 rats into four equal groups— normal control, ginger treated, alcohol treated, and alcohol plus ginger treated. Ginger was given to the alcohol treated group for 30 days. The researchers found that the ginger was able to reverse the damage caused by the alcohol, and the "antioxidant status [returned] to normal levels." Additionally, "degenerative changes in renal cells with alcohol treatment were minimized." The researchers concluded that "alcohol-induced nephrotoxicity was attenuated by ginger extract treatment, thus ginger can [be] used as a regular nutrient to protect the renal cells."[3]

Cardiovascular Benefit

In a study published in 2010 in *Inflammopharmacology,* researchers from Egypt evaluated the ability of ginger to lower elevated levels of cholesterol in rats. The researchers began by dividing 48 rats into six groups of 8 rats. One group, which consisted of rats eating the standard diet, served as the control. The rats in the five remaining groups were all fed a high-cholesterol diet. One of these groups served as the high-cholesterol control. Three groups were also fed different amounts of aqueous infusion of ginger (100, 200, and 400 mg/kg). The rats in the last group had atorvastatin (0.18 mg/kg), a medication used to treat elevated levels of serum cholesterol, added to their diets. The researchers found that after two and four weeks of treatment, the rats in the three groups that received the three different doses of ginger had significant decreases in all lipid profile parameters.[4]

Helps Prevent Cataracts in People with Diabetes

In a study published in 2010 in *Molecular Vision,* researchers from India investigated the ability of ginger to prevent cataracts in people with diabetes. The researchers began by setting aside one group of rats to serve as the control and inducing diabetes in three additional groups of rats. For two months, two of these three groups of rats were fed a diet that included 0.5% or 3% ginger. The progression of cataracts was monitored through the use of slit-lamp biomicroscope. The researchers found that "the feeding of ginger not only delayed the onset but also the progression of cataract in rats." They concluded that foods such as ginger "may be explored for the prevention or delay of diabetic complications."[5]

Treatment for Pregnancy-Related Nausea and Vomiting

In a single-blind, randomized, clinical trial published in 2009 in *The Journal of Alternative and Complementary Medicine,* researchers from Iran wanted to determine if ginger would be of assistance to pregnant women who are dealing with nausea and vomiting. The cohort consisted of 67 pregnant women who were complaining of nausea and vomiting. Women in the experimental group took four 250-mg ginger capsules each day for four days; the women in the control group took placebos. The researchers found that the women taking ginger had a higher rate of nausea improvement than the women on the placebos—85% versus 56%. The decrease in vomiting times among the ginger users was also significantly greater than the women on placebos—50% versus 9%. The researchers concluded that "ginger is an effective herbal remedy for decreasing nausea and vomiting during pregnancy."[6]

Treatment for Chemotherapy-Induced Nausea and Vomiting

In a randomized, double-blind study published in 2011 in *Pediatric Blood & Cancer,* researchers from India wanted to learn if ginger would help children and young adults experiencing nausea and vomiting from chemotherapy for bone sarcoma (a type of bone cancer). The researchers divided their group of 60 patients with bone sarcoma into two groups. In addition to their regular medications, the members of one group also took ginger root powder capsules, and the members of the second group took placebos. The findings were notable. The members of the control group experienced far more acute moderate to severe nausea and vomiting than the members of the ginger group. However, the researchers noted that even though the ginger reduced the severity of nausea and vomiting, "it did not eliminate them." Still, they wrote that "ginger root powder may be used as an add-on therapy in patients receiving chemotherapy with high emetogenic potential."[7]

In a study presented to the 2009 annual meeting of the American Society of Clinical Oncology, researchers from several United States cities evaluated the ability of ginger to bring relief to 644 patients who experienced nausea after undergoing one cycle of chemotherapy. Most of the participants were women who were dealing with breast cancer. In addition to their regular antinausea medications, the participants were randomly assigned to receive a placebo or 0.5, 1.0, or 1.5 g of ginger in a capsule once a day for six days, starting three days before the first day of a cycle of chemotherapy. During the first four days of a chemotherapy cycle, the participants rated their nausea on a seven point scale—a rating of 1 meant no nausea and a rating of seven meant the severest level of nausea. The researchers found that at the end of the first day, the patients who took the two lowest amounts of ginger rated their nausea either 1 or 2. That meant they had little or no nausea. On the other hand, at the end of the first day, the patients on the placebo rated their nausea either 4 or 5. Surprisingly, the higher dose of ginger worked, but not as well as the lower doses. The benefits continued for the four days of the study.[8]

Different results were obtained from a randomized, double-blind, placebo-controlled study published in 2009 in *Supportive Care in Cancer*. Researchers from Michigan investigated the use of ginger in 162 patients who had experienced nausea and vomiting during at least one previous round of chemotherapy. The patients, who were all taking medications to prevent nausea and vomiting, received either a placebo or 1.0 or 2.0 g ginger for three days. The researchers found that the participants failed to obtain any benefit from the ginger. They noted that there "was no significant difference between either of the ginger doses compared to placebo in the prevalence of acute or delayed nausea or vomiting."[9]

Is Ginger Beneficial?
Ginger does appear to be useful for a number of medical problems. Moreover, for the vast majority of people, it seems to be well-tolerated.

Notes
1. The George Mateljan Foundation Website. www.whfoods.com.
2. Wang, H. M., C. Y. Chen, H. A. Chen, at al. December 2010. "*Zingiber officinale* (Ginger) Compounds Have Tetracycline-Resistance Modifying Effects against Clinical Extensively Drug-Resistant *Acinetobacter baumannii*." *Phytotherapy Research* 24(12): 1825–1830.
3. Shanmugam, K. R., S. M. Korivi, N. Kesireddy, et al. May 2011. "Ginger Feeding Protects against Renal Oxidative Damage Caused by Alcohol Consumption in Rats." *Journal of Renal Nutrition* 21(3): 263–270.

4. ElRokh, El-Sayed M., Nemet A. Z. Yassin, Siham M. A. El-Shenawy, et al. December 2010. "Antihypercholesterolaemic Effect of Ginger Rhizome (*Zingiber officinale*) in Rats." *Inflammopharmacology* 18(6): 309–315.
5. Saraswat, M., P. Suryanarayana, P. Y. Reddy, et al. August 2010. "Antiglycating Potential of *Zingiber officinalis* and Delay of Diabetic Cataract in Rats." *Molecular Vision* 16: 1525–1537.
6. Ozgoli, Giti, Marjan Goli, and Masoumeh Simbar. March 2009. "Effects of Ginger Capsules on Pregnancy, Nausea, and Vomiting." *The Journal of Alternative and Complementary Medicine* 15(3): 243–246.
7. Pillai, A. K., K. K. Sharma, Y. K. Gupta, and S. Bakhshi. February 2011. "Anti-Emetic Effect of Ginger Powder versus Placebo as an Add-On Therapy in Children and Young Adults Receiving High Emetogenic Chemotherapy." *Pediatric Blood & Cancer* 56(2): 234–238.
8. American Society of Clinical Oncology Website. www.asco.org.
9. Zick, Suzanna M., Mack T. Ruffin, Julia Lee, et al. May 2009. "Phase II Trial of Encapsulated Ginger as a Treatment for Chemotherapy-Induced Nausea and Vomiting." *Supportive Care in Cancer* 17(5): 563–572.

References and Resources

Magazines, Journals, and Newspapers

ElRokh, El-Sayed M., Nemat A. Z. Yassin, Siham M. A. El-Shenawy, et al. December 2010. "Antihypercholesterolaemic Effect of Ginger Rhizome (*Zingiber officinale*) in Rats." *Inflammopharmacology* 18(6): 309–315.

Ozgoli, Giti, Marjan Goli, and Masoumeh Simbar. March 2009. "Effects of Ginger Capsules on Pregnancy, Nausea, and Vomiting." *The Journal of Alternative and Complementary Medicine* 15(3): 243–246.

Pillai, A. K., K. K. Sharma, Y. K. Gupta, and S. Bakhshi. February 2011. "Anti-Emetic Effect of Ginger Powder versus Placebo as an Add-On Therapy in Children and Young Adults Receiving High Emetogenic Chemotherapy." *Pediatric Blood & Cancer* 56(2): 234–238.

Saraswat, M., P. Suryanarayana, P. Y. Reddy, et al. August 2010. "Antiglycating Potential of *Zingiber officinalis* and Delay of Diabetic Cataract in Rats." *Molecular Vision* 16: 1525–1537.

Shanmugam, K. R., S. M. Korivi, N. Kesireddy, et al. May 2011. "Ginger Feeding Protects against Renal Oxidative Damage Caused by Alcohol Consumption in Rats." *Journal of Renal Nutrition* 21(3): 263–270.

Wang, H. M., C. Y. Chen, H. A. Chen, et al. December 2010. "*Zinigiber officinale* (Ginger) Compounds Have Tetracycline-Resistance Modifying Effects against Clinical Extensively Drug-Resistant *Acinetobacter baumannii*." *Phytotherapy Research* 24(12): 1825–1830.

Zick, Suzanna M., Mack T. Ruffin, Julia Lee, et al. May 2009. "Phase II Trial of Encapsulated Ginger as a Treatment for Chemotherapy-Induced Nausea and Vomiting." *Supportive Care in Cancer* 17(5): 563–572.

Websites
American Society of Clinical Oncology. www.asco.org.
The George Mateljan Foundation. www.whfoods.com.

Ginkgo 🌿

Scientifically known as *Ginkgo biloba,* ginkgo leaves and seeds have been used for thousands of years for a vast array of medical concerns. Probably best known as a treatment for circulatory disorders, such as poor circulation in the legs, and memory problems, such as dementia, ginkgo contains flavonoids and terpenoids, chemicals that have strong antioxidant properties. Like other antioxidants, they fight free radicals, compounds that damage cells in the body.[1] But, it is important to review what the researchers have learned.

Improves Cognition

In a 26-page article published in 2009 in *Human Psychopharmacology,* a researcher from Germany reviewed a total of 29 published clinical trials on ginkgo extracts. The review only included randomized, double-blind, and placebo-controlled studies of the chronic administration of ginkgo for more than four weeks. In total, there were 2,414 participants who were either healthy older adults or people showing the first signs of cognitive decline. The researcher found "consistent evidence that chronic administration [of ginkgo] improves selective attention, some executive processes and long-term memory for verbal and non-verbal material." Moreover, "in spite of possible biases which cannot be ruled out in some trials, predominantly complex measures of memory, attention and intelligence improved."[2]

In a randomized, double-blind, multicenter trial published in 2011 the *International Journal of Geriatric Psychiatry,* researchers from Germany, Israel, and the Ukraine examined the efficacy and safety of ginkgo treatments for people with dementia who have presented with neuropsychiatric features. The cohort consisted of 410 outpatients with mild to moderate dementia. For 24 weeks, the subjects took either 240 mg of ginkgo or a placebo. By the end of the trial, those taking ginkgo had a marked improvement in their symptoms. "Active treatment was significantly superior to placebo in improving patients' cognitive performance, neuropsychiatric symptoms, functional abilities, and overall condition." As a result, "the distress perceived by caregivers due to patients' aberrant behaviours was alleviated."[3]

On the other hand, in a randomized, double-blind, placebo-controlled clinical trial published in 2009 in *JAMA: The Journal of the American Medical Association,* researchers from multiple locations in the United States had different results. The cohort consisted of 3,069 people, between the ages of 72 and 96, who lived in the community. A little more than half of the participants were placed on twice daily doses of 120 mg of ginkgo, and a little less than half were placed on an identical-appearing placebo. The median follow-up was 6.1 years. Still, the researchers found no proof that ginkgo was making a difference in the lives of the elders. According to the researchers, there was "no evidence that *G biloba* slows the rate of cognitive decline in older adults."[4]

Reduces Pain and Inflammation

In a study published in 2011 in *Anesthesia & Analgesia,* researchers from the United Kingdom induced pain and inflammation in the paws of rats. Then, they treated some of the rats with ginkgo extract and other rats with diclofenac, a nonsteroidal anti-inflammatory drug that is often used for arthritis. These treatments were injected into the paws and the spinal cord. Ginkgo was found to be just as effective as diclofenac in reducing pain. The researchers concluded that ginkgo "acts both at the site of inflammation and centrally at the spinal cord level to inhibit inflammation and thermal hyperalgesia [increased sensitivity to pain] and may be useful in the treatment of inflammatory pain."[5]

Migraine Prevention

In an open-label prospective trial published in 2010 in *Neurological Sciences,* researchers from Milan, Italy, and Pensacola, Florida tested the ability of Ginkgolide B, an herbal product made from ginkgo tree leaves, to help children who suffer from migraines. The cohort consisted of 24 children and teens, 12 males and 12 females, between the ages of 8 and 18, who suffered from migraines without aura. For three months, the young subjects were treated twice each day with Ginkgolide B 80 mg, coenzyme Q10 20 mg, vitamin B2 1.6 mg, and magnesium 300 mg. When compared to the prestudy baseline, the researchers found, "the number of monthly migraine attacks was substantially reduced after three months of treatment with Ginkgolide B." Furthermore, the researchers added that "the treatment was well tolerated and the compliance was good." No one experienced a worsening of his or her condition. The researchers concluded that "this treatment could be a good option for patients suffering from migraine without aura in particular for young patients, where therapies without side effects are needed."[6]

In another study published in 2011 in *Neurological Sciences*, researchers from Naples, Italy also studied the use of ginkgo for 119 "school-aged patients" with migraines without aura. They took supplements comparable to those in the previous study for three months. And, these supplements also provided "effective and safe" relief to the subjects in this study. The researchers concluded that "in childhood headache management, the use of alternative treatments must be considered not to evoke a placebo effect, but as soft therapy without adverse reactions."[7]

May Be Useful for Vitiligo Vulgaris

In a study published in 2011 in *BMC Complementary and Alternative Medicine*, researchers from Canada reviewed the use of ginkgo for vitiligo vulgaris, a disorder in which patches of skin lose their pigmentation. The cohort initially consisted of 12 participants between the ages of 12 and 35 years. Everyone had a first visit and three follow-up visits; everyone took one 60-mg capsule twice daily. Eleven participants completed the 12-week trial. The researchers noted that the progression of the disorders stopped in all the participants. And, while they maintained that their finding were not conclusive, "they did provide preliminary evidence that ginkgo may have a role in the management of vitiligo." Should people with this disorder begin ginkgo supplementation? The researchers commented that they recommend "any attempt to use ginkgo in the management of vitiligo should be carefully monitored by a health care practitioner, given that there are still many questions about the correct dose, its true effectiveness, interactions with other conditions or therapies, and possible adverse reactions."[8]

Helps with Symptoms of Tardive Dyskinesia

In a double-blind study published in 2011 in *The Journal of Clinical Psychiatry*, researchers from China wanted to learn if ginkgo would help people with schizophrenia who are experiencing tardive dyskinesia, involuntary movements of the tongue, lips, face, trunk, and extremities caused by long-term treatment with certain antipsychotic medications. The cohort consisted of 157 male inpatients with diagnosed schizophrenia. They were all randomly assigned to receive either 12 weeks of treatment with 240 mg ginkgo per day (78 patients) or a placebo (79 patients). Of the 157 patients, 152 completed the study. During the treatment period, the researchers found that ginkgo group had "a highly significantly therapeutic effect." Moreover, this positive effect "continued for at least 6 months after the medication had been discontinued." According to the researchers, these actions may be the result of ginkgo's "antioxidant and free-radical scavenging activities." The researchers concluded that "the potential usefulness of the extract in the treatment of TD [tardive dyskinesia] has clinical importance, as it has only rare and transitory side effects in relatively high doses."[9]

Is Ginkgo Beneficial?

Ginkgo is one of the most readily available and well-studied herbs. And, it seems to be useful for a wide variety of health concerns. Ginkgo may well be an herb that should be discussed with health care providers.

Notes

1. University of Maryland Medical Center Website. www.umm.edu.
2. Kaschel, Reiner. July 2009. "*Ginkgo biloba*: Specificity of Neuropsychological Improvement—a Selective Review in Search of Differential Effects." *Human Psychopharmacology: Clinical & Experimental* 24(5): 345–370.
3. Ihl, R., N. Bachinskaya, A. D. Korczyn, et al. November 2011. "Efficacy and Safety of a Once-Daily Formulation of *Ginkgo biloba* Extract EGb 761 in Dementia with Neuropsychiatric Features: A Randomized Controlled Trial." *International Journal of Geriatric Psychiatry* 26(11): 1186–1194.
4. Snitz, Beth E., Ellen S. O'Meara, Michelle C. Carlson, et al. December 2009. "*Ginkgo biloba* for Preventing Cognitive Decline in Older Adults: A Randomized Trial." *JAMA: The Journal of the American Medial Association* 302(24): 2663–2670.
5. Thorpe, Laura Biddlestone, Michelle Goldie, and Sharron Dolan. May 2011. "Central and Local Administration of *Ginkgo Biloba* Extract EGb 761® Inhibits Thermal Hyperalgesia and Inflammation in the Rat Carrageenan Model." *Anesthesia & Analgesia* 112(5): 1226–1231.

6. Usai, S., L. Grazzi, F. Andrasik, and G. Bussone. June 2010. "An Innovative Approach for Migraine Prevention in Young Age: A Preliminary Study." *Neurological Sciences* 31(Supplement 1): S181–S183.
7. Esposito, M., and M. Carotenuto. February 2011. "Ginkgolide B Complex Efficacy for Brief Prophylaxis of Migraine in School-Aged Children: An Open-Label Study." *Neurological Sciences* 32(1): 79–81.
8. Szczurko, O., N. Shear, A. Taddio, and H. Boon. March 2011. "*Ginkgo biloba* for the Treatment of Vitiligo Vulgaris: An Open Label Pilot Clinical Trial." *BMC Complementary and Alternative Medicine* 11: 21.
9. Zhang, W.F., Y.L. Tan, X.Y. Zhang, et al. May 2011. "Extract of *Ginkgo biloba* Treatment for Tardive Dyskinesia in Schizophrenia: A Randomized, Double-Blind, Placebo-Controlled Trial." *The Journal of Clinical Psychiatry* 72(5): 615–621.

References and Resource

Magazines, Journals, and Newspapers

Esposito, M., and M. Carotenuto. February 2011. "Ginkgolide B Complex Efficacy for Brief Prophylaxis of Migraine in School-Aged Children: An Open-Label Study." *Neurological Sciences* 32(1): 79–81.

Ihl, R., N. Bachinskaya, A.D. Korczyn, et al. November 2011. "Efficacy and Safety of a Once-Daily Formulation of *Ginkgo biloba* Extract EGb 761 in Dementia with Neuropsychiatric Features: A Randomized Controlled Trial." *International Journal of Geriatric Psychiatry* 26(11):1186–1194.

Kaschel, Reiner. July 2009. "*Ginkgo biloba*: Specificity of Neuropsychological Improvement—A Selective Review in Search of Differential Effects." *Human Psychopharmacology: Clinical & Experimental* 24(5): 345–370.

Snitz, Beth E., Ellen S. O'Meara, Michelle C. Carlson, et al. December 2009. "*Ginkgo biloba* for Preventing Cognitive Decline in Older Adults: A Randomized Trial." *JAMA: The Journal of the American Medical Association* 302(24): 2663–2670.

Szczurko, O.N. Shear, A. Taddio, and H. Boon. March 2011. "*Ginkgo biloba* for the Treatment of Vitiligo Vulgaris: An Open Label Pilot Clinical Trial." *BMC Complementary and Alternative Medicine* 11: 21.

Thorpe, Laura Biddlestone, Michelle Goldie, and Sharron Dolan. May 2011. "Central and Local Administration of *Ginkgo biloba* Extract EGb 761® Inhibits Thermal Hyperalgesia Inflammation in the Rat Carregeenan Model." *Anesthesia & Analgesia* 112(5): 1226–1231.

Usai, S., L. Grazzi, F. Andrasik, and G. Bussone. June 2010. "An Innovative Approach for Migraine Prevention in Young Age: A Preliminary Study." *Neurological Sciences* 31 (Supplement 1): S181–S183.

Zhang, W.E., Y.L. Tan, X.Y. Zhang, et al. May 2011. "Extract of *Ginkgo biloba* Treatment for Tardive Dyskinesia in Schizophrenia: A Randomized,

Double-Blind, Placebo-Controlled Trial." *The Journal of Clinical Psychiatry* 72(5): 615–621.

Website
University of Maryland Medical Center. www.umm.edu.

Ginseng ❦

There are two main types of ginseng—American (*Panax quinquefolius*) and Asian or Korean (*Panax ginseng*). They both belong to the species *Panax* and have a similar chemical composition. Some researchers focus on one type of ginseng; other researchers tend to lump the two together. For the purposes of this entry, American and Asian or Korean ginseng will be combined and termed ginseng. (Siberian ginseng is an entirely different herb, and it will not be discussed in this entry.)

Ginseng is said to boost the immune system, support cardiovascular health, foster weight loss, assist those with type 2 diabetes, improve mental performance and physical endurance, reduce stress, enhance well-being, kill cancer cells, and improve menopausal symptoms.[1] Is ginseng really able to solve so many disparate health concerns? It is important to review what researchers have learned.

Prevention and/or Treatment of Human Lung Cancer
In a study published in 2010 in the *Journal of Medicinal Food,* researchers from Korea wanted to determine if ginseng could play a role in the prevention and/or treatment of human lung cancer. They began by inoculating mice with human lung cancer cells. This established a human tumor xenograft (tissue graft) model. Next, the mice were divided into five groups. Two groups became the positive and negative controls. Three different doses of lipid-soluble ginseng extract were administered orally to the mice in the other three groups. After 15 days of treatment, the researchers found that "the oral administration of the lipid-soluble extract of red ginseng showed a potent anticancer effect in nude mice bearing human lung cancer cells in a dose-dependent manner without any apparent toxicity." And, they concluded that "a lipid-soluble extract of red ginseng could be considered as a nontoxic potential anticancer supplement for prevention of cancer as well as for growth inhibition of tumors in the initial stage."[2]

Fatigue Relief for Cancer Patients

In 2007, researchers based at the Mayo Clinic in Minnesota presented a study on the use of ginseng to relieve fatigue in people with cancer at the annual meeting of the American Society of Clinical Oncology. The researchers enrolled 282 patients with various types of cancer to participate in this eight-week randomized, placebo-controlled trial. All the participants were either currently receiving cancer treatment (chemotherapy or radiation therapy) or had recently completed treatment. They were assigned to one of four groups—placebo (no ginseng), 750 mg of ginseng per day, 1,000 mg of ginseng per day, or 2,000 mg of ginseng per day. The participants were surveyed about their fatigue at the beginning of the study, at the end of four weeks, and at the end of eight weeks. When compared to the participants taking 750 mg of ginseng, the participants taking 1,000 and 2,000 mg had lower levels of fatigue. The researchers concluded that the two higher doses of ginseng "may be effective for alleviating cancer related fatigue."[3]

Provides Gastric Ulcer Protection

In a study published in 2010 in *BMC Complementary and Alternative Medicine,* researchers from Japan assessed the ability of ginseng to provide a degree of protection from gastric ulcers. After putting aside some mice to serve as the controls, the researchers began by treating mice with three different doses of ginseng. One hour later, they used two different compounds (hydrochloride/ethanol and indomethacin) to induce stomach ulcers in the mice. The researchers found that when compared to the placebo, the two larger doses of ginseng significantly inhibited the ability of both compounds to form gastric ulcers. And, they concluded that ginseng "may be a powerful remedy for gastric mucosal lesions."[4]

Weight Loss

In a study published in 2010 in *Cytotechnology,* researchers from Japan investigated the ability of ginseng to assist with weight loss. For eight weeks, they fed mice one of four diets—a low-fat diet with 4% fat, a high-fat diet with 40% fat, a high-fat diet supplemented with 0.8% ginseng, or a high-fat diet supplemented with 1.6% ginseng. By the end of the trial, the researchers found that the weight gain of the mice on the high-fat diet was significantly higher than the weight gain of the mice on the low-fat diet.

However, when compared to the mice on the high-fat diet, the body weight of the mice eating the high-fat diet supplemented with 1.6% ginseng was significantly reduced. Meanwhile, the mice eating the high-fat diet with 0.8% ginseng lost more weight than those on the high-fat diet, "but the difference was not significant." The researchers concluded that ginseng "may prevent the development of obesity and hyperlipidemia in HFD [high fat diet]-induced obese mice."[5]

Treatment for Allergic Rhinitis

In a double-blind, placebo-controlled study published in 2011 in *Allergy, Asthma & Immunology Research,* researchers from Korea attempted to learn if fermented ginseng could bring relief to people suffering from allergic rhinitis, a medical condition that is caused by an allergy and has symptoms similar to those experienced with a cold. The researchers recruited 66 people who had been experiencing allergic rhinitis for two years. They were divided into two groups. For four weeks, the members of one group took fermented ginseng, and the members of the other group took a placebo. Fifty-nine people completed the study. The researchers found that the people taking ginseng had significant improvements in nasal congestion. And, they concluded that fermented ginseng may "be safely used as a health food to treat allergic rhinitis [and] can improve both nasal symptoms and overall quality of life."[6]

Does Not Appear to Improve Endurance

In a randomized, double-blind, placebo-controlled study published in 2011 in the *Indian Journal of Medicinal Research,* researchers from Malaysia and India examined ginseng's ability to increase endurance. Their cohort consisted of nine male subjects between the ages of 20 and 40. They were all "heat adapted recreational runners" or runners who had experience navigating in the hot and humid environment of Malaysia. One hour before exercising on a treadmill, the runners were given 200 mg of ginseng or a placebo. The researchers found no difference between the endurance of the runners who ingested ginseng or a placebo. They concluded that supplementation with ginseng "did not affect the endurance running performance and other selected physiological parameters in the heat."[7] However, one can not help but wonder if conclusions may be drawn from such a small number of men in a single study. Most likely, more evidence is needed.

Ginseng May Induce Oxidative Stress

In a double-blind, parallel study published in 2009 in the *Journal of the American College of Nutrition,* researchers from Madison, Wisconsin, wanted to determine if ginseng could provide postmenopausal women with a degree of antioxidant protection. Twelve female subjects (between the ages of 55 and 75) were told to consume two capsules, each containing 500 mg of ginseng, every day for four months. At the same time, a group of 13 female control subjects, who were about the same ages, consumed two placebo capsules. Before and after the supplementation, each subject walked on a treadmill for 30 minutes. The researchers found that "ginseng supplementation had no effects on heart rate, blood pressure, plasma blood glucose, or lactate concentration at rest or immediately after exercise tests." Nevertheless, results of blood and urine tests indicated that the women on ginseng experienced oxidative stress, a harmful condition in which there are an excess number of free radicals in the body.[8] The ginseng did not provide the protection the researchers had predicted. Yet, as in the previously noted study, one can not help but speculate if serious conclusions should be drawn from such a small study.

Is Ginseng Beneficial?

Ginseng may well be beneficial for some people with certain health problems. But, the research literature mentions numerous potential side effects and medications with which ginseng should not be mixed. For example, ginseng may cause high blood pressure and should not be combined with blood-thinning medications. Before beginning ginseng supplementation, it is important to have a discussion with a healthcare provider.

Notes

1. University of Maryland Medical Center Website. www.umm.edu.
2. Lee, Sung Dong, Song-Kyu Park, Eun Sil Lee, et al. February 2010. "A Lipid-Soluble Red Ginseng Extract Inhibits the Growth of Human Lung Tumor Xenografts in Nude Mice." *Journal of Medicinal Food* 13(1): 1–5.
3. American Society of Clinical Oncology Website. www.asco.org.
4. Oyagi, Arsushi, Kenjirou Ogawa, Mamoru Kakino, and Hideaki Hara. August 2010. "Protective Effects of a Gastrointestinal Agent Containing Korean Red Ginseng on Gastric Ulcer Models in Mice." *BMC Complementary and Alternative Medicine* 10: 45+.

5. Lee, Young-Sil, Byung-Yoon Cha, Kohji Yamaguchi, et al. August 2010. "Effects of Korean White Ginseng Extracts on Obesity in High-Fat Diet-Induced Obese Mice." *Cytotechnology* 62(4): 367–376.
6. Jung, J.W., H.R. Kang, G.E. Ji, et al. April 2011. "Therapeutic Effects of Fermented Red Ginseng in Allergic Rhinitis: A Randomized, Double-Blind, Placebo-Controlled Study." *Allergy, Asthma & Immunology Research* 3(2): 103–110.
7. Ping, Fadzel Wong Chee, Chen Chee Keong, and Amit Bandyopadhyay. January 2011. "Effects of Acute Supplementation of *Panax Ginseng* on Endurance Running in a Hot & Humid Environment." *Indian Journal of Medical Research* 133(1): 96–102.
8. Dickman, J.R., R.T. Koenig, and L.L. Ji. April 2009. "American Ginseng Supplementation Induces an Oxidative Stress in Postmenopausal Women." *Journal of the American College of Nutrition* 28(2): 219–228.

References and Resources

Magazines, Journals, and Newspapers

Dickman, J.R., R.T. Koenig, and L.L. Ji. April 2009. "American Ginseng Supplementation Induces an Oxidative Stress in Postmenopausal Women." *Journal of the American College of Nutrition* 28(2): 219–228.

Jung, J.W., H.R. Kang, G.E. Ji, et al. April 2011. "Therapeutic Effects of Fermented Red Ginseng in Allergic Rhinitis: A Randomized, Double-Blind, Placebo-Controlled Study." *Allergy, Asthma & Immunology Research* 3(2): 103–110.

Lee, Sung Dong, Song-Kyu Park, Eun Sil Lee, et al. February 2010. "A Lipid Soluble Red Ginseng Extract Inhibits the Growth of Human Lung Tumor Xenografts in Nude Mice." *Journal of Medicinal Food* 13(1): 1–5.

Lee, Young-Sil, Byung-Yoon Cha, Kohji Yamaguchi, et al. August 2010. "Effects of Korean White Ginseng on Obesity in High-fat Diet-Induced Obese Mice." *Cytotechnology* 62(4): 367–376.

Oyagi, Atsushi, Kenjirou Ogawa, Mamoru Kakino, and Hideaki Hara. August 2010. "Protective Effects of a Gastrointestinal Agent Containing Korean Red Ginseng on Gastic Ulcer Models in Mice." *BMC Complementary and Alternative Medicine* 10: 45+.

Ping, Fadzel Wong Chee, Chen Chee Keong, and Amit Bandyopadhyay. January 2011. "Effects of Acute Supplementation of *Panax ginseng* on Endurance Running in a Hot & Humid Environment." *Indian Journal of Medical Research* 133(1): 96–102.

Websites

American Society of Clinical Oncology. www.asco.org.

University of Maryland Medical Center. www.umm.edu.

Gotu Kola 🦌

Scientifically known as *Centella asiatica,* gotu kola has been considered a medicinal herb in India, China, and Indonesia for thousands of years. In ancient times, it was used to heal wounds and skin conditions and to improve mental clarity. Historically, gotu kola has also been thought to be an effective treatment for stomach ulcers, mental fatigue, diarrhea, epilepsy, hepatitis, syphilis, fever, and asthma. Today, gotu kola is more often used for chronic venous insufficiency, a condition in which blood pools in the legs, and as an ointment for minor skin wounds.[1] Gotu kola is sold in a wide variety of forms, including capsules, creams, powders, liquids, and teas, and is grown in many parts of the world, including Japan, China, Australia, South Africa, Madagascar, Sri Lanka, and India.[2] It is important to review what researchers have learned.

Wound Healing

In a study published in 2010 in the *Journal of the Medical Association of Thailand,* a researcher from Pathumthani, Thailand, enrolled 200 patients who had diabetes-related foot ulcers. The patients were then randomly divided into one of two groups. The members of one group took daily doses of gotu kola, and the members of the second group took a placebo. The same investigator examined the wounds at days 7, 14, and 21. In the end, 170 people completed the study and were included in the results. When compared to the placebo group, gotu kola was found to promote wound healing. Patients taking gotu kola had improved wound healing and less scar tissue.[3]

A few years earlier, in a study published in 2006 in *The International Journal of Lower Extremity Wounds,* researchers from Manipal, India, evaluated the ability of gotu kola to aid in wound healing in Wistar Albino rats. The researchers divided 24 rats into four groups of 6. The first group of rats served as the control. Their wounds were treated with normal saline. The second group of rats had their wounds treated with gotu kola extract. The wounds of the third group of rats were treated with dexamethasone, a glucocorticoid that suppresses wound healing. The final group of rats had wounds treated with dexamethasone and gotu kola extract. The researchers found that gotu kola extract promoted healing. Moreover, wound healing in the steroid-treated group of rats was significantly better when treated with gotu kola. The researchers concluded that it is probably the antioxidant properties of gotu kola leaf extract that "influenced the faster wound healing demonstrated in this rat model."[4]

Generalized Anxiety Disorder

In a study published in 2010 in the *Nepal Medical College Journal,* researchers from India investigated the role that gotu kola may play in treating people with generalized anxiety disorder. For 60 days, 18 men and 15 women, with an average age of 33 years, took 500-mg capsules of gotu kola twice each day. The researchers found that gotu kola "reduced stress, attenuated anxiety, negated depression and enhanced adjustment and attention in patients without any side effects like vertigo, nausea and dizziness or mental weakness."[5]

Improvement in Cognition and Mood

In a study published in 2008 in the *Journal of Ethnopharmacology,* researchers from Thailand wanted to determine if gotu kola could improve the cognitive functioning of older men and women. The cohort consisted of 4 men and 24 females, with a mean age of 65.05. All the participants were in good health. For two months, the subjects took either 250 mg, 500 mg, or 750 mg of gotu kola once per day. The researchers found that the highest dose of gotu kola improved both memory and mood. And, they concluded that their findings "suggest the potential of *Centella asiatica* to attenuate the age-related decline in cognitive function and mood disorder in the healthy elderly."[6]

Alzheimer's Disease

In a study published in 2009 in *Phytotherapy Research,* researchers from Texas noted that "one of the distinguishing neurological features of Alzheimer's disease" is the "deposition of amyloid β [beta] peptide into plaques in the brain parenchyma and cerebral blood vessels." In other words, the brains of people with Alzheimer's disease have been found to contain certain types of pathologic lesions known as amyloid plaques, and there is a cerebrovascular accumulation of amyloid β. These plaques are believed to be responsible "for the memory loss and behavioral changes associated with Alzheimer's disease." Locating these plaques during an autopsy is one of the ways that people have been diagnosed with Alzheimer's disease following death.

The researchers investigated whether the long-term treatment of mice bred to have an increased production of amyloid β peptide with gotu kola could reduce the prevalence of these pathologic lesions. And, that is exactly what the researchers learned. Using gotu kola over an extended period of time decreased the levels of amyloid β peptides. The researchers wrote that their "study shows that *Centella asiatica* treatment alters amyloid β pathology in the PSAPP Alzheimer's disease mouse model after prolonged treatment. . . . It was shown that CaE [gotu kola extract] displayed antioxidant properties . . . providing multiple mechanisms to alter pathology in [the] Alzheimer's brain."[7]

Protection Against Damage from Radiation

In a study published in 2009 in the *Journal of Pharmacy and Pharmacology,* researchers from India attempted to determine if gotu kola could protect DNA and membranes against damage from gamma radiation. After conducting both in vitro and in vivo trials, the researchers found that gotu kola reduced radiation-induced damage to DNA and membranes. "*Centella asiatica* extract rendered radioprotection to DNA and membranes against radiation exposure, both in vitro and in vivo."[8]

Cardiovascular Health

Mixed results were obtained in a study published in 2009 in the *Journal of Food Science*. Researchers from Malaysia wanted to learn the role that gotu kola could play on the lipid metabolism of rats with oxidative stress. At the end of the 25-week trial, the researchers determined that compared to the rats fed a control diet, the rats fed gotu kola powder had significantly lowered serum low-density lipoprotein (LDL; "bad" cholesterol). Additionally, when compared to the control rats, the rats fed gotu kola powder or extract had significantly higher high-density lipoprotein (HDL; "good" cholesterol) and lower triglyceride levels. However, the total cholesterol levels of the rats fed gotu kola powder or extract were significantly higher than the control rats.[9]

Skin Antiaging Properties

In a randomized, double-blind study that was published in 2008 in *Experimental Dermatology,* researchers from France examined the skin antiaging properties of madecassoside, a compound extracted from gotu kola.

The researchers noted that madecassoside supports collagen, which is found in abundance in the skin, and it controls inflammation. The cohort consisted of 20 female volunteers with photoaged skin. For six months, the volunteers applied a preparation containing 5% vitamin C and 0.1% madecassoside. After six months, the researchers observed "a significant improvement of the clinical score for deep and superficial wrinkles, suppleness, firmness, roughness and skin hydration." Additionally, "two-thirds of the subjects showed an improvement." The researchers concluded that their "results reveal a functional and structural remodeling of chronically sun-damaged skin."[10]

Is Gotu Kola Beneficial?

Gotu kola appears to have a number of beneficial properties. It would probably be of most use to those who are dealing with severe memory concerns, such as those associated with Alzheimer's disease. Unfortunately, at present, people dealing with Alzheimer's disease have only a limited range of traditional treatments. But, it may well have many other uses.

Notes

1. University of Maryland Medical Center Website. www.umm.edu.
2. Drugs.com Website. www.drugs.com.
3. Paocharoen, V. December 2010. "The Efficacy and Side Effects of Oral *Centella asiatica* Extract for Wound Healing Promotion in Diabetic Wound Patients." *Journal of the Medical Association of Thailand* 93 (Supplement 7): S166–S170.
4. Shetty, Somashekar, S. L. Udupa, A. L. Udopa, and N. Somayaji. September 2006. "Effect of *Centella asiatica* L. (Umbelliferae) on Normal and Dexamethasone-Suppressed Wound Healing in Wistar Albino Rats." *The International Journal of Lower Extremity Wounds* 5(3): 137–143.
5. Jana, U., T. K. Sur, L. N. Maity, et al. March 2010. "A Clinical Study on the Management of Generalized Anxiety Disorder with *Centella asiatica*." *Nepal Medical College Journal* 12(1): 8–11.
6. Wattanathorn, Jintanaporn, Lugkana Mator, Supaporn Muchimapura, et al. March 2008. "Positive Modulation of Cognitive and Mood in the Healthy Elderly Volunteer Following the Administration of *Centella asiatica*." *Journal of Ethnopharmacology* 116(2): 325–332.
7. Dhanasekaran, Muralikrishnan, Leigh A. Holcomb, Angie R. Hitt, et al. January 2009. "*Centella asiatica* Extract Selectively Decreases Amyloid β Levels in Hippocampus of Alzheimer's Disease Animal Model." *Phytotherapy Research* 23(1): 14–19.

8. Joy, J., and C. K. Nair. July 2009. "Protection of DNA and Membranes from Gamma-Radiation Induced Damages by *Centella asiatica.*" *Journal of Pharmacy and Pharmacology* 61(7): 941–947.

9. Hussin, M., A. A. Hamid, S. Mohamad, et al. March 2009. "Modulation of Lipid Metabolism by *Centella asiatica* In Oxidative Stress Rats." *Journal of Food Science* 74(2): H72–H78.

10. Haftek, Marek, Sophie Mac-Mary, Marie-Aude Le Bitoux, et al. November 2008. "Clinical, Biometric and Structural Evaluation of the Long-Term Effects of Topical Treatment with Ascorbic Acid and Madecassoside in Photoaged Human Skin." *Experimental Dermatology* 17(11): 946–952.

References and Resources

Magazines, Journals, and Newspapers

Dhanasekaran, Muralikrishnan, Leigh A. Holcomb, Angie R. Hitt, et al. January 2009. "*Centella asiatica* Extract Selectively Decreases Amyloid β Levels in Hippocampus of Alzheimer's Disease Animal Model." *Phytotherapy Research* 23(1): 14–19.

Haftek, Marek, Sophie Mc-Mary, Marie-Aude Le Bitoux, et al. November 2008. "Clinical, Biometric and Structural Evaluation of the Long-Term Effects of a Topical Treatment with Ascorbic Acid and Madecassoside in Photoaged Human Skin." *Experimental Dermatology* 17(11): 946–952.

Hussin, M., A. A. Hamid, S. Mohamad, et al. March 2009. "Modulation of Lipid Metabolism by *Centella asiatica* in Oxidative Stress Rats." *Journal of Food Science* 74(2): H72–H78.

Jana, U., T. K. Sur, L. N. Maity, et al. March 2010. "A Clinical Study on the Management of Generalized Anxiety Disorder with *Centella asiatica.*" *Nepal Medical College Journal* 12(1): 8–11.

Joy, J., and C. K. Nair. July 2009. "Protection of DNA and Membranes from Gamma-Radiation Induced Damages by *Centella asiatica.*" *Journal of Pharmacy and Pharmacology* 61(7): 941–947.

Paocharoen, V. December 2010. "The Efficiency and Side Effects of Oral *Centella asiatica* Extract for Wound Healing Promotion in Diabetic Wound Patients." *Journal of the Meidcal Association of Thailand* 93 (Supplement 7): S166–S170.

Shetty, Somashekar, S. L. Udupa, A. L. Udopa, and N. Somayaji. September 2006. "Effect of *Centella asiatica* L. (Umbelliferae) on Normal and Dexamethasone-Suppressed Wound Healing in Wistar Albino Rats." *The International Journal of Lower Extremity Wounds* 5(3): 137–143.

Wattanathorn, Jintanaporn, Lugkana Mator, Supaporn Muchimapura, et al. March 2008. "Positive Modulation of Cognition and Mood in the Healthy Elderly Volunteer Following the Administration of *Centella asiatica.*" *Journal of Ethnopharmacology* 116(2): 325–332.

Websites
Drugs.com. www.drugs.com.
University of Maryland Medical Center. www.umm.edu.

Grape Seed Extract 🍇

Since ancient times, people have used grapes for medicinal purposes. So, it should surprise no one that grape seed extract, *Vitis vinifera,* is now considered an effective preventive agent and treatment for a number of medical problems such as several types of cancer, hypertension (high blood pressure), type 2 diabetes, and Alzheimer's disease. It may even be useful for weight loss. But, what have the researchers learned?

Colorectal Cancer

The results of in vitro and in vivo studies on grape seed extract were published in 2006 in *Clinical Cancer Research.* In their in vitro studies, researchers at the University of Colorado Health Sciences Center exposed two different types of human colorectal cancer cells to varying amounts of grape seed extract. They found that the inhibition of cell growth was dose- and time-dependent. Thus, the most benefit was obtained when the highest amount of grape seed was used for the longest period of time. In fact, when the highest dose was used for the longest period of time—two days—there was a stunning 92% decrease in live cells.

In the in vivo portion of the trial, the researchers implanted mice with advanced human colorectal cells and fed them 200 mg/kg of body weight of grape seed every day for eight weeks. When compared to a control group of mice, the researchers found that the volume of the tumor in the grape seed–eating mice was reduced by 44%. The researchers noted that grape seed extract "may be an effective chemopreventive agent against colorectal cancer."[1]

Lung Cancer

In a study published in 2009 in *Clinical Cancer Research,* Alabama researchers studied the in vitro and in vivo uses of grape seed extract against human nonsmall cell lung cancer. The researchers found that grape seed extract inhibited the growth of 10 different lung cancer cell lines. Additionally, grape seed extract had a similar effect on lung cancer cells in mice. At the same time, grape seed extract did not kill or stunt the growth of normal cells. Though the studies are preliminary, the researchers noted that grape seed extract may be able to play a role in the prevention and treatment of lung cancer.[2]

Skin Cancer

In 2007, during the national meeting of the American Chemical Society, the organization held a one-day symposium entitled "Natural Products, Diets and Cancer Prevention." Santosh K. Katiyar, Ph.D., a researcher at the University of Alabama in Birmingham, Alabama described some of his work on grape seed extract and skin cancer. Dr. Katiyar explained that he and his colleagues divided hairless mice into two groups. One group was fed a standard diet with two different levels of grape seed extract supplementation. Meanwhile, the control group was fed just a standard diet. To increase their risk for skin cancer, all the mice were exposed to ultraviolet light.

The findings were notable. The mice that were fed the grape seed extract had up to 65% fewer tumors than the mice in the control group. Furthermore, the tumors in mice that were fed grape seed extract were up to 78% smaller than those seen in the control group. Dr. Katiyar noted that grape seed extract appears to prevent ultraviolet light from suppressing the immune system. And, he stated that the regular supplementation of diets with grape seed extract may well be useful in the prevention of skin cancer.[3]

Leukemia

In a laboratory study published in 2009 in *Clinical Cancer Research,* researchers from the University of Kentucky and China exposed leukemia cells to varying amounts of grape seed extract for different periods of time. As in the research results on colorectal cancer, the death of leukemia cells was dose- and time-dependent. So, the higher doses of grape seed extract resulted in larger numbers of dead leukemia cells. While grape seed extract killed leukemia cells, it did not have any effect on normal cells.[4]

Blood Pressure

In a study published in 2009 in *Metabolism,* researchers from California and Illinois divided 27 adults with metabolic syndrome into one of three groups. (Metabolic syndrome is a cluster of health problems, including excess belly fat, high blood pressure, high cholesterol, insulin resistance, and inflammation that raises the risk for heart disease and type 2 diabetes.) While one group took placebos, the other subjects, between the ages of 25 and 80, took either 150 or 300 mg/day of grape seed extract. At the end of the four-week trial, the researchers found that the subjects in both the grape seed groups had reductions in both systolic and diastolic blood pressures. The researchers concluded that "the present study has demonstrated that an extract of grape seed lowers blood pressure in subjects with metabolic syndrome."[5]

Type 2 Diabetes

In a study published in 2009 in *Diabetic Medicine,* United Kingdom researchers examined the effect grape seed extract had on 32 subjects with type 2 diabetes who were at high risk for cardiovascular disease. For four weeks, the participants took either a placebo or 600 mg of grape seed extract every day. The researchers found that the subjects who took grape seed extract had significantly improved markers of inflammation and glycemia, thus reducing their risk for cardiovascular disease. They noted that grape seed extract "may have a therapeutic role in decreasing cardiovascular risk."[6]

Weight Loss

In a randomized, double-blind, crossover study published in 2004 in the *European Journal of Clinical Nutrition,* Dutch researchers attempted to determine if grape seed extract could play a role in weight loss. Fifty-one subjects between the ages of 18 and 65 took 300-mg grape seed extract supplements three times daily 30 to 60 minutes before breakfast, lunch, and dinner. The researchers provided the breakfasts, which the subjects ate at home. Meanwhile, lunches and dinners were consumed at the restaurant affiliated with Maastricht University. After a washout period of three weeks, the subjects repeated the trial. During the second trial, they took placebos.

The researchers found no difference in the 24-hour energy intake between the grape seed extract and the placebo groups. However, in the 23 subjects who had a higher-than-average energy requirement, the subjects taking grape seed extract had a 4% lower energy intake than the subjects taking the placebo. The researchers concluded that their findings suggest that "grape seed could be effective in reducing 24 h EI [24-hour energy intake] in normal to overweight dietary unrestrained subjects, and could, therefore, play a significant role in body-weight management."[7]

Alzheimer's Disease

In a study published in 2008 in *The Journal of Neuroscience*, researchers from New York and California supplemented the diet of mice genetically modified to develop a condition similar to Alzheimer's disease with grape seed extract. A separate group of mice that also had this condition received a placebo. At the end of five months, the mice reached the age in which they would normally begin to develop Alzheimer-like symptoms. However, the researchers found that the mice that were on grape seed extract had lower levels of brain indicators of Alzheimer's disease—amyloid beta accumulation and plaque formation. They also demonstrated lower levels of cognitive decline and improved spatial memory. The researchers speculated that grape seed extract may be able to prevent or delay Alzheimer's disease and reduce the rate of cognitive deterioration. "Our study suggests that grape seed-derived polyphenolics may be useful agents to prevent or treat AD [Alzheimer's disease]."[8]

Is Grape Seed Extract Beneficial?

Maybe. It certainly appears to have some excellent properties.

Notes

1. Kaur, Manjinder, Rana P. Singh, Mallikarjuna, et al. October 2006. "Grape Seed Extract Inhibits *In Vitro* and *In Vivo* Growth of Human Colorectal Carcinoma Cells." *Clinical Cancer Research* 12(20): 6194–6202.
2. Akhtar, Suhail, Syed M. Meeran, Nandan Katiyar, and Santosh K. Katiyar. February 2009. "Grape Seed Proanthocyanidins Inhibit the Growth of Human Non-Small Cell Lung Cancer Xenografts by Targeting Insulin-Like Growth Factor Binding Protein-3, Tumor Cell Proliferation, and Angiogenic Factors." *Clinical Cancer Research* 15: 821–831.
3. Reuters Website. www.reuters.com; Medical News Today Website. www.medicalnewstoday.com.
4. Gao, Ning, Amit Budhraja, Senping Cheng, et al. January 2009. "Induction of Apoptosis in Human Leukemia Cells by Grape Seed Extract Occurs via Activation of c-Jun NH_2-Terminal Kinase." *Clinical Cancer Research* 15(1): 140–149.

5. Sivaprakasapillai, Brahmesh, Indika Edirisinghe, Jody Randolph, et al. December 2009. "Effect of Grape Seed Extract on Blood Pressure in Subjects with Metabolic Syndrome." *Metabolism* 58(12): 1743–1746.

6. Kar, P., D. Laight, H. K. Rooprai, et al. May 2009. "Effects of Grape Seed Extract in Type 2 Diabetic Subjects in High Cardiovascular Risk: A Double Blind Randomized Placebo Controlled Trial Examining Metabolic Markers, Vascular Tone, Inflammation, Oxidative Stress and Insulin Sensitivity." *Diabetic Medicine* 26(5): 526–531.

7. Vogels, N., I.M.T. Nijs, and M. S. Westerterp-Plantenga. 2004. "The Effect of Grape-Seed Extract on 24 H Energy Intake in Humans." *European Journal of Clinical Nutrition* 58: 667–673.

8. Wang, Jun, Lap Ho, Wei Zhao, et al. June 2008. "Grape-Derived Polyphenolics Prevent Aß Oligomerization and Attenuate Cognitive Deterioration in a Mouse Model of Alzheimer's Disease." *The Journal of Neuroscience* 28(25): 6388–6392.

References and Resources

Magazines, Journals, and Newspapers

Akhtar, Suhail, Syed M. Meeran, Nandan Katiyar, and Santosh K. Katiyar. February 2009. "Grape Seed Proanthocyanidins Inhibit the Growth of Non-Small Cell Lung Cancer Xenografts by Targeting Insulin-Like Growth Factor Binding Protein-3, Tumor Cell Proliferation, and Angiogenic Factors." *Clinical Cancer Research* 15: 821–831.

Gao, Ning, Amit Budhraja, Senping Cheng, et al. January 2009. "Induction of Apoptosis in Human Leukemia Cells by Grape Seed Extract Occurs via Activation of c-Jun NH_2-Terminal Kinase." *Clinical Cancer Research* 15(1): 140–149.

Kar, P., D. Laight, H. K. Rooprai, et al. May 2009. "Effects of Grape Seed Extract in Type 2 Diabetic Subjects at High Cardiovascular Risk: A Double Blind Randomized Placebo Controlled Trial Examining Metabolic Markers, Vascular Tone, Inflammation, Oxidative Stress and Insulin Sensitivity." *Diabetic Medicine* 26(5): 526–531.

Kaur, Manjinder, Rana P. Singh, Mallikarjuna Gu, et al. October 2006. "Grape Seen Extract Inhibits *In Vitro* and *In Vivo* Growth of Human Colorectal Carcinoma Cells." *Clinical Cancer Research* 12(20): 6194–6202.

Sivaprakasapillai, Brahmesh, Indika Edirisinghe, Jody Randolph, et al. December 2009. "Effect of Grape Seed Extract on Blood Pressure in Subjects with Metabolic Syndrome." *Metabolism* 58(12): 1743–1746.

Vogels, N., I.M.T. Nijs, and M. S. Westerterp-Plantenga. 2004. "The Effects of Grape-Seed Extract on 24 H Energy Intake in Humans." *European Journal of Clinical Nutrition* 58: 667–673.

Wang, Jun, Lap Ho, Wei Zhao, et al. June 2008. "Grape-Derived Polypheno-lics Prevent Aß Oligomerization of Attenuate Cognitive Deterioration in a Mouse Model of Alzheimer's Disease." *The Journal of Neuroscience* 28(25): 6388–6392.

Websites

Medical News Today. www.medicalnewstoday.com.

Reuters. www.reuters.com.

H

Hawthorn

Hawthorn is probably best known as a treatment for cardiovascular disease. In fact, according to the National Center for Complementary and Alternative Medicine, a division of the National Institutes of Health, hawthorn fruit "has been used for heart disease since the first century."[1] An article in a 2006 issue of *Better Nutrition* stated that "hawthorn is one of the oldest known medicinal plants in Europe."[2] More recently, hawthorn, scientifically known as *Crataegus laevigata* or *Crataegus oxyacantha,* has been used for other cardiac problems such as heart failure and coronary artery disease. Some consider hawthorn an effective treatment for digestive and kidney problems. It is important to review what the researchers have learned.

Lowering Lipid Levels
In a study published in 2009 in *The American Journal of Chinese Medicine,* researchers from Australia selected six mice to be in Group A. They would be fed a normal mouse diet. Meanwhile, for eight weeks, the researchers fed a larger group of mice a high-cholesterol diet. Of this larger group of mice, the 18 that developed high blood lipid levels and atherosclerotic lesion plaque were then chosen to be part of a trial. These mice were randomly assigned to one of three groups. Each group had six mice. Group B mice continued to be fed a high-cholesterol diet. Group C mice were fed a high-cholesterol diet and Simvastatin, a medication designed to raise good cholesterol (high-density lipoprotein; HDL) and lower bad cholesterol (low-density lipoprotein; LDL) and triglycerides. Group D was fed a high-cholesterol diet and a hawthorn fruit compound. At the end of eight

weeks, the researchers observed notable results. When compared to the mice in Group A, the Group B mice had significantly higher levels of blood lipids. The researchers commented that this finding "confirmed the validity of Group A and Group B controls in this study." When the researchers compared Groups C and D to Group B, they found cardiovascular benefits from both the medication and hawthorn—"a significant reduction in triglyceride and in the ratio between low-density lipoprotein cholesterol (LDL-C) and serum cholesterol." Moreover, the mice in Group D had a reduction in LDL levels (another cardiac benefit) that was not seen in the Group C mice. The researchers concluded that hawthorn "can be considered for the treatment of hyperlipidemia and prevention of atherosclerosis."[3] While the numbers of mice in the study were small, the findings are nevertheless important. Hawthorn may support cardiovascular health.

In a randomized study published in 2006 in the *British Journal of General Practice,* researchers from the United Kingdom began by explaining that it is not uncommon for their health care providers to use hawthorn in conjunction with prescribed medications to treat high blood pressure (hypertension). The researchers then noted that in this trial they investigated the effect of treating patients with type 2 diabetes and hypertension with hawthorn. The cohort consisted of 79 patients with type 2 diabetes. For 16 weeks, 39 people took a daily dose of 1,200 mg hawthorn; 40 people took a placebo. At the end of the trial, the researchers noted "a significant group difference in mean diastolic blood pressure reductions." (Diastolic pressure is the number on the bottom. It measures pressure while the heart is relaxed.) The people taking hawthorn "showed greater reductions" than those on the placebo. No such difference was observed in systolic blood pressures.[4] (Systolic pressure is the number on the top. It measures pressure while the heart is contracting.)

Improvements in Obesity and Dyslipidemia
In a study published in 2009 in the *Journal of Ethnopharmacology,* researchers from Taiwan investigated the use of hawthorn for obesity and dyslipidemia (elevated levels of cholesterol and triglycerides in the blood). After feeding hamsters high-fat diets, the hamsters became obese and developed high levels of blood cholesterol and triglycerides. The researchers then placed some of the hamsters on hawthorn supplements; other hamsters that were not given hawthorn served as controls. When compared to the controls, the hamsters on hawthorn had "markedly reduced" levels of food

intake, body weight, and weights of brown and white adipose (fat) tissue. The hamsters on hawthorn had lower levels of total cholesterol, triglyceride, LDL (bad) cholesterol and high levels of HDL (good) cholesterol. The researchers concluded that hawthorn has the potential to reduce obesity and improve cholesterol and triglyceride levels.[5]

Chronic Heart Failure

A study published in 2008 in the *Cochrane Database of Systematic Reviews* combined the results of 10 randomized, controlled trials that compared the effects of adding hawthorn extract or placebo to conventional therapies for chronic heart failure. The trials included a total of 855 patients. The results of the meta-analysis indicated that adding hawthorn to the heart failure treatment had the following effects: improved heart workload, reduced consumption of oxygen by the heart, increased patient tolerance for exercise, with less shortness of breath and fatigue. Side effects were "infrequent, mild and transient." Only a few people reported "nausea, dizziness, and cardiac and gastrointestinal complaints." The report concluded that "there is significant benefit in symptom control and physiologic outcomes from hawthorn as an adjunctive treatment for chronic heart failure."[6]

Meanwhile, in a randomized, double-blind, placebo-controlled multicenter study published in 2008 in the *European Journal of Heart Failure,* researchers from Germany, Poland, and Boston, Massachusetts, reviewed the efficacy and safety of including hawthorn to the treatment of patients with heart failure. The trial consisted of 2,681 patients in 156 centers in 13 European countries. The patients received either a placebo or twice-daily pills containing hawthorn in a "moderately high" dose. Eighteen months after the study began, the lives of the people taking hawthorn were extended by four months. However, after two years, about the same number of people from both groups had died. Still, according to the researchers, the trial determined that hawthorn was safe to use for people with heart failure, and it "can potentially reduce the incidence of sudden cardiac death."[7]

A year later, in 2009, the same journal published different results from researchers in Ann Arbor and Dearborn, Michigan. Their randomized, double-blind, placebo-controlled study included 120 ambulatory patients aged 18 or older with heart failure. In addition to their regular medications, the patients were given placebos or 450 mg of hawthorn, taken twice daily. After finding that "there were significantly more adverse events reported in the hawthorn group . . . although most were non-cardiac," the researchers questioned the safety of treating people with heart failure with hawthorn. They concluded that "hawthorn provides no symptomatic or functional benefit when given with standard medical therapy to patients with heart failure."[8]

Sedating Effects on Central Nervous System

In a study published in 2010 in *Pharmaceutical Biology,* researchers from Turkey examined the effect that hawthorn seed extracts and pulp had on the central nervous systems (brain and spinal cord) of mice. The researchers found that both forms of hawthorn triggered decreases in levels of activity among the mice. Moreover, "exploratory behaviors of animals suggested CNS [central nervous system] depressant activities of both extracts." The researchers concluded that their "findings seem to support the traditional use of this plant to treat stress, nervousness, sleep disorders, and pain control."[9]

Is Hawthorn Beneficial?

From the research, it is evident that hawthorn may well be beneficial to some people. People with more serious health concerns, such as heart failure, should use hawthorn with caution and only after discussing it with their healthcare provider. Since a 2010 article in *Archives of Pathology & Laboratory Medicine* warns that hawthorn may compromise the effectiveness of digoxin, a cardiac medication, people on digoxin should not use hawthorn.[10]

Notes

1. National Center for Complementary and Alternative Medicine Website. http://nccam.nih.gov.
2. Ackerson, Amber D. February 2006. "Hawthorn: This Berry-Bearing Herb May Help Keep Your Heart Pumping Strong." *Better Nutrition* 68(2): 12.
3. Xu, H., H.E. Xu, and D. Ryan. 2009. "A Study of the Comparative Effects of Hawthorn Fruit Compound and Simvastatin on Lowering Blood Lipid Levels." *The American Journal of Chinese Medicine* 37(5): 903–908.
4. Walker, Ann F., Georgios Marakis, Eleanor Simpson, et al. June 2006. "Hypotensive Effects of Hawthorn for Patients with Diabetes Taking Prescription Drugs: A Randomised Controlled Trial." *British Journal of General Practice* 56(527): 437–443.
5. Kuo, D.H., C.H. Yeh, P.C. Shieh, et al. July 2009. "Effect of Shanzha, a Chinese Herbal Product, on Obesity and Dyslipidemia in Hamsters Receiving High-fat Diet." *Journal of Ethnopharmacology* 124(3): 544–550.

6. Guo, Ruoling, Max H. Pittler, and Edzard Ernst. 2008. "Hawthorn Extract for Treating Chronic Heart Failure." *Cochrane Database of Systematic Reviews* (Issue 1): Art No.: CD005312 DOI: 10.1002/14651858.CD005312.pub2.

7. Holubarsch, C. J., W. S. Colucci, T. Meinertz, et al. December 2008. "The Efficacy and Safety of Crataegus Extract WS 1442 in Patients with Heart Failure: The SPICE Trial." *European Journal of Heart Failure* 10(12): 1255–1263.

8. Zick, Suzanna M., Bonnie Montyka Vautaw, Brenda Gillespie, and Keith D. Aaronson. 2009. "Hawthorn Extract Randomized Blinded Chronic Heart Failure (HERB CHF) Trial." *European Journal of Heart Failure* 11(10): 990–999.

9. Can, O. D., U. D. Ozkay, N. Oztürk, and Y. Oztürk. August 2010. "Effects of Hawthorn Seed and Pulp Extracts on the Central Nervous System." *Pharmaceutical Biology* 48(8): 924–931.

10. Dasgupta, A., L. Kidd, B. J. Poindexter, and R. J. Bick. August 2010. "Interference of Hawthorn on Serum Digoxin Measurements by Immunoassays and Pharmacodynamic Interaction with Digoxin." *Archives of Pathology & Laboratory Medicine* 134(8): 1188–1192.

References and Resources

Magazines, Journals, and Newspapers

Ackerson, Amber D. February 2006. "Hawthorn: This Berry-Bearing Herb May Help Keep Your Heart Pumping Strong." *Better Nutrition* 68(2): 12.

Can, O. D., U. D. Ozkay, N. Oztürk, and Y. Oztürk. August 2010. "Effects of Hawthorn Seed and Pulp Extracts on the Central Nervous System." *Pharmaceutical Biology* 48(8): 924–931.

Dasgupta, A., L. Kidd, B. J. Poindexter, and R. J. Bick. August 2010. "Interference of Hawthorn on Serum Digoxin Measurements by Immunoassays and Pharmacodynamic Interaction with Digoxin." *Archives of Pathology & Laboratory Medicine* 134(8): 1188–1192.

Guo, Ruoling, Max H. Pittler, and Edzard Ernst. 2008. "Hawthorn Extract for Treating Chronic Heart Failure." *Cochrane Database of Systematic Reviews* (Issue 1): Art No.: CD005312 DOI: 10.1002/14651858.CD005312.pub2.

Holubarsch, C. J., W. S. Colucci, T. Meinertz, et al. December 2008. "The Efficacy of Crataegus Extract WS 1442 in Patients with Heart Failure: The SPICE Trial." *European Journal of Heart Failure* 10(12): 1255–1263.

Kuo, D. H., C. H. Yeh, P. C. Shieh, et al. July 2009. "Effect if Shanzha, a Chinese Herbal Product, on Obesity and Dyslipidemia in Hamsters Receiving High-Fat Diet." *Journal of Ethnopharmacology* 124(3): 544–550.

Walker, Ann F., Georgios Marakis, Eleanor Simpson, et al. June 2006. "Hypotensive Effects of Hawthorn for Patients with Diabetes Taking Prescription Drugs: A Randomized Controlled Trial." *British Journal of General Practice* 56(527): 437–443.

Xu, H., Xu H. E., and D. Ryan. 2009. "A Study of the Comparative Effects of Hawthorn Fruit Compound and Simvastatin on Lowering Blood Lipid Levels." *The American Journal of Chinese Medicine* 37(5): 903–908.

Zick, Suzanna M., Bonnie Montyka Vautaw, Brenda Gillespie, and Keith D. Aaronson. 2009. "Hawthorn Extract Randomized Blinded Chronic Heart Failure (HERB CHF) Trial." *European Journal of Heart Failure* 11(10): 990–999.

Website
National Center for Complementary and Alternative Medicine. http://nccam.nih.gov.

Hibiscus ❦

Scientifically known as *Hibiscus sabdariffa,* hibiscus is native to sections of North Africa and Southeast Asia. Today, it is primarily grown in Thailand, China, Mexico, and the Sudan.

Hibiscus is said to be useful for a wide variety of medical problems. These include hypertension (high blood pressure), nervous restlessness, respiratory infections, constipation, and the retention of fluids.[1] Is hibiscus really an effective treatment for all such disparate concerns? It is important to review what researchers have learned.

Hypertension (High Blood Pressure)
In a randomized, double-blind, placebo-controlled trial published in 2010 in *The Journal of Nutrition,* Boston researchers examined the antihypertensive properties of hibiscus tea in humans. The cohort consisted of 65 pre- and mildly hypertensive adults between the ages of 30 and 70. None of the participants took blood pressure–lowering medication. For six weeks, all participants either drank three 240-mL servings per day of brewed hibiscus tea or a placebo, while they ate their usual diets. At the end of the trial, the researchers found that "the change in SBP [systolic blood pressure] among participants who consumed hibiscus tea was greater than in participants who consumed the placebo beverage." They concluded that the "daily consumption of hibiscus tea, in an amount readily incorporated into the diet, lowers BP [blood pressure] in pre- and mildly hypertensive adults and may prove an effective component of the dietary changes recommended for people with these conditions."[2]

In a double-blind, randomized, controlled trial published in 2009 in the *Journal of Human Hypertension,* researchers from Yazd, Iran compared the antihypertensive effectiveness of two types of tea—hibiscus tea and black tea. While the cohort initially consisted of 60 people who had diabetes and mild hypertension, 53 subjects actually completed the study. None of the participants took medication for elevated blood pressure or cholesterol. After being randomly assigned to one of the two tea groups, the participants were told to drink their tea two times each day for one month.

The researchers found that the participants in the hibiscus group experienced significant reductions in their systolic blood pressure. They concluded that consuming hibiscus tea two times a day "has positive effects on BP [blood pressure] in type II diabetic patients."[3]

And, in a randomized, double-blind, and controlled study published two years earlier, in 2007, in *Planta Medica,* researchers from Mexico treated 168 participants between the ages of 25 and 61 with either hibiscus or lisinopril, a medication for high blood pressure, for four weeks. The researchers found that both groups displayed reductions in blood pressure. But, the group taking lisinopril had a more significant decrease. Still, the researchers added, hibiscus "exerted important antihypertensive effectiveness with a wide margin of tolerability and safety."[4]

Lowering Lipid Levels of the Blood

In a study published in 2007 in *Nutrition Research,* researchers from Taiwan investigated the ability of hibiscus to lower cholesterol levels of human subjects. The four-week trial included 42 volunteers who ranged in age from 18 to 75. Subjects were randomly divided into one of three groups. The members of the first group took one hibiscus capsule with each meal; the members of the second group took two capsules with each meal; and the members of the third group took three capsules with each meal. After two weeks, when compared to baseline values, the "serum cholesterol levels were found to be lower in all groups." Similar observations were seen after four weeks. But, the most improvement was seen in the members of the second group. "It is important to note that the serum cholesterol level for 71% of the group II volunteers was significantly lowered with a mean reduction of 12%."[5]

In a four-week study published in 2010 in *Acta Poloniae Pharmaceutica,* researchers from India compared the use of three different doses of hibiscus to atorvastatin (a cholesterol-lowering medication also known as Lipitor) in rats with elevated levels of cholesterol. Hibiscus was given at 100, 200, and 300 mg/kg orally and atorvastatin was administered at 10 mg/kg orally. Although the hibiscus dose of 100 mg/kg did not result in a significant reduction in cholesterol levels, the two other higher doses did. The higher doses also resulted in significant reductions in serum triglyceride levels and low-density lipoprotein (LDL; "bad") cholesterol levels. Hibiscus did not trigger any significant changes in high-density lipoprotein (HDL; "good") cholesterol levels. The 300-mg/kg appeared to be more effective than the 200-mg/kg dose, but less effective than atorvastatin. The researchers concluded that hibiscus has been "shown to possess hypolipidemic and hypocholesterolemic activity."[6]

On the other hand, in a randomized, double-blind, placebo-controlled study published in 2010 in *BMC Complementary and Alternative Medicine,* researchers from Bangalore, India, placed 60 people with elevated levels of LDL "bad" cholesterol but no history of coronary heart disease in one of two groups. The subjects in the experimental group took 1 g of hibiscus extract for 90 days, while the placebo group took a similar amount of maltodextrin, a food additive. The subjects were also given dietary and physical activity advice on controlling their blood lipids. Interestingly, the researchers found that "while body weight, serum LDL cholesterol, and triglycerides levels decreased in both groups, there were no significant differences between the experimental and placebo group." And, they concluded that a dose of 1 g per day of hibiscus "did not appear to have a blood lipid lowering effect."[7]

Weight Control

In a study published in 2009 in the *Journal of Biomedicine and Biotechnology,* researchers from Mexico examined the effect of hibiscus extract on fat absorption and excretion and body weight in rats. Rats were fed either a regular diet (control group) or a regular diet that included 5%, 10%, or 15% hibiscus extract. The researchers found that the body weight gain in the 10% and 15% hibiscus extract groups was significantly less than in the control group. The consumption of food in the experimental groups decreased as the doses increased. But, it was only statistically significant in the 15% group. The researchers theorized that hibiscus extract "at the intermediate and greater concentrations used in this experiment could be considered possible antiobesity agents."[8]

Is Hibiscus Beneficial?

While hibiscus does appear to have some cardiovascular benefits, a study published in 2010 in *Pharmaceutical Biology* should warn women who are pregnant or nursing babies to avoid this herb. The study, which was completed in Nigeria on rats, was designed to examine whether the consumption of hibiscus during lactation would affect the onset of puberty. On the first postnatal day, the lactating rats were randomly grouped into one of three groups. One group received tap water; a second group had 0.6-g aqueous hibiscus extract/100 mL; and the third group had 1.8-g aqueous hibiscus extract/100 mL. The rats drank these fluids throughout lactation. The weights of the offspring were recorded at several different times, including the onset of puberty. The researchers found that the mothers on hibiscus had decreased maternal fluid and food intake. Furthermore, when compared to the female offspring who were fed water without hibiscus, the female offspring fed hibiscus exhibited a delayed onset of puberty.[9] Could this also occur in humans? If so, what would be the consequences? At present, it is not clear. Those who may be at risk should simply refrain from using this herb.

Notes

1. American Botanical Council Website. www.abc.harbalgram.org.
2. McKay, Diane L., C.-Y. Oliver Chen, Edward Saltzman, and Jeffrey B. Blumberg. February 2010. "*Hibiscus sabdariffa* L. Tea (Tisane) Lowers Blood Pressure in Prehypertensive and Mildly Hypertensive Adults." *The Journal of Nutrition* 140(2): 298–303.
3. Mozaffari-Khosravi, H., B.-A. Jalali-Khanabadi, M. Afkhami-Ardekani, et al. January 2009. "The Effect of Sour Tea (*Hibiscus sabdariffa*) on Hypertension in Patients with Type II Diabetes." *Journal of Human Hypertension* 23(1): 48–54.
4. Herrera-Arellano, Armando, Judith Miranda-Sánchez, Pedro Ávila-Castro, et al. 2007. "Clinical Effects Produced by a Standardized Herbal Medicinal Products of *Hibiscus sabdariffa* on Patients with Hypertension. A Randomized, Double-Blind, Lisinopril-Controlled Clinical Trial." *Planta Medica* 73(1): 6–12.
5. Lin, Tzu-Li, Hui-Hsuan Lin, Chang-Che Chen, et al. March 2007. "*Hibiscus sabdariffa* Extract Reduces Serum Cholesterol in Men and Women." *Nutrition Research* 27(3): 140–145.
6. Gosain, S., R. Ircchiaya, P. C. Sharma, et al. March–April 2010. "Hypolipidemic Effect of Ethanolic Extract from the Leaves of *Hibiscus sabdariffa* L. in Hyperlipidemic Rats." *Acta Poloniae Pharmaceutica* 67(2): 179–184.

7. Kuriyan, Rebecca, Divya R. Kumar, R. Rajendran, and Anura V. Kurpad. June 2010. "An Evaluation of the Hypolipidemic Effect of an Extract of *Hibiscus sabdariffa* Leaves in Hyperlipidemic Indians: A Double Blind, Placebo Controlled Trial." *BMC Complementary and Alternative Medicine* 10: 27.
8. Carvajal-Zarrabal, O., P. M. Hayward-Jones, Z. Orta-Flores, et al. 2009. "Effect of *Hibiscus sabdariffa* L. Dried Calyx Ethanol Extract on Fat Absorption-Excretion, and Body Weight Implication in Rats." *Journal of Biomedicine and Biotechnology* Article ID: 394592, 5 pages. DOI: 10.1155/2009/394592.
9. Iyare, E. E., O. A. Adegoke, and U. I. Nwagha. October 2010. "Mechanism of Delayed Puberty in Rats Whose Mothers Consumed *Hibiscus sabdariffa* during Lactation." *Pharmaceutical Biology* 48(10): 1170–1176.

References and Resources

Magazines, Journals, and Newspapers

Carvajal-Zarrabal, O., P. M. Hayward-Jones, Z. Orta-Flores, et al. 2009. "Effect of *Hibiscus sabdariffa* L. Dried Calyx Ethanol Extract on Fat absorption-Excretion, and Body Weight Implications in Rats." *Journal of Biomedicine and Biotechnology* Article ID 394592, 5 pages. DOI: 10.1155/2009/394592.

Gosain, S., R. Ircchiaya, P. C. Sharma, et al. March–April 2010. "Hypolipidemic Effect of Ethanolic Extract from the Leaves of *Hibiscus sabdariffa* L. in Hyperlipidemic Rats." *Acta Poloniae Pharmaceutica* 67(2): 179–184.

Herrera-Arellano, Armando, Judith Miranda-Sánchez, Pedro Ávila-Castro, et al. 2007. "Clinical Effects Produced by a Standardized Herbal Medicinal Product of *Hibiscus sabdariffa* on Patients with Hypertension: A Randomized, Double-Blind, Lisinopril-Controlled Clinical Trial." *Planta Medica* 73(1): 6–12.

Iyare, E. E., O. A. Adegoke, and U. I. Nwagha. October 2010. "Mechanism of Delayed Puberty in Rats Whose Mothers Consumed *Hibiscus sabdariffa* during Lactation." *Pharmaceutical Biology* 48(10): 1170–1176.

Kuriyan, Rebecca, Divya R. Kumar, R. Rajendran, and Anura V. Kurpad. June 2010. "An Evaluation of the Hypolipidemic Effects of an Extract of *Hibiscus sabdariffa* Leaves in Hyperlipidemic Indians: A Double Blind, Placebo Controlled Trial." *BMC Complementary and Alternative Medicine* 10: 27.

Lin, Tzu-Li, Hui-Hsuan Lin, Chang-Che Chen, et al. March 2007. "*Hibiscus sabdariffa* Extract Reduces Serum Cholesterol in Men and Women." *Nutrition Research* 27(3): 140–145.

McKay, Diane L., C.-Y. Oliver Chen, Edward Saltzman, and Jeffrey B. Blumberg. February 2010. "*Hibiscus sabdariffa* L. Tea (Tisane) Lowers Blood Pressure in Prehypertensive and Mildly Hypertensive Adults." *The Journal of Nutrition* 140(2): 298–303.

Mozaffari-Khosravi, H., B. A. Jalali-Khanabadi, M. Afkhami-Ardekani, et al. January 2009. "The Effects of Sour Tea (*Hibiscus sabdariffa*) on Hypertension in Patients with Type II Diabetes." *Journal of Human Hypertension* 23(1): 48–54.

Website
American Botanical Council. www.abc.herbalgram.org.

Horse Chestnut 🌰

Also known as horse chestnut seed extract, and buckeye, horse chestnut has been used for hundreds of years for a variety of different medical problems.

Horse chestnut is probably best known as a treatment for chronic venous insufficiency (CVI), a syndrome in which people have leg swelling, varicose veins, leg pain, itching, and skin ulcers. However, horse chestnut, scientifically known as *Aesculus hippocastanum,* is also said to be effective for other problems.[1] It is interesting to see what the researchers have learned.

Chronic Venous Insufficiency

In a meta-analysis published in 2002 in *International Angiology,* researchers from Munich, Germany, and Boston reviewed a number of studies on the use of oral horse chestnut to treat CVI. After a systematic review of the literature, the researchers identified 13 randomized control trials that included 1,051 people and 3 observational studies that included 10,725 people. The researchers found that in the randomized control trials, when compared to the placebos, horse chestnut reduced leg volume, pain, edema, and itching. The observational studies "showed significant effectiveness regarding pain, edema, and leg fatigue/heaviness." The researchers concluded that horse chestnut "appears to be an effective and safe treatment for" CVI.[2]

An analysis of four clinical studies on the use of horse chestnut (Aesculaforce) for CVI was published in 2006 in *Advances in Therapy.* The researchers determined that the clinical trials found that horse chestnut resulted in a "reduction in lower leg edema and the subjective alleviation of leg pain, heaviness, and itching." They noted that horse chestnut "offers a real alternative in the treatment of patients with mild to moderate venous insufficiency."[3]

A study published in 2002 in *Phytotherapy Research* compared treating CVI with Venostasin, which contains horse chestnut, to treating the condition with Pycnogenol, which has French maritime pine bark extract.

For four weeks, 40 people who had been diagnosed with CVI were treated every day with either 600 mg of Venostasin or 360 mg of Pycnogenol. While Pycnogenol was found to result in a significant reduction in the circumference of the lower limbs and significantly improve the subjective symptoms, Venostasin "only moderately but not significantly reduced the circumference of the lower limbs and marginally improved symptoms."[4]

Venous Leg Ulcers
In a prospective triple-blind, randomized, placebo-controlled trial published in 2006 in the *Journal of Wound Care,* researchers from South Australia treated 54 people with venous leg ulcers with either horse chestnut or a placebo. At the end of 12 weeks, the researchers observed that the "difference between groups in the number of healed leg ulcers and change in wound surface area, depth, volume, pain and exudates was not statistically significant." However, the researchers added that when compared to the wounds treated with the placebo, the horse chestnut did have a significant effect on wound slough and the number of dressing changes.[5]

In a second article on this same study published in 2006 in *Ostomy Wound Management,* the same researchers analyzed the cost effectiveness of treating venous leg ulcers with the conventional therapy of dressings and compression and horse chestnut versus treating them only with conventional therapy. The researchers noted that when they calculated all the costs associated with treatment, such as horse chestnut, dressing materials, travel, staff salaries, and infrastructure for each patient, horse chestnut therapy combined with conventional therapy was found to be more cost effective. When horse chestnut was used, fewer dressing changes were required, which meant that fewer nursing visits were needed.[6]

Antiaging
In a study published in 2006 in the *Journal of Cosmetic Science,* Japanese researchers tested a gel formation that included 3% of horse chestnut on 40 healthy female volunteers. For nine weeks, three times each day, the gel was applied topically to the skin around the eyes. After six weeks, when compared to the controls, "significant decreases in the wrinkle scores at the corners of the eye or in the lower eyelid skin were observed." Similar results were obtained after the full nine weeks. The researchers concluded

that the findings "suggest that an extract of horse chestnuts can generate contraction forces in fibroblasts [cells that give rise to connective tissue] and is a potent anti-aging ingredient."[7]

The possible science behind these antiaging benefits was noted years before in an 1999 article published in the *International Journal of Cosmetic Science*. United Kingdom researchers wrote that horse chestnut contains aescins, which have "potent anti-inflammatory compounds." Furthermore, they noted that horse chestnut has "one of the highest 'active-oxygen' scavenging abilities of 65 different plants tested."[8]

Inner Ear Disturbances

In a randomized, clinical study published in 2008 in *Phytomedicine: International Journal of Phytotherapy & Phytopharmacology,* German researchers investigated whether a combination of aescin, found in horse chestnut, and troxerutin, a natural bioflavonoid, could aid people dealing with hearing problems associated with inner ear disturbances. The cohort consisted of 68 people. Thirty-four people received the therapy; 34 received the placebo. Both were administered orally. At the end of the trial, which continued for 40–44 days, two-thirds of the men and women who had taken the aescin and troxerutin experienced significant improvements in their hearing. In the control group, only six people had notable improvements in their hearing. The researchers commented that the medications were "well-tolerated."[9]

Potential Treatment for Lymphedema

In a prospective clinical study published in 2009 in the *Australian Journal of Medical Herbalism,* Australian researchers recruited 15 normal female volunteers between the ages of 50 and 60. None of the women had a history of breast cancer, lymphedema (swelling caused by lymph accumulating in tissue), radiation therapy, chemotherapy, or chest surgery. Tests were conducted to determine each woman's bilateral upper limb rate of lymphatic drainage. The women were then placed on three months of a twice-daily daily herbal supplement that contained horse chestnut, butcher's broom, and Ginkgo biloba. At the end of three months, the volunteers were tested to determine if their rate of lymphatic drainage had changed. The researchers observed that the combination of herbs had "the potential to accelerate lymphatic drainage in the normal population."[10]

Reduce Varicocele-Associated Male Infertility

In a study published in 2010 in *Phytomedicine: International Journal of Phytotherapy & Phytopharmacology,* researchers from Columbia, Missouri, and China divided 219 men who had varicocele-associated infertility into three groups: control, surgery, and aescin. When compared to the men in the control group, the men who had surgery and the men who took aescin for two months had improvements in factors that increase fertility, such as sperm density and sperm mobility. The researchers concluded that aescin "is a safe and effective drug to improve sperm quality in Chinese male patients with varicocele-associated infertility."[11]

Is Horse Chestnut Beneficial?

It certainly appears to have some benefits. However, since it may lower blood sugar and/or increase bleeding, people with diabetes, hypoglycemia, or bleeding disorders should not use this herb. In addition, there have been reports of liver and kidney toxicity.

Notes

1. National Center for Complementary and Alternative Medicine Website. www.nccam.nih.gov.
2. Siebert, U., M. Brach, G. Sroczynski, and K. Überla. December 2002. "Efficacy, Routine Effectiveness, and Safety of Horse Chestnut Seed Extract in the Treatment of Chronic Venous Insufficiency. A Meta-Analysis of Randomized Controlled Trials and Large Observational Studies." *International Angiology* 21(4): 305–315.
3. Suter, Andy, Silvia Bommer, and Jordan Rachner. January 2006. "Treatment of Patients with Venous Insufficiency with Fresh Plant Horse Chestnut Seed Extract: A Review of Five Clinical Studies." *Advances in Therapy* 23(1): 179–190.
4. Koch, Rainer. 2002. "Comparative Study of Venostasin® and Pycnogenol® in Chronic Venous Insufficiency." *Phytotherapy Research* 16(S1): 1–5.
5. Leach, M. J., J. Pincombe, and G. W. Foster. April 2006. "Clinical Efficacy of Horse Chestnut Seed Extract in the Treatment of Venous Ulceration." *Journal of Wound Care* 15(4): 159–167.
6. Leach, M. J., J. Pincombe, and G. Foster. April 2006. "Using Horse Chestnut Seed Extract in the Treatment of Venous Leg Ulcers: A Cost–Benefit Analysis." *Ostomy Wound Management* 52(4): 68–70, 72–74, 76–78.
7. Fujimura, Tsutomu, Kazue Tsukahara, Shigeru Moriwaki, et al. September–October 2006. "A Horse Chestnut Extract, which Induces Contraction Forces in Fibroblasts, Is a Potent Anti-Aging Ingredient." *Journal of Cosmetic Science* 57(5): 369–376.

8. Wilkinson, J.A., and A.M. Brown. December 1999. "Horse Chestnut—*Aesculus hippocastanum*: Potential Applications in Cosmetic Skin-Care Products." *International Journal of Cosmetic Science* 21(6): 437–447.

9. Siegers, C.P., S. Syed Ali, and M. Tegtmeier. March 2008. "Aescin and Troxerutin as a Successful Combination for the Treatment of Inner Ear Perfusion Disturbances." *Phytomedicine: International Journal of Phytotherapy & Phytopharmacology* 15(3): 160–163.

10. Wheat, Janelle, Geoffrey Currie, Hosen Kiat, and Kerry Bone. Fall 2009. "Improving Lymphatic Drainage with Herbal Preparations: A Potentially Novel Approach to Management of Lymphedema." *Australian Journal of Medical Herbalism* 21(3): 66–70.

11. Fang, Yujiang, Lei Zhao, Feng Yan, et al. March 2010. "Escin Improves Sperm Quality in Male Patients with Varicocele-Associated Infertility." *Phytomedicine: International Journal of Phytotherapy & Phytopharmacology* 17(3–4): 192–196.

References and Resources

Magazines, Journals, and Newspapers

Baumann, Leslie S. January 2006. "Horse Chestnut." *Skin & Allergy News* 37(1): 16.

Fang, Yujiang, Lei Zhao, Feng Yan, et al. March 2010. "Escin Improves Sperm Quality in Male Patients with Varicocele-Associated Infertility." *Phytomedicine: International Journal of Phytotherapy & Phytopharmacology* 17(3–4): 192–196.

Fujimura, Tsutomu, Kazue Tsukahara, Shigeru Moriwaki, et al. September–October 2006. "A Horse Chestnut Extract, which Induces Contraction Forces in Fibroblasts, Is a Potent Anti-Aging Ingredient." *Journal of Cosmetic Science* 57(5): 369–376.

Koch, Rainer. 2002. "Comparative Study of Venostasin® and Pycnogenol® in Chronic Venous Insufficiency." *Phytotherapy Research* 16(S1): 1–5.

Leach, M.J., J. Pincombe, and G. Foster. April 2006. "Using Horse Chestnut Seed Extract in the Treatment of Venous Leg Ulcers: A Cost–Benefit Analysis." *Ostomy Wound Management* 52(4): 68–70, 72–74, 76–78.

Leach, M.J., J. Pincombe, and G.W. Foster. April 2006. "Clinical Efficacy of Horse Chestnut Seed Extract in the Treatment of Venous Ulceration." *Journal of Wound Care* 15(4): 159–167.

Rathbun, Suman W., and Angelia C. Kirkpatrick. 2007. "Treatment of Chronic Venous Insufficiency." *Current Treatment Options in Cardiovascular Medicine* 9: 115–126.

Sego, Sherril. December 2006. "Horse Chestnut Seed Extract." *Clinical Advisor* 9(12): 100–101.

Siebert, U., M. Brach, G. Sroczynski, and K. Überla. December 2002. "Efficacy, Routine Effectiveness and Safety of Horse Chestnut Seed Extract in the

Treatment of Chronic Venous Insufficiency. A Meta-Analysis of Randomized Controlled Trials and Large Observational Studies." *International Angiology* 21(4): 305–315.

Siegers, C. P., S. Syed Ali, and M. Tegtmeier. March 2008. "Aescin and Troxerutin as a Successful Combination for the Treatment of Inner Ear Perfusion Disturbances." *Phytomedicine: International Journal of Phytotherapy & Phytopharmacology* 15(3): 160–163.

Suter, Andy, Silvia Bommer, and Jordan Rechner. January 2006. "Treatment of Patients with Venous Insufficiency with Fresh Plant Horse Chestnut Seed Extract: A Review of Five Clinical Studies." *Advances in Therapy* 23(1): 179–190.

Wheat, Janelle, Geoffrey Curie, Hosen Kiat, and Kerry Bone. Fall 2009. "Improving Lymphatic Drainage with Herbal Preparations: A Potentially Novel Approach to Management of Lymphedema." *Australian Journal of Medical Herbalism* 21(3): 66–70.

Wilkinson, J. A., and A. M. Brown. December 1999. "Horse Chestnut—*Aesculus hippocastanum*: Potential Applications in Cosmetic Skin-Care Products." *International Journal of Cosmetic Science* 21(6): 437–447.

Website

National Center for Complementary and Alternative Medicine. www.nccam.nih.gov.

K

Kudzu 🌱

Scientifically known by several names, including *Pueraria lobata* and *Pueraria mirifica,* kudzu has been used in Chinese medicine for many centuries. It is said to be helpful for a wide variety of medical concerns, including menopausal symptoms, alcoholism, diabetes, fever, the common cold, and neck or eye pain.[1] But, it is important to review what researchers have learned.

Treating Alcohol Abuse and Dependence

In a double-blind, placebo-controlled, crossover study published in 2011 in *Alcoholism: Clinical & Experimental Research,* researchers from McLean Hospital in Belmont, Massachusetts, examined the effect of kudzu on 12 healthy adult men and women who consumed moderate amounts of alcohol. For nine days, the volunteers were treated with either kudzu extract or a matched placebo. On days eight and nine, they received a medium- or high-alcohol challenge. The researchers found that the pretreatment with kudzu had little effect on the participants' behavioral, physical, or cognitive performance. They wrote that "a relatively short-term treatment with kudzu failed to have a significant effect on alcohol-induced intoxication and other psychomotor and cognitive effects." Still, the researchers observed that the volunteers pretreated with kudzu had elevated levels of skin temperature, heart rate, and blood ethanol levels. They hypothesized that the elevated levels of blood ethanol "might increase the rewarding effects of the first drink consumed, especially when the higher doses are consumed, and the desire for subsequent drinks might be delayed."[2]

In another study published in 2009 in *Alcoholism: Clinical & Experimental Research,* researchers from several locations in the United States and Australia identified compounds found in kudzu, especially daidzin, that reduce the intake of alcohol in animals. How is this accomplished? The researchers explained that daidzin inhibits the action of aldehyde dehydrogenase 2 (ALDH-2). (ALDH-2 is a liver enzyme that breaks down alcohol into acetaldehyde.) As a result, acetaldehyde levels accumulate. This causes people to feel ill and flushed. So, to avoid these uncomfortable symptoms, people tend to drink less alcohol.

In the study, the researchers produced a kudzu-like compound, which they called CVT-10216, and they tested it on rats that had been bred to drink moderate to large amounts of alcohol. The results are noteworthy. The researchers found that CVT-10216, a selective reversible inhibitor of ALDH-2, increased the levels of acetaldehyde in the rats and reduced heavy drinking even "when alcohol is continually available." They concluded that "it is possible that selective reversible inhibitors of ALDH-2 might lead to the development of a novel therapeutic agent to help human alcoholics successfully reduce excessive drinking."[3]

And, in a crossover study published a few years earlier, in 2005, also in *Alcoholism: Clinical & Experimental Research,* researchers from Belmont, Cambridge, and Watertown, Massachusetts, placed 14 heavier drinking men and women on either a kudzu extract or placebo for seven days. Then, the participants were provided with an opportunity to drink their preferred brand of beer in a "naturalistic laboratory setting." The participants were not aware that a scale measured the changing volume in their beer mugs. Eleven participants completed the study. Of these, eight participants drank fewer beers when taking kudzu than when they were on the placebo. During the 90 minutes drinking sessions, the participants averaged 1 1/2 beers while taking kudzu and 2 1/2 beers while taking the placebo. The researchers concluded that "kudzu extract may be a useful adjunct in managing excessive alcohol consumption in a population of moderately heavy drinkers."[4]

Improve Symptoms of Metabolic Syndrome

In a study published in 2009 in the *Journal of Agriculture and Food Chemistry,* researchers from Alabama and Iowa tested the use of kudzu for treating stroke-prone spontaneously hypertensive rats (SP-SHR). Such rats have increased risk of metabolic syndrome and its symptoms, such as obesity, high blood pressure, and impaired glucose and insulin metabolism.

For two months, all the rats were fed a polyphenol-free diet. Then, for two months, a small amount of kudzu was added to the diet of some SP-SHR rats. At the same time, other SP-SHR rats, which served as the controls, had no kudzu. When compared to the control rats, the rats that ate kudzu had lower levels of cholesterol, blood pressure, blood sugar, and insulin. No side effects were observed. The researchers concluded that "because the supplement appears to have no adverse or toxic effects on these dietary levels in rats, it may be useful to consider the use of kudzu polyphenols as complements to strategies used to reduce metabolic disorders."[5]

Relief for Menopausal Symptoms

In a randomized, double-blind trial published in 2011 in the *Archives of Gynecology and Obstetrics,* researchers from Thailand examined the use of two different doses of kudzu (25 and 50 mg) on 52 women who had undergone hysterectomies and were experiencing menopausal symptoms. For six months, half the women took 25 mg and the other half took 50 mg. The researchers found that both doses "were effective and not significantly different." Moreover, "both [doses] were safe for the treatment of menopausal symptoms in women who had undergone hysterectomy."[6]

Cardiovascular Health in Older Women

In a randomized, double-blind, placebo-controlled trial published in 2008 in *The Tohoku Journal of Experimental Medicine,* researchers from Japan and Thailand studied the effects kudzu had on serum lipid parameters in postmenopausal women. The researchers began by dividing 23 women into two groups. For two months, 12 women were treated with kudzu and 11 with a placebo. When it was determined that four of the women on placebo were not postmenopausal, their results were eliminated. Still, the researchers found that the treatment with kudzu resulted in significant increases in concentrations of high-density lipoprotein (HDL; "good" cholesterol) and significant decreases in concentrations of low-density lipoprotein (LDL; "bad" cholesterol). The researchers concluded that kudzu "has a beneficial effect on lipid metabolism in postmenopausal women."[7]

Perimenopausal Symptoms Such as Hot Flashes and Night Sweats

In a study published in 2007 in the *Journal of the Medical Association of Thailand,* researchers from Thailand wanted to learn if kudzu was useful against symptoms of perimenopause, such as hot flashes and night sweats. At the start, 71 women were enrolled. But, 11 were excluded for failing to complete the initial work-up and follow-up. The remaining women were randomly assigned to take kudzu or conjugated equine estrogen (the medication found in the hormone-replacement drug Premarin). At the end of the 60-day trial, the researchers conducted tests on the women that evaluated their levels of estrogen. These included measures of the female hormone estradiol, the follicle stimulating hormone (FSH), and the luteinizing hormone (LH). The researchers found that the women taking supplemental kudzu and the women on conjugated equine estrogen had similar results. Apparently, kudzu contains phytoestrogens, which are plant compounds that mimic and support human estrogens. And, kudzu had "estrogenic effects as similar as CEE [conjugated equine estrogen]." Kudzu alleviated the symptoms of perimenopause without any of the negative side effects associated with hormone replacement therapy. The researchers concluded that kudzu should be viewed as an effective supplement to address the symptoms of perimenopause.[8]

Is Kudzu Beneficial?

One cannot help but be intrigued by this herb, which grows in abundance in the southeast areas of the United States. And, kudzu may well be an effective treatment for a number of different medical concerns. For most people, kudzu is safe. However, because it contains phytoestrogens, people with estrogen receptor–positive breast cancer and people taking the breast cancer medication tamoxifen should avoid kudzu. It should also not be used by anyone on a medication to treat diabetes.

Notes

1. Memorial Sloan-Kettering Cancer Center Website. www.mskcc.org.
2. Penetar, David M., Robert R. MacLean, Jane F. McNeil, and Scott E. Lukas. April 2011. "Kudu Extract Treatment Does Not Increase the Intoxicating Effects of Acute Alcohol in Human Volunteers." *Alcoholism: Clinical & Experimental Research* 35(4): 726–743.
3. Arolfo, M. P., D. H. Overstreet, L. Yao, et al. November 2009. "Suppression of Heavy Drinking and Alcohol Seeking by a Selective ALDH-2 Inhibitor." *Alcoholism: Clinical & Experimental Research* 33(11): 1935–1944.
4. Lukas, S. E., D. Penetar, J. Berko, et al. May 2005. "An Extract of the Chinese Herbal Root Kudzu Reduces Alcohol Drinking by Heavy Drinkers in a

Naturalistic Setting." *Alcoholism: Clinical & Experimental Research* 29(5): 756–762.

5. Peng, N., J.K. Prasain, Y. Dai, et al. August 2009. "Chronic Dietary Kudzu Isoflavones Improve Components of Metabolic Syndrome in Stroke-Prone Spontaneously Hypertensive Rats." *Journal of Agriculture and Food Chemistry* 57(16): 7268–7273.

6. Virojchaiwong, P., Suvithayasiri, and A. Itharat. 2011. "Comparison of *Pueraria mirifica* 25 and 50 mg for Menopausal Symptoms." *Archives of Gynecology and Obstetrics* 284(2): 411–419.

7. Okamura, S., Y. Sawada, T. Satoh, et al. December 2008. "*Pueraria mirifica* Phytoestrogens Improve Dyslipidemia in Postmenopausal Women Probably by Activating Estrogen Receptor Subtypes." *The Tohoku Journal of Experimental Medicine* 216(4): 341–351.

8. Chandeying, V., and M. Sangthawan. September 2007. "Efficacy Comparison of *Pueraria mirifica* (PM) against Conjugated Equine Estrogen (CEE) with/ without Medroxyprogesterone Acetate (MPA) in the Treatment of Climacteric Symptoms in Perimenopausal Women: Phase III Study." *Journal of the Medical Association of Thailand* 90(9): 1720–1726.

References and Resources

Magazines, Journals, and Newspapers

Arolfo, M.P., D.H. Overstreet, L. Yao, et al. November 2009. "Suppression of Heavy Drinking and Alcohol Seeking by a Selective ALDH-2 Inhibitor." *Alcoholism: Clinical & Experimental Research* 33(11): 1935–1944.

Chandeying, V., and M. Sangthawan. September 2007. "Efficacy Comparison of *Pueraria mirifica* (PM) against Conjugated Equine Estrogen (CEE) with/ without Medroxyprogesterone Acetate (MPA) in the Treatment of Climacteric Symptoms in Perimenopausal Women: Phase III Study." *Journal of the Medical Association of Thailand* 90(9): 1720–1726.

Lukas, S.E., D. Penetar, J. Berko, et al. May 2005. "An Extract of the Chinese Herbal Root Kudzu Reduces Alcohol Drinking by Heavy Drinkers in a Naturalistic Setting." *Alcoholism: Clinical & Experimental Research* 29(5): 756–762.

Okamura, S., Y. Sawada, T. Satoh, et al. December 2008. "*Pueraria mirifica* Phytoestrogens Improve Dyslipidemia in Postmenopausal Women Probably by Activating Estrogen Receptor Subtypes." *The Tohoku Journal of Experimental Medicine* 216(4): 341–351.

Penetar, David M., Robert R. MacLean, Jane F. McNeil, and Scott E. Lukas. April 2011. "Kudzu Extract Treatment Does Not Increase the Intoxicating Effects of Acute Alcohol in Human Volunteers." *Alcoholism: Clinical & Experimental Research* 35(4): 726–743.

Peng, N., J.K. Prasain, Y. Dai, et al. August 2009. "Chronic Dietary Kudzu Isoflavones Improve Components of Metabolic Syndrome in Stroke-Prone

Spontaneously Hypertensive Rats." *Journal of Agriculture and Food Chemistry* 57(16): 7268–7273.

Virojchaiwong, P., V. Suvithayasiri, and A. Itharat. 2011. "Comparison of *Pueraria mirifica* 25 and 50 mg for Menopausal Symptoms." *Archives of Gynecology and Obstetrics* 284(2): 411–419.

Website
Memorial Sloan-Kettering Cancer Center. www.mskcc.org.

L

Lavender 🌿

Native to the Mediterranean region, lavender was used in ancient Egypt to mummify bodies. Historically, lavender was also an antiseptic and considered beneficial for psychiatric disorders. Today, lavender, which is scientifically known as *Lavendula angustifolia,* is said to be helpful for anxiety, restlessness, insomnia, headaches, gastrointestinal distress, and hair loss. In addition, lavender is frequently used in aromatherapy.[1] But, what have the researchers learned?

Anxiety

In a multicenter, double-blind, randomized study published in 2010 in *Phytomedicine: International Journal of Phytotherapy and Phytopharmacology,* German researchers compared treating generalized anxiety disorder (GAD) with either lavender oil (silexan) or Lorazepam, a benzodiazepine or antianxiety prescription medication also known as Ativan. Why would they seek an alternative treatment such as lavender? The benzodiazepine medications are known to induce sedation and have a high risk of drug abuse.

For six weeks, adults with GAD took either Silexan or Lorazepam. During this time, the researchers used the Hamilton Anxiety Rating Scale and other measurement tools to assess the subjects' levels of anxiety. The researchers found that "silexan is as effective as lorazepam in adults with GAD." Moreover, "since lavender oil showed no sedative effects in our study and has no potential for drug abuse, silexan appears to be an effective and well tolerated alternative to benzodiazepines for amelioration of generalized anxiety."[2]

Earlier, in 2007, *Phytomedicine: International Journal of Phytotherapy and Phytopharmacology* published another study in which U.K. researchers compared the treatment of rats with lavender oil to the treatment of them with chlordiazepoxide (an antianxiety medication also known as Librium). To do this, they completed a variety of experiments. In one experiment, the researchers exposed the rats to varying amounts of lavender oil (0.1–1.0) for 30 minutes before conducting an open-field test, a common measure of general activity and exploratory behavior in mice and rats. They also exposed the rats to the same amounts of lavender oil for one hour and injected rats with chlordiazepoxide (10 mg/kg i.p.) before the open-field test. The researchers found that the higher doses of lavender oil had effects that were similar to chlordiazepoxide. "Together, these experiments suggest that lavender oil does have anxiolytic (preventing or reducing anxiety) effects in the open field, but that a sedative effect can occur at the highest doses."[3]

In a cluster randomized–controlled trial published in 2010 in *Community Dentistry and Oral Epidemiology*, London researchers assessed the anxiety levels of 340 patients waiting for scheduled dental appointments while exposing them either to the aroma of lavender or no scent. The researchers found that the patients exposed to lavender had significantly lower levels of anxiety. However, the lavender had no impact on "future anxiety-provoking thoughts." As a result, the researchers wrote that lavender "should be perceived as a means of 'on-the-spot' reduction of anxiety and not as an anxiety treatment." They concluded that the use of lavender in a dental setting is "a low cost, simple intervention for alleviating affective components of dental patient anxiety."[4]

In a double-blind study published in 2009 in *Human Psychopharmacology: Clinical and Experimental*, U.K. researchers attempted to determine if anxiety triggered by a scary film clip could be alleviated by an orally administered capsule containing 100 or 200 µL of lavender oil or a placebo. The cohort consisted of 97 subjects. At the beginning of the study, the subjects viewed a "neutral film." That was followed by an "anxiety provoking" film. The study ended with a "light hearted recovery film clip." The researchers found that lavender oil had an anti-anxiety effect on humans under "conditions of low anxiety." However, they noted that "these effects may not extend to conditions of high anxiety."[5]

In a randomized controlled, blind study published in 2009 in the *Journal of PeriAnesthesia Nursing*, Minnesota researchers investigated whether aromatherapy made from lavender and ginger essential oils could reduce the distress of 94 children, with and without disabilities, in a perianesthesia setting. The control group received an intervention that contained jojoba oil. The researchers found that "the mean distress level was lower for the children in the essential oil group." However, the results were not statistically significant.[6]

Insomnia

In a single-blind, randomized, crossover study published in 2005 in *The Journal of Alternative & Complementary Medicine,* U.K. researchers attempted to learn if lavender oil could help people with mild insomnia. The cohort consisted of five men and five women, who were divided into two groups. During the first week, no treatments were given. Then, for one week, the people in the first group received lavender oil. After a washout week, they took almond oil for a week. The second group began with one week of almond oil. After their washout week, they took lavender oil for a week. The researchers found that the "women and younger volunteers with milder insomnia improved more than others." Yet, though the study came close, it was not statistically significant.[7]

In a study published on 2009 in *Phytomedicine: International Journal of Phytotherapy and Phytopharmacology,* Brazilian researchers wanted to determine what happened to mice when they inhaled linalool, a liquid commonly found in essential oils such as lavender. For 60 minutes, they placed mice in an inhalation chamber saturated with 1% or 3% linalool. The mice in both groups slept for longer periods of time, and none of the mice had any disruption in motor coordination. The researchers concluded that "linalool inhaled for one hour seems to induce sedation without impairment in motor abilities, a side effect shared by most psycholeptic [calming] drugs."[8]

Caveats

A study published in 2007 in the *New England Journal of Medicine* reported that a pediatric endocrinologist at the University of Colorado at Denver and Health Science Center's School of Medicine diagnosed three young boys, ages 4, 7, and 10, with prepubertal gynecomastia, a rare condition in which boys develop enlarged breast tissue prior to puberty. Researchers at the National Institute of Environmental Health Sciences later confirmed what the pediatric endocrinologist suspected. All three boys had repeatedly used products, such as soaps, skin lotions, and shampoos, containing lavender oil and/or tea tree oil. Lavender and tea tree oil have weak estrogenic and antiandrogenic (reduces male hormones) activities that probably led to a hormone imbalance. Not long after these products were discontinued, the condition either subsided or resolved. The researchers concluded "that repeated topical exposure to lavender and tea tree oils probably caused prepubertal gynecomastia in these boys."[9]

In a study published in 2008 in *Psychoneuroendocrinology,* researchers, primarily from the Ohio State University, monitored the effects of lavender and lemon aromatherapy treatments on 56 volunteers—21 men and 35 women. Since it has no odor, water served as the control. The subjects participated in three half-day sessions. Researchers reviewed blood pressure, heart rate, blood biochemistry, healing ability, reaction to pain, and the results of psychological testing of mood and stress. While lemon oil was found to enhance mood, lavender oil did not. Neither lemon nor lime improved immune status or reduced stress or pain. On occasion, water scored better than lavender.[10]

In a study published in 2010 in *Contact Dermatitis,* Swedish researchers noted that although pure linalool tends not to be allergenic, when it is exposed to air, the oxidized result is allergenic. In fact, the researchers commented that oxidized linalool "is an important allergen."[11] As has been noted, linalool is found naturally in lavender and other oils. So, people who are allergic to oxidized linalool will, most likely, react to the use of any lavender oil.

Is Lavender Beneficial?

From the research, it appears that lavender may well help mild to moderate anxiety that continues for a relatively short period of time. The same may well be true for insomnia. Right now, there is little research to support the other claims.

Notes

1. National Center for Complementary and Alternative Medicine Website. www .nccam.nih.gov.
2. Woelk, H., and S. Schläfke. February 2010. "A Multi-Center, Double-Blind, Randomised Study of the Lavender Oil Preparation Silexan in Comparison to Lorazepam for Generalized Anxiety Disorder." *Phytomedicine: International Journal of Phytotherapy and Phytopharmacology* 17(2): 94–99.

3. Shaw, D., J.M. Annett, B. Doherty, and J.C. Leslie. September 2007. "Anxiolytic Effects of Lavender Oil Inhalation on Open-Field Behaviour in Rats." *Phytomedicine: International Journal of Phytotherapy and Phytopharmacology* 14(9): 613–620.

4. Kritsidima M., T. Newton, and K. Asimakopoulou. February 2010. "The Effects of Lavender Scent on Dental Patient Anxiety Levels: A Cluster Randomised-Controlled Trial." *Community Dentistry and Oral Epidemiology* 38(1): 83–87.

5. Bradley, B.F., S.L. Brown, S. Chu, and R.W. Lea. June 2009. "Effects of Orally Administered Lavender Essential Oil on Responses to Anxiety-Provoking Film Clips." *Human Psychopharmacology: Clinical and Experimental* 24(4): 319–330.

6. Nord, D., and J. Belew. October 2009. "Effectiveness of the Essential Oils in Lavender and Ginger in Promoting Children's Comfort in a Perianesthesia Setting." *Journal of PeriAnesthesia Nursing* 24(5): 307–312.

7. Lewith, George T., Anthony Dean Godfrey, and Philip Prescott. August 2005. "A Single-Blinded, Randomized Pilot Study Evaluating the Aroma of *Lavandula augustifolia* as a Treatment for Mild Insomnia." *The Journal of Alternative & Complementary Medicine* 11(4): 631–637.

8. Linck, Viviane de Moura, Adriana Lourenço da Silva, Micheli Figueiró, et al. April 2009. "Inhaled Linalool-Induced Sedation in Mice." *Phytomedicine: International Journal of Phytotherapy and Phytopharmacology* 16(4): 303–307.

9. Henley, Derek V., Natasha Lipson, Kenneth S. Korach, and Clifford A. Bloch. February 2007. "Prepubertal Gynecomastia Linked to Lavender and Tea Tree Oils." *New England Journal of Medicine* 356(5): 479–485.

10. Kiecolt-Glaser, Janice K., Jennifer E. Graham, William B. Malarkey, et al. April 2008. "Olfactory Influences on Mood and Autonomic, Endocrine, and Immune Function." *Psychoneuroendocrinology* 33(3): 328–339.

11. Christensson, J.B., M. Matura, B. Gruvberger, et al. January 2010. "Linalool—a Significant Contact Sensitizer after Air Exposure." *Contact Dermatitis* 62(1): 32–41.

References and Resources

Magazines, Journals, and Newspapers

Bradley, B.F., S.L. Brown, S. Chu, and R.W. Lea. June 2009. "Effects of Orally Administered Lavender Essential Oil on Responses to Anxiety-Provoking Film Clips." *Human Psychopharmacology: Clinical and Experimental* 24(4): 319–330.

Christensson, J.B., M. Matura, B. Gruvberger, et al. January 2010. "Linalool—A Significant Contact Sensitizer after Air Exposure." *Contact Dermatitis* 62(1): 32–41.

Henley, Derek V., Natasha Lipson, Kenneth S. Korach, and Clifford A. Bloch. February 2007. "Prepubertal Gynecomastia Linked to Lavender and Tea Tree Oils." *New England Journal of Medicine* 356(5): 479–485.

Kiecolt-Glaser, Janice K., Jennifer E. Graham, William B. Malarkey, et al. April 2008. "Olfactory Influences on Mood an Autonomic, Endocrine, and Immune Function." *Psychoneuroendocrinology* 33(3): 328–339.

Kritsidima, M., T. Newton, and K. Asimakopoulou. February 2010. "The Effects of Lavender Scent on Dental Patient Anxiety Levels: A Cluster Randomized-Controlled Trial." *Community Dentistry and Oral Epidemiology* 38(1): 83–87.

Lewith, George T., Anthony Dean Godfrey, and Philip Prescott. August 2005. "A Single-Blinded, Randomized Pilot Study Evaluating the Aroma of *Lavendula augustifolia* as a Treatment for Mild Insomnia." *The Journal of Alternative & Complementary Medicine* 11(4): 631–637.

Linck, Viviane de Moura, Adriana Lourenço da Silva, Micheli Figueiró, et al. April 2009. "Inhaled Linalool-Induced Sedation in Mice." *Phytomedicine: International Journal of Phytotherapy and Phytopharmacology* 16(4): 303–307.

Nord, D., and J. Belew. October 2009. "Effectiveness of the Essential Oils Lavender and Ginger in Promoting Children's Comfort in a Perianesthesia Setting." *Journal of PeriAnesthesia Nursing* 24(5): 307–312.

Shaw, D., J.M. Annett, B. Doherty, and J.C. Leslie. September 2007. "Anxiolytic Effects of Lavender Oil Inhalation on Open-Field Behaviour in Rats." *Phytomedicine: International Journal of Phytotherapy and Phytopharmacology* 14(9): 613–620.

Woelk, H., and S. Schläfke. February 2010. "A Multi-Center, Double-Blind, Randomised Study of the Lavender Oil Preparation Silexan in Comparison to Lorazepam for Generalized Anxiety Disorder." *Phytomedicine: International Journal of Phytotherapy and Phytopharmacology* 17(2): 94–99.

Website
National Center for Complementary and Alternative Medicine. www.nccam.nih.gov.

Lemon Balm 🌿

Scientifically known as *Melissa officinalis,* lemon balm has been used medically for at least 2,000 years. Traditionally, it was thought to be effective for anxiety and other nervous system complaints. However, by the Middle Ages, lemon balm was widely used in Europe. A 2011 article in the *Journal of Primary Health Care* noted that in 1696 the London Dispensary said that lemon balm helped "renew youth, strengthen the brain, relieve languishing nature and prevent baldness." Today, lemon balm may also be used topically for oral and genital herpes simplex.[1] But, it is important to review what researchers have learned.

Anti-anxiety

In a study published in 2010 in *Phytomedicine: International Journal of Phytotherapy & Phytopharmacology,* researchers from France and New Jersey fed lemon balm to mice with laboratory-induced heightened anxiety levels. The results were dramatic. The researchers found that lemon balm had an effect similar to benzodiazepine drugs, a group of anti-anxiety prescription medications. The researchers determined that lemon balm enhanced the level of gamma-aminobutyric acid (GABA), a neurotransmitter that regulates emotions and calms the central nervous system. And, they concluded that their findings support the use of lemon balm for anxiety and nervous disorders.[2]

In a randomized, double-blind, placebo-controlled study published in 2004 in *Psychosomatic Medicine,* researchers from the United Kingdom gave 18 healthy volunteers (mean age 29.11) two separate single doses of lemon balm extract (300 mg, 600 mg) or a placebo on different days— separated by seven-day washout periods. While the subjects completed a test known for "increasing negative ratings of mood and engendering physiological responses concomitant with increased stress," the researchers assessed their mood and cognitive performance.

They found that lemon balm "ameliorated the negative change in mood associated" with the test. This improvement in mood was most evident with the 600-mg dose. "This dose was associated both with significantly improved calmness and significantly decreased alertness in comparison to placebo."[3]

May or May Not Help with the Agitation
Associated with Alzheimer's Disease

In a randomized, double-blind, placebo-controlled, parallel group trial published in 2011 in *Dementia and Geriatric Cognitive Disorders,* researchers from the United Kingdom evaluated the use of lemon balm, donepezil (also known as Aricept, a treatment for dementia), or a placebo to treat agitated elders from three psychiatric centers who had "probable or possible

Alzheimer's disease." The initial 114 participants were placed in one of three treatment groups: placebo medication and active lemon balm aromatherapy, or active medication and placebo aromatherapy, or placebo medication and placebo aromatherapy. After 4 weeks, the cohort had dropped to 94 participants, and after 12 weeks, the number was down to 81. The researchers found that both the lemon balm aromatherapy and the donepezil were "well tolerated." Interestingly, "there were no significant differences between aromatherapy, donepezil and placebo at week four and week 12, but importantly there were substantial improvements in all three groups." As a result of these findings, the researchers wrote that "there is no evidence that Melissa aromatherapy is superior to placebo or donepezil in the treatment of agitation in people with Alzheimer's disease." However, they then added, "the sizeable improvement in the placebo group emphasizes the potential non-specific benefits of touch and interaction in the treatment of people with Alzheimer's disease."[4]

Useful for Dyssomnia (Nervous Sleep Disturbance) in Children

In a multicenter, nonrandomized, noncontrolled trial published in 2006 in *Phytomedicine: International Journal of Phytotherapy & Phytopharmacology,* researchers from Germany tested the ability of a combination of lemon balm and valerian to be of assistance to children with dyssomnia. The cohort consisted of 918 children with dyssomnia. The mean age of the subjects was 8.4, and the mean duration of treatment was 31.9 days. The researchers found that more than 80% of the subjects experienced some degree of improvement. And, they concluded that this combination of herbs "might be an interesting alternative to chemical psychotropic drugs in the therapy of restlessness and dyssomnia in younger children."[5]

Treatment for Herpes Simplex Virus Type 1 and/or Type 2

In a study published in 2008 in *Phytomedicine: International Journal of Phytotherapy & Phytopharmacology,* researchers from Heidelberg, Germany investigated the antiviral ability of lemon balm essential oil on herpes simplex virus type 1 (the type of herpes found in cold sores on the lips) and herpes simplex virus type 2 (genital herpes, which is sexually transmitted). The researchers found that the lemon balm resulted in significant reductions in both types of herpes virus without being toxic to host cells. The researchers concluded that lemon balm essential oil "might be suitable for topical treatment of herpetic infections."[6]

In a study published in 2008 in *Natural Product Research,* researchers from Italy examined the ability of lemon balm to treat the lesions of type 2 herpes simplex virus. When the researchers tested lemon balm leaf extract on herpes cells, they found that even at a very safe dose the extract reduced the toxic effects of the virus. How was that accomplished? The researchers wrote that their findings "suggest that the extract does not prevent the entry of virus in the cells, but it acts after penetration of the virus in the host cell." The researchers noted that the rosmarinic acid found in lemon balm is most likely the cause of this effect. They concluded that their findings "support the use of lemon balm for treating Herpes simplex lesions."[7]

Useful for People with Diabetes
In a study published in 2010 in the *British Journal of Nutrition,* researchers from Korea evaluated the ability of lemon balm to lower glucose levels in mice with type 2 diabetes. For six weeks, the mice that served as controls were fed regular mouse food; the treatment mice were fed the regular food with lemon balm essential oil. When compared to the control mice, the researchers found that the mice that were fed lemon balm essential oil had significantly increased serum insulin concentrations and reduced levels of plasma glucose. They concluded that lemon balm "administered at low concentrations is an efficient hypoglycaemic agent."[8]

Protective against Low-Dose Radiation
In a study published in 2011 in *Toxicology and Industrial Health,* researchers from Iran wanted to learn if radiology staff members exposed to low-levels of radiation over an extended period of time would benefit from infusions of lemon balm. The cohort consisted of 55 members of a radiology staff—20 males and 35 females. For 30 days, they drank the lemon balm infusions twice daily. The researchers learned that "the oral administration of Lemon balm infusion may be helpful for the protection of the radiology staff against radiation induced oxidative stress and improve antioxidant defense system, especially enzymatic defense, due to antioxidant properties."[9]

Is Lemon Balm Beneficial?

Like so many other herbs, lemon balm appears to have a number of different benefits. It may well be an herb that should be discussed with a health care provider.

Notes

1. Rasmussen, Phil. June 2011. "Lemon Balm—*Melissa officinalis*; Also Known as Lemon Balm, Bee Balm, Garden Balm. Melissa, Melissengeist." *Journal of Primary Health Care* 3(2): 165–166.
2. Ibarra, Alvin, Nicolas Feuillere, Marc Roller, et al. May 2010. "Effects of Chronic Administration of *Melissa officinalis* L. Extract on Anxiety-Like Reactivity and on Circadian and Exploratory Activities in Mice." *Phytomedicine: International Journal of Phytotherapy & Phytopharmacology* 17(6): 397–403.
3. Kennedy, David O., Wendy Little, and Andrew B. Scholey. 2004. "Attenuation of Laboratory-Induced Stress in Humans after Acute Administration of *Melissa officinalis* (Lemon Balm)." *Psychosomatic Medicine* 66: 607–613.
4. Burns, A., E. Perry, C. Holmes, et al. 2011. "A Double-Blind Placebo-Controlled Randomized Trial of *Melissa officinalis* Oil and Donepezil for the Treatment of Agitation in Alzheimer's Disease." *Dementia and Geriatric Cognitive Disorders* 31(2): 158–164.
5. Müller, S. F., and S. Klement. 2006. "*Melissa officinalis* and *Valeriana officinalis* Combination in Treatment of Childhood Dyssomnia." *Phytomedicine: International Journal of Phytotherapy & Phytopharmacology* 13: 383–387.
6. Schnitzler, P., A. Schuhmacher, A. Astani, and J. Reichling. September 2008. "*Melissa officinalis* Oil Affects Infectivity of Enveloped Herpes Viruses." *Phytomedicine: International Journal of Phytotherapy & Phytopharmacology* 15(9): 734–740.
7. Mazzanti, G., L. Battinelli, C. Pompeo, et al. 2008. "Inhibitory Activity of *Melissa officinalis* L. Extract on Herpes Simplex Virus Type 2 Replication." *Natural Product Research* 22(16): 1433–1440.
8. Chung, M.J., S.Y. Cho, M.J. Bhuiyan, et al. July 2010. "Anti-Diabetic Effects of Lemon Balm (*Melissa officinalis*) Essential Oil on Glucose- and Lipid-Regulating Enzymes in Type 2 Diabetic Model." *British Journal of Nutrition* 104(2): 180–188.
9. Zeraatpishe, A., S. Oryan, M.H. Bagheri, et al. April 2011. "Effects of *Melissa officinalis* L. on Oxidative Status and DNA Damage in Subjects Exposed to Long-Term Low-Dose Ionizing Radiation." *Toxicology and Industrial Health* 27(3): 205–212.

References and Resources

Magazines, Journals, and Newspapers

Burns, A., E. Perry, C. Holmes, et al. 2011. "A Double-Blind Placebo-Controlled Randomized Trial of *Melissa officinalis* Oil and Donepezil for the Treatment of Agitation in Alzheimer's Disease." *Dementia and Geriatric Cognitive Disorders* 31(2): 158–164.

Chung, M.J., S.Y. Cho, M.J. Bhuiyan, et al. July 2010. "Anti-Diabetic Effects of Lemon Balm (*Melissa officinalis*) Essential Oil on Glucose- and Lipid-Regulating Enzymes in Type 2 Diabetic Mice." *British Journal of Nutrition* 104(2): 180–188.

Ibarra, Alvin, Nicolas Feuillere, Marc Roller, et al. May 2010. "Effects of Chronic Administration of *Melissa officinalis* L. Extract on Anxiety-Like Reactivity and on Circadian and Exploratory Activities in Mice." *Phytomedicine: International Journal of Phytotherapy & Phytopharmacology* 17(6): 397–403.

Kennedy, David O., Wendy Little, and Andrew B. Scholey. 2004. "Attenuation of Laboratory-Induced Stress in Humans after Acute Administration of *Melissa officinalis* (Lemon Balm)." *Psychosomatic Medicine* 66: 607–613.

Mazzanti, G., L. Battinelli, C. Pompeo, et al. 2008. "Inhibitory Activity of *Melissa officinalis* L. Extract on Herpes Simplex Virus Type 2 Replication." *Natural Product Research* 22(16): 1433–1440.

Müller, S.F., and S. Klement. 2006. "A Combination of Valerian and Lemon Balm Is Effective in the Treatment of Restlessness and Dyssomnia in Children." *Phytomedicine: International Journal of Phytotherapy & Phytopharmacology* 13: 383–387.

Rasmussen, Phil. June 2011. "Lemon Balm—*Melissa officinalis*; Also Known as Lemon Balm, Bee Balm, Garden Balm, Melissa, Melissengeist." *Journal of Primary Health Care* 3(2): 165–166.

Schnitzler, P., A. Schuhmacher, A. Astani, and J. Reichling. September 2008. "*Melissa officinalis* Oil Affects Infectivity of Enveloped Herpes Viruses." *Phytomedicine: International Journal of Phytotherapy & Phytopharmacology* 15(9): 734–740.

Sego, Sherril. March 2009. "Alternative Meds Update: What You Should Know About the Herbs and Supplements Patients Use." *Clinical Advisor* 12(3): 51–52.

Zeraatpishe, A., S. Oryan, M.H. Bagheri, et al. April 2011. "Effects of *Melissa officinalis* L. on Oxidative Status and DNA Damage in Subjects Exposed to Long-Term Low-Dose Ionizing Radiation." *Toxicology and Industrial Health* 27(3): 205–212.

Website
University of Maryland Medical Center. www.umm.edu.

Licorice Root 🌱

Scientifically known as *Glycyrrhiza glabra,* licorice root has been used as a medicinal herb for thousands of years. Also known as sweet root, licorice root has been considered useful for a wide variety of medical problems. These include treating obesity, upper respiratory infections such as colds and coughs, skin conditions such as psoriasis, indigestion, and liver disease.[1] It is important to review what researchers have learned.

Weight Loss

In a randomized, double-blind, placebo-controlled study published in 2009 in *Obesity Research & Clinical Practice,* researchers from Japan wanted to learn if licorice root could play a role in weight loss. The cohort consisted of 84 healthy men and women between the ages of 40 and 60; there were 56 men and 28 women. All the women were postmenopausal; all the subjects were moderately overweight. Each subject was randomly placed into one of four groups. The members of the first group took three placebo tablets each day; the members of the second group took one 300-mg licorice flavonoid oil (LFO) capsules each day and two placebos; the members of the third group took two 300-mg LPO capsules each day and one placebo; and the members of the fourth group took three 300-mg LPO capsules each day and no placebos. The researchers found that LFO "safely reduced body weight in overweight subjects by reducing total body fat." In fact, the highest dose—900 mg/day—"reduced body weight, body fat mass, visceral fat area, and serum LDL-cholesterol." The researchers concluded that "supplementing with LFO (at least 300 mg/day, preferably 900 mg/day) may contribute to the prevention or ameliorate obesity and probably to prevent obesity-induced metabolic syndrome, when combined with lifestyle modifications including moderate caloric restriction and moderate exercise."[2]

On the other hand, an article published in 2011 in *Lipids in Health and Disease* described two randomized, double-blinded studies completed at the University of Memphis in Memphis, Tennessee. The first included 22 men and women between the ages of 20 and 53. Though they exercised two to four days per week, they were all overweight. The second study included 23 athletic men between the ages of 19 and 35. In both studies, the participants were treated with either LFO or a placebo for eight weeks. The subjects in the second study also consumed a supplemental meal prior to bedtime. This was "an attempt to induce an acute state of overfeeding and body weight/fat gain."

In the first study, the researchers found no statistically significant differences "in anthropometric [human-body measurements] or biochemical markers of health and adiposity" between the men and women who received the supplementation and those who took placebos. In the second study, the subjects on LFO "did experience less overall fat gain." But, the results were not statistically significant. Still, the researchers noted that LFO "may provide some benefit to certain individuals engaged in a period of overfeeding."[3]

Psoriasis

In a pilot, open parallel study published in 2010 in *Giornale Italiano di Dermatologia e Venereologia,* researchers from Italy compared the use of mometasone furoate ointment (topical steroid used to reduce inflammation) containing licorice root and milk protein to the same ointment without these added ingredients on treating psoriasis. The cohort consisted of 40 people with psoriasis. Twenty people were randomly assigned to receive the ointment alone, and another 20 people used the ointment with licorice roots and milk protein. Clinical assessments were made at baseline, at two weeks, and at four weeks, when the study ended. All the participants completed the study and showed improvement in their psoriasis. However, when compared to the group who used only mometasone furoate ointment, the people who used the ointment with the added ingredients had "significantly greater improvement of desquamation [shedding of the outer skin], surface area affected, and subjective symptoms . . . observed at week four."[4]

Bronchial Asthma

In a study published in 2010 in *Clinical Biochemistry,* researchers from Egypt wanted to determine if an herbal combination of licorice root, boswellia, and turmeric root could provide relief from those dealing with bronchial asthma. The researchers divided the cohort, which consisted of 63 people with bronchial asthma, into two groups. The people in the first group took a soft capsule, which contained the herbs, three times a day for four weeks; the people in the second group took a placebo. During the trial, several different bronchial asthma tests were evaluated. The researchers found that the herbal combination has a significant effect in improving the symptoms of bronchial asthma. They noted that the herbs had "a pronounced effect in the management of bronchial asthma."[5]

Oral Health

In a study published in 2011 in the *International Journal of Oral Science,* researchers based in Los Angeles, California, conducted two pilot trials, with identical protocols, to determine the ability of sugar-free licorice root lollipops to kill cavity-causing bacteria in the mouth. The studies began with an initial screening. The 26 subjects were then told to suck on two lollipops per day for the next 10 days. After 10 days, the subjects returned for a second screening. The researchers learned that the lollipops were safe "and their antimicrobial activities are stable in the formulations intended for delivery." They concluded that the use of two lollipops per day for 10 days "led to a marked reduction of cavity-causing bacteria in [the] oral cavity among most of the human subjects tested."[6]

The year earlier, in 2010, a study on the use of licorice lollipops was published in the *European Archives of Paediatric Dentistry*. In this trial, researchers from Michigan investigated the use of sugar-free lollipops containing licorice root extract on a preschool population. The children were placed in one of three groups—high, medium, and low risk of caries (cavities). Then, for three weeks, each child consumed a lollipop in the morning and the afternoon. At the end of the study, the researchers were able to analyze the data obtained on 66 children (12 low risk, 37 moderate risk, and 17 high risk). The researchers found that the use of the lollipops significantly reduced the amount of bacteria that causes cavities. And, they concluded that "a potential for simple effectives caries [cavities]-prevention for high-risk children has been demonstrated."[7]

Prevention of Stomach Ulcers

In a study published in 2009 in the *Journal of Ethnopharmacology*, researchers from Germany wanted to understand how licorice root is able prevent stomach ulcers caused by *Helicobacter pylori*. During their experiments, in which they used human stomach tissue, the researchers found that licorice root "significantly inhibited the adhesion of *Helicobacter pylori* to human stomach tissue." And, they concluded that licorice root aqueous extract may "be assessed as a strong antiadhesive preparation against *Helicobacter pylori*."[8]

Is Licorice Root Beneficial?

From the research review, it is evident that licorice root may benefit some people. But, it is an herb that should be used with a good deal of caution. People with high blood pressure, cardiovascular disease, diabetes, kidney or liver disease, and problems with fluid retention should not use licorice root. Women who are pregnant or nursing should avoid this herb. Since licorice roots reacts with a host of different medications, such as ace inhibitors and diuretics, before taking this herb, it should be discussed with a medical provider. Finally, it is best not to use licorice root for more than four to six weeks.

Notes

1. University of Maryland Medical Center Website. www.umm.edu.
2. Tominaga, Yuji, Kaku Nakagawa, Tatsumasa Mae, et al. August 2009. "Licorice Flavonoid Oil Reduces Total Body Fat and Visceral Fat in Overweight Subjects: A Randomized, Double-Blind, Placebo-Controlled Study." *Obesity Research & Clinical Practice* 3(3): 169–178.
3. Bell, Zach W., Robert E. Canale, and Richard J. Bloomer. 2011. "A Dual Investigation of the Effect of Dietary Supplementation with Licorice Flavonoid Oil on Anthropometric and Biochemical Markers of Health and Adiposity." *Lipids in Health and Disease* 10: 29.
4. Cassano, N., R. Mantegazza, S. Battaglini, et al. December 2010. "Adjuvant Role of a New Emollient Cream in Patients with Palmer and/or Plantar Psoriasis: A Pilot Randomized Open-Label Study." *Giornale Italiano di Dermatologia e Venereologia* 145(6): 789–792.
5. Houssen, M.E., A. Ragab, A. Mesbah, et al. July 2010. "Natural Anti-Inflammatory Products and Leukotriene Inhibitors as Complementary Therapy for Bronchial Asthma." *Clinical Biochemistry* 43(10–11): 887–890.
6. Hu, C.H., J. He, R. Eckert, et al. January 2011. "Development and Evaluation of a Safe and Effective Sugar-Free Herbal Lollipop that Kills Cavity-Causing Bacteria." *International Journal of Oral Science* 3(1): 13–20.
7. Peters, M.C., J.A. Tallman, T.M. Braun, and J.J. Jacobson. December 2010. "Clinical Reduction of *S. mutans* in Pre-School Children Using a Novel Liquorice Root Extract Lollipop: A Pilot Study." *European Archives of Paediatric Dentistry* 11(6): 274–278.
8. Wittschier, N., G. Faller, and A. Hensel. September 2009. "Aqueous Extracts and Polysaccharides from Liquorice Roots (*Glycyrrhiza glabra* L.) Inhibit Adhesion of *Helicobacter Pylori* to Human Gastric Mucosa." *Journal of Ethnopharmacology* 125(2): 218–223.

References and Resources

Magazines, Journals, and Newspapers

Bell, Zach W., Robert E. Canale, and Richard J. Bloomer. 2011. "A Duel Investigation of the Effect of Dietary Supplementation with Licorice Flavonoid Oil on Anthropometric and Biochemical Markers of Health and Adiposity." *Lipids in Health and Disease* 10: 29.

Cassano, N., R. Mantegazza, S. Battaglini, et al. December 2010. "Adjuvant Role of a New Emollient Cream in Patients with Palmar and/or Plantar Psoriasis: A Pilot Randomized Open-Label Study." *Giornale Italiano di Dermatologia e Venereologia* 145(6): 789–792.

Houssen, M. E., A. Ragab, A. Mesbah, et al. July 2010. "Natural Anti-Inflammatory Products and Leukotriene Inhibitors as Complementary Therapy for Bronchial Asthma." *Clinical Biochemistry* 43(10–11): 887–890.

Hu, C. H., J. He, R. Eckert, et al. January 2011. "Development and Evaluation of a Safe and Effective Sugar-Free Herbal Lollipop that Kills Cavity-Causing Bacteria." *International Journal of Oral Science* 3(1): 13–20.

Peters, M. C., J. A. Tallman, T. M. Braun, and J. J. Jacobson. December 2010. "Clinical Reduction of *S. mutans* in Pre-School Children Using a Novel Liquorice Root Extract Lollipop: A Pilot Study." *European Archives of Paediatric Dentistry* 11(6): 274–278.

Tominaga, Yuji, Kaku Nakagawa, Tatsumasa Mae, et al. August 2009. "Licorice Flavonoid Oil Reduces Total Body Fat and Visceral Fat in Overweight Subjects: A Randomized, Double-Blind, Placebo-Controlled Study." *Obesity Research & Clinical Practice* 3(3): 169–178.

Wittschier, N., G. Faller, and A. Hensel. September 2009. "Aqueous Extracts and Polysaccharides from Liquorice Roots (*Glycyrrhiza glabra* L.) Inhibit Adhesion of *Helicobacter pylori* to Human Gastric Mucosa." *Journal of Ethnopharmacology* 125(2): 218–223.

Website

University of Maryland Medical Center. www.umm.edu.

M

Milk Thistle 🌱

Scientifically known as *Silybum marianum,* milk thistle, which is native to the Mediterranean region, has been used for about 2,000 years for a wide variety of medical problems. Most often, milk thistle is considered an herb that supports the liver. But, it is also said to be an effective herb for lowering cholesterol levels, reducing insulin resistance, and slowing or stopping the growth of certain types of cancer cells. The most active ingredient in milk thistle is silymarin, which is actually a group of flavonoids—silibinin, silidianin, and silicristin.[1] In fact, milk thistle and silymarin, silibinin, silidianin, and silicristin are often used interchangeably. Is milk thistle a truly effective herb? It is important to review what the researchers have learned.

Liver and Kidney Protection

In a study published in 2010 in *Toxicology International,* researchers from India evaluated the ability of silymarin and *Terminalia chebula,* an Ayurvedic herb also known as Haritaki, to protect the liver and kidneys against experimentally induced acetaminophen toxicity (*N*-acetyl-*p*-aminophenol; APAP) in rats. The researchers began by dividing 24 rats into four groups, each with 6 rats. For the first three days of the trial, the rats in all four groups were given high doses of acetaminophen. That triggered liver and kidney toxicity symptoms, such as elevation in serum triglycerides, total cholesterol, blood urea nitrogen, serum creatinine, and transaminase elevation (an indicator that the liver is injured). The second part of the trial continued for 10 days. During this time, the first group of rats was fed distilled water; the second group of rats was fed 25 mg/kg of silymarin; the third group was fed 125 mg/kg of *T. chebula*; and the final group of rats was fed a combination of silymarin and *T. chebula,* at the previously noted doses. The researchers found that both herbs significantly reversed the toxicity caused by the high levels of acetaminophen. And, they concluded that "silymarin and *T. chebula* exhibit good hepato- and nephro-protections against APAP toxicity."[2]

Liver Protection

In a study published in 2011 in *Evidence-Based Complementary and Alternative Medicine,* researchers from Quebec, Canada, explored the use of silibinin to treat nonalcoholic steatohepatitis (NASH), a progressive liver disease related to metabolic syndrome, obesity, and diabetes. The researchers investigated the use of silibinin in an experimental rat NASH model. They began by dividing 20 rats into three groups. Consisting of six rats, the first group served as the control. These rats were fed a standard liquid diet for 12 weeks. The six rats in the second group were fed a high-fat diet for 12 weeks. Meanwhile, the eight rats in the third group were fed a high-fat liquid diet for 12 weeks. But, during the final five weeks of the trial, they were fed 200 mg/kg/day of silibinin. The researchers found that silibinin was notably effective in mitigating some of the problems associated with NASH. For example, silibinin "was very efficient in reversing the progression of NASH." The researchers wrote that their "study clearly confirms that silibinin . . . is efficient at improving injuries caused by a chronic liver disease. It also demonstrates for the first time that a therapeutic treatment with silibinin . . . is effective in reversing steatosis [fatty liver disease], oxidative stress, and insulin resistance in an *in vivo* rat model of diet-induced NASH."[3]

In a study published in 2009 in the *International Journal of Biological Sciences,* researchers from New Orleans, Louisiana, and Egypt investigated the ability of silymarin and garlic extract to protect the liver against hepatotoxicity—damage caused by drugs, chemicals, or other agents. The researchers began by pretreating male albino rats with silymarin or garlic or both for one week. Then, the animals were treated with two chemicals designed to trigger liver toxicity. At the end of six weeks, the researchers found that the "administration of garlic or silymarin significantly reduced the liver toxicity." However, the "combined administration was more effective in preventing the development of hepatotoxicity." They concluded that "silymarin and garlic have synergistic effects, and could be used as hepatoprotective agents against hepatotoxicity."[4]

Hepatitis

In a randomized, placebo-controlled, blinded trial published in 2009 in *Phytomedicine: International Journal of Phytotherapy and Phytopharmacology,* researchers from the University of Maryland School of Medicine in Baltimore and Egypt treated 105 patients with acute clinical hepatitis (inflammation of the liver) with either 140 mg of silymarin three times a day or a vitamin placebo. The trial continued for four weeks. After the supplementation was discontinued, there were four additional weeks of follow-up. The researchers found that the patients treated with silymarin experienced a quicker resolution to their acute hepatitis symptoms, such as dark urine and jaundice. The researchers concluded that silymarin had definite benefits. "Despite a modest sample size and multiple etiologies for acute clinical hepatitis, our results suggest that standard recommended doses of silymarin are safe and may be potentially effective in improving symptoms of acute clinical hepatitis."[5]

In a study published in 2011 in *Alimentary Pharmacology and Therapeutics,* researchers from several locations in the United States assessed the use of silymarin on the progression of liver disease in 1,049 patients with hepatitis C. The researchers found that "among the patients with advanced hepatitis-C related liver disease is associated with reduced progression from fibrosis to cirrhosis." But, the researchers also learned that among these patients, silymarin did not alter the clinical outcomes. "Nevertheless," the researchers wrote, "our results provide support for conducting additional studies of silymarin, including intervention trials with defined dosage regimens and standard silymarin product."[6]

Liver Cancer

In a study published in 2009 in *Cell Proliferation,* researchers from India, Italy, and Mexico examined the ability of a variety of doses of silymarin to inhibit the growth of human liver cancer cells. The researchers found that silymarin did indeed impair the growth of human liver cancer cells "in a dose-dependent manner." So, "inhibition was directly proportional to dose." The higher the dose, the greater the inhibition. Furthermore, the researchers noted that silymarin both prevents cell proliferation and induces apoptosis or cell death.[7]

Colon Cancer

In an in vitro study published in 2011 in *Cancer Chemotherapy and Pharmacology,* researchers from Milan, Italy, examined the ability of silymarin, when used as a pretreatment for the anticancer drugs doxorubicin or paclitaxel, to destroy two different cell lines of colon cancer. One of the tested colon cell lines was resistant to several different types of drug therapy. The researchers learned that "silymarin had similar antiproliferative activity against both cell lines." They concluded that their "findings confirm activity of silymarin against colon carcinoma, including multi-drug-resistant types, at relatively high but clinically achievable concentrations."[8]

Alzheimer's Disease

In a study published in 2009 in the *British Journal of Pharmacology,* researchers from China and Japan triggered memory impairment and the accumulation of oxidative stress in the brains of mice by injecting amyloid beta peptide. After feeding different doses of silibinin to the mice for the next several days, the researchers conducted memory tests on the mice. They noted that silibinin may alleviate the memory deficits caused by the amyloid beta peptide. Additionally, "silibinin is well tolerated and largely free of adverse effects and has few negative drug interactions."[9]

Is Milk Thistle Beneficial?

Milk thistle appears to have a number of beneficial qualities, particularly for those who are at increased risk for liver problems. It may well be useful to discuss this herb with your health care provider.

Notes

1. University of Maryland Medical Center Website. www.umm.edu.
2. Gopi, K., A. Reddy, K. Jyothi, and B. Kumar. July–December 2010. "Acetaminophen-Induced Hepato- and Nephrotoxicity and Amelioration by Silymarin and *Terminalia chebula* in Rats." *Toxicology International* 17(2): 64–66.
3. Haddad, Y., D. Vallerand, A. Brault, and P. S. Haddad. 2011. "Antioxidant and Hepatoprotective Effects of Silibinin in a Rat Model of Nonalcoholic Steatophepatitis." *Evidence-Based Complementary and Alternative Medicine* Article ID 647903: 10 pages. DOI: 10.1093/ecam/nep164.

4. Shaarawy, S. M., A. A. Tohamy, S. M. Elgendy, et al. August 2009. "Protective Effects of Garlic and Silymarin on NDEA-Induced Rats Hepatotoxicity." *International Journal of Biological Sciences* 5(6): 549–557.

5. El-Kamary, S. S., M. D. Shardell, M. Abdel-Hamid, et al. May 2009. "A Randomized Controlled Trial to Assess the Safety and Efficacy of Silymarin on Symptoms, Signs and Biomarkers of Acute Hepatitis." *Phytomedicine: International Journal of Phytotherapy and Phytopharmacology* 16(5): 391–400.

6. Freedman, N. D., T. M. Curto, C. Morishima, et al. January 2011. "Silymarin Use and Live Disease Progression in the Hepatitis C Antiviral Long-Term Treatment against Cirrhosis Trial." *Alimentary Pharmacology and Therapeutics* 33(1): 127–137.

7. Ramakrishnan, G., L. Lo Muzio, C. M. Elinos-Báez, et al. April 2009. "Silymarin Inhibited Proliferation and Induced Apoptosis in Hepatic Cancer Cells." *Cell Proliferation* 42(2): 229–240.

8. Colombo, V., M. Lupi, F. Falcetta, et al. 2011. "Chemotherapeutic Activity of Silymarin Combined with Doxorubicin or Paclitaxel in Sensitive and Multidrug-Resistant Colon Cancer Cells." *Cancer Chemotherapy and Pharmacology* 67: 369–379.

9. Lu, P., T. Mamiya, L. L. Lu, et al. August 2009. "Silibinin Prevents Amyloid Beta Peptide-Induced Memory Impairment and Oxidative Stress in Mice." *British Journal of Pharmacology* 157(7): 1270–1277.

References and Resources

Magazines, Journals, and Newspapers

Colombo, V., M. Lupi, F. Falcetta, et al. 2011. "Chemotherapeutic Activity of Silymarin Combined with Doxorubicin or Paclitaxel in Sensitive and Multidrug-Resistant Colon Cancer Cells." *Cancer Chemotherapy and Pharmacology* 67: 369–379.

El-Kamary, S. S., M. D. Shardell, M. Abdel-Hamid, et al. May 2009. "A Randomized Controlled Trial to Assess the Safety and Efficacy of Silymarin on Symptoms, Signs and Biomarkers of Acute Hepatitis." *Phytomedicine: International Journal of Phytotherapy and Phytopharmacology* 16(5): 391–400.

Freedman, N. D., T. M. Curto, C. Morishima, et al. January 2011. "Silymarin Use and Liver Disease Progression in the Hepatitis C. Antiviral Long-Term Treatment against Cirrhosis Trial." *Alimentary Pharmacology and Therapeutics* 33(1): 127–137.

Gopi, K., A. Reddy, K. Jyothi, and B. Kumar. July–December 2010. "Acetaminophen-Induced Hepato- and Nephrotoxicity and Amelioration by Silymarin and *Terminalia chebula* in Rats." *Toxicology International* 17(2): 64–66.

Haddad, Y., D. Vallerand, A. Brault, and P. S. Haddad. 2011. "Antioxidant and Hepatoprotective Effects of Silibinin in a Rat Model of Nonalcoholic

Steatophepatitis." *Evidenced-Based Complementary and Alternative Medicine* Article ID 647903: 10 pages. DOI: 10.1093/ecam/nep164.

Lu, P., T. Mamiya, L. L. Lu, et al. August 2009. "Silibinin Prevents Amyloid Beta Peptide-Induced Memory Impairment and Oxidative Stress in Mice." *British Journal of Pharmacology* 157(7): 1270–1277.

Ramakrishnan, G., L. Lo Muzio, C. M. Elinos-Báez, et al. April 2009. "Silymarin Inhibited Proliferation and Induced Apoptosis in Hepatic Cancer Cells." *Cell Proliferation* 42(2): 229–240.

Shaarawy, S. M., A. A. Tohamy, S. M. Elgendy, et al. August 2009. "Protective Effects of Garlic and Silymarin on NDEA-Induced Rats Hepatotoxicity." *International Journal of Biological Sciences* 5(6): 549–557.

Websites

National Center for Complementary and Alternative Medicine. www.nccam.nih.gov.

University of Maryland Medical Center. www.umm.edu.

N

Noni 🐨

Scientifically known as *Morinda citrifolia,* noni grows in many areas of the world, including the tropical regions of the Pacific Ocean. Historically, noni is probably best known as an important part of Polynesian folk medicine. For centuries, Polynesians used noni to treat joint pain and skin conditions. Today, noni is often considered to be an herb that supports overall health. But, people sometimes view noni as a component of the treatment for diabetes, cardiovascular disease, cancer, and other chronic illnesses.[1] It is important to review what researchers have learned.

Arthritis Pain Relief
In a study published in 2010 in *Phytotherapy Research,* German researchers tested the ability of noni to provide relief from painful inflammatory conditions, such as arthritis, in a standardized animal model. In one test, known as the hot plate test, the researchers placed mice that had been fed noni in their drinking water on a specially designed hot plate. By observing their reaction to the heat, the researchers were able to determine the effectiveness of noni. The researchers found that noni "reduced the pain sensitivity comparably to the central analgesic drug tramadol." This is a striking finding. Tramadol is an opiate pain medication used to relieve moderate to severe pain. The researchers concluded that their work "supported the hypothesis of the beneficial effects of noni fruit juice on painful inflammatory diseases, such as arthritis, suggested by its use in ethnic folk medicine and recent epidemiological observation."[2]

Prevention of Esophageal Cancer

In a study published in 2010 in *Pharmaceutical Research,* researchers from Columbus, Ohio investigated the ability of several types of fruits, including noni, to prevent chemically induced esophageal cancer in rats. To induce esophageal cancer in rats, they were treated with a chemical for five weeks. Then, they were placed on a diet containing 5% of noni or six other types of fruit such as black or red raspberries. The researchers found that all seven types of fruit were "about equally effective" in inhibiting the growth of esophageal cancer. They also all were instrumental in increasing the levels of serum antioxidants.[3]

Cognitive Functioning

In a study published in 2010 in *Physiology & Behavior,* researchers from Japan wanted to determine if supplementation with noni juice could attenuate stress-induced impairment of cognitive functioning of mice. To accomplish this goal, they divided 40 mice into four groups of 10 each. While one group served as the control, the mice in the other three groups were subjected to eight hours of chronic restraint stress (CRS) six days a week for six weeks. One of the three groups received noni supplementation, and one other group received vitamin E supplementation. From their tests on the mice, the researchers learned that "the administration of noni fruit juice protects brains from stress-induced impairment of cognitive function."[4]

Cardiovascular Health Benefits

In a study published in 2010 in *Lipids in Health and Disease,* researchers from Pakistan and Saudi Arabia wanted to learn if extracts of noni fruit, leaves, and roots could improve lipid and triglyceride levels in rats. In addition to feeding the rats the various forms of noni, some rats were fed a compound (triton) that alters serum lipid levels and other rats were fed a high-fat diet. The researchers found that "all three extracts caused reduction in total cholesterol and triglyceride level in triton-induced dyslipidemia [abnormal concentration of lipids in the blood]." In the rats fed high-fat diets, the three extracts caused "significant reduction in total cholesterol, triglyceride, low density lipoprotein-cholesterol (LDL-C) ["bad" cholesterol] . . . and TC/HDL ratio." Noni roots also resulted in an increase in high-density lipoprotein (HDL) cholesterol "good" cholesterol.

The researchers concluded that their findings support "the medicinal use of *Morinda citrifolia* in dyslipidemia."[5]

Provides Brain and Serum Insulin Protection

In a study published in 2010 in the *Journal of Natural Medicines,* researchers from Japan evaluated the protective effect of noni juice in brain damage caused by ischemic stress (insufficient blood supply) in mice. The researchers began by adding noni to the drinking water of some mice. Other mice, in the control group, did not have any noni. The mice were then subjected to middle cerebral artery occlusion (blockage). The researchers found that the ingestion of noni had a "protective effect on neuronal cell death and on behavioral abnormality." Moreover, the intake of noni "suppressed the deterioration of learning and memory." Additionally, the researchers observed that noni treatment significantly increased serum insulin levels to a greater degree than the control group.[6]

Useful for Postoperative Nausea and Vomiting

In a randomized, double-blind, placebo-controlled trial published in 2010 in the *Journal of the Medical Association of Thailand,* researchers from Thailand evaluated the ability of noni to reduce or prevent postoperative nausea and vomiting in patients considered to be at high risk for these problems. One hundred patients between the ages of 18 and 65 were randomly assigned to take a placebo or 150, 300, or 600 mg of noni extract one hour before surgery. The researchers found that the 600-mg dose was the minimum dose of noni extract required to reduce the incidence of postoperative nausea during the early postoperative period (between zero and six hours following surgery). At the same time, the incidence of postoperative nausea and vomiting during the other time periods "was not statistically different for all three noni doses compared to the placebo group."[7]

Cancer Prevention

In a study published in 2010 in *The Southeast Asian Journal of Tropical Medicine and Public Health,* researchers from Thailand examined the anticancer properties of Thai noni leaves. The researchers tested the noni against four different types of cancer cells. Though noni showed varying abilities to kill the different cancer cells, it did appear to be particularly effective against epidermoid (lung) and cervical cells. The researchers wrote that noni leaf extract "may have potential as a functional food for chemoprevention against epidermoid and cervical cancers."[8]

Protection from UVB Rays

In a study published in 2009 in the *Journal of Natural Medicines,* researchers from Utah (United States) wondered if noni would protect the skin from UVB rays from the sun. Their cohort consisted of 25 adults (3 males and 22 females) between the ages of 21 and 58. All the volunteers had sun-sensitive skin; they had skin that burned easily and tanned within the first 30 to 45 minutes of sun exposure. The researchers selected several sites on the backs of the volunteers; most were treated with noni, a few were not. Fifteen minutes after the extract was applied, the test sites were exposed to increasing amounts of UVB radiation. Evaluations were made 22 to 24 hours after exposure. The researchers found that "the UVB dose required to induce erythema [skin that is red] at the protected sites was almost 3.5 times greater than the MED [minimal erythemal dose] of untreated skin."[9]

Is Noni Beneficial?

A review of the research on noni cannot help but leave that impression that this herb has a number of benefits. Yet, the literature also contains a few indications that noni may not be safe. To address this concern, researchers from Utah conducted a single-center, double-blind, placebo-controlled study that was published in 2009 in *Pacific Health Dialogue.* For 28 days, 96 healthy volunteers, between the ages of 18 and 64, were randomly assigned to take either a placebo or three different doses of Tahitian noni (30, 300, or 750 mL). The researchers found that "during the trial, those in the noni groups experienced 20 to 50% fewer total adverse events than those in the placebo group." And, they concluded that "drinking up to 750 mL Tahitian noni juice per day is safe."[10]

Notes

1. National Center for Complementary and Alternative Medicine Website. www .nccam.nit.gov.
2. Basar, S., K. Uhlenhut, P. Högger, et al. January 2010. "Analgesic and Anti-inflammatory Activity of *Morinda citrifolia* L. (Noni) Fruit." *Phytotherapy Research* 24(1): 38–42.

3. Stoner, G.D., L.S. Wang, C. Seguin, et al. June 2010. "Multiple Berry Types Prevent N-Nitrosomethylbenzylamine-Induced Esophageal Cancer in Rats." *Pharmaceutical Research* 27(6): 1138–1145.

4. Muto, J., L. Hosung, A. Uwaya, et al. September 2010. *"Morinda citrifolia* Fruit Reduces Stress-Induced Impairment of Cognitive Function Accompanied by Vasculature Improvement in Mice." *Physiology & Behavior* 101(2): 211–217.

5. Mandukhail, S.U., N. Aziz, and A.H. Gilani. August 2010. "Studies on Antidyslipidemic Effects of *Morinda citrifolia* (noni) Fruits, Leaves, and Root Extracts." *Lipids in Health and Disease* 9: 88.

6. Harada, S., W. Fujita-Hamabe, K. Kamiya, et al. October 2010. *"Morinda citrifolia* Fruit Juice Prevents Ischemic Neuronal Damage through Suppression of the Development of Post-Ischemic Glucose Intolerance." *Journal of Natural Medicines* 64(4): 468–473.

7. Prapaitrakool S., and A. Itharat. December 2010. *"Morinda citrifolia* Linn. for Prevention of Postoperative Nausea and Vomiting." *Journal of the Medical Association of Thailand* 93 (Supplement 7): S204–S209.

8. Thani, Wasina, Omboon Vallisuta, Pongpan Siripong, et al. March 2010. "Anti-Proliferative and Antioxidative Activities of Thai Noni/Yor (*Morinda citrifolia* Linn.) Leaf Extract." *The Southeast Asian Journal of Tropical Medicine and Public Health* 41(2): 482–489.

9. West, Brett J., Shixin Deng, Afa K. Palu, and C. Jarakae Jensen. July 2009. *"Morinda citrifolia* Linn (Rubiaceae) Leaf Extracts Mitigate UVB-Induced Erythema." *Journal of Natural Medicines* 63(3): 351–354.

10. West, B.J., L.D. White, C.J. Jensen, and A.K. Palu. November 2009. "A Double-Blind Clinical Safety Study of Noni Fruit Juice." *Pacific Health Dialogue* 15(2): 21–32.

References and Resources

Magazines, Journals, and Newspapers

Basar, S., K. Uhlenhut, P. Högger, et al. January 2010. "Analgesic and Antiinflammatory Activity of *Morinda citrifolia* L. (Noni) Fruit." *Phytotherapy Research* 24(1): 38–42.

Harada, S., W. Fujita-Hamabe, K. Kamiya, et al. October 2010. *"Morinda citrifolia* Fruit Juice Prevents Ischemic Neuronal Damage through Suppression of the Development of Post-Ischemic Glucose Intolerance." *Journal of Natural Medicines* 64(4): 468–473.

Mandukhail, S.U., N. Aziz, and A.H. Gilani. August 2010. "Studies on Antidyslipidemic Effects of *Morinda citrifolia* (Noni) Fruit, Leaves and Root Extract." *Lipids in Health and Disease* 9: 88.

Muto, J., L. Hosung, A. Uwaya, et al. September 2010. *"Morinda citrifolia* Fruit Reduces Stress-Induced Impairment of Cognitive Function Accompanied by Vasculature Improvement in Mice." *Physiology & Behavior* 101(2): 211–217.

Prapaitrakool, S., and A. Itharat. December 2010. "*Morinda citrifolia* Linn. For Prevention of Postoperative Nausea and Vomiting. *Journal of the Medical Association of Thailand* 93 (Supplement 7): S204–S209.

Stoner, G. D., L. S. Wang, C. Seguin, et al. June 2010. "Multiple Berry Types Prevent N-Nitrosomethylbenzylamine-Induced Esophageal Cancer in Rats." *Pharmaceutical Research* 27(6): 1138–1145.

Thani, Wasina, Omboon Vallisuta, Pongpan Siripong, et al. March 2010. "Anti-Proliferative and Antioxidative Activities of Thai Noni/Yor (*Morinda citrifolia* Linn.) Leaf Extract." *The Southeast Asian Journal of Tropical Medicine and Public Health* 41(2): 482–489.

West, Brett J., Shixin Deng, Afa K. Palu, and C. Jarakae Jensen. July 2009. "*Morinda citrifolia* Linn. (Rubiaceae) Leaf Extracts Mitigate UVB-Induced Erythema." *Journal of Natural Medicines* 63(3): 351–354.

West, Brett J., L. D. White, C. J. Jensen, and A. K. Palu. November 2009. "A Double-Blind Clinical Study of Non Fruit Juice." *Pacific Health Dialogue* 15(2): 21–32.

Website

National Center for Complementary and Alternative Medicine. www.nccam.nih.gov.

Olive Leaf Extract 🌿

Scientifically known as *Olea europaea,* olive leaf extract has been used since biblical days for many different medicinal purposes. These include treating fevers, skin rashes, malaria, healing wounds, and curing infections. Today, olive leaf extract is also thought to be useful for a wide variety of cardiovascular concerns. It is known that olive leaf extracts are filled with natural antioxidants, such as the flavonoids, apigenin, luteolin, chrysoeriol, hesperidin, rutin, quercetin, and kaempferol. However, the most abundant component in olive leaf extract is oleuropein, which has powerful anti-fungal and antibacterial properties.[1] But, it is important to review what researchers have learned.

High Blood Pressure (Hypertension)

In a randomized, double-blind, parallel, and active-controlled clinical study published in 2011 in *Phytomedicine: International Journal of Phytotherapy & Phytopharmacology,* researchers from Indonesia and Switzerland compared the antihypertensive effect and tolerability of olive leaf extract and Captopril, a medication used for elevated levels of blood pressure, in people with stage 1 hypertension. The initial cohort included 232 participants between the ages of 25 to 60 with stage 1 hypertension (systolic blood pressure 140–159 mmHg and/or diastolic blood pressure 90–99 mmHg). Following a four-week period in which the participants received no treatment, they had eight weeks in which they were treated with either one 500 mg of olive leaf extract (Benolea) twice each day or 12.5 to 25 mg Captopril twice each day. One hundred and sixty-two people completed the trial. Both the people taking olive leaf extract and those on

Captopril experienced significant improvements in levels of systolic and diastolic blood pressure. In fact, the reductions in the two groups were not significantly different. The researchers concluded that olive leaf extract "at the dosage regimen of 500 mg twice daily was similarly effective in lowering systolic and diastolic blood pressures in subjects with stage 1 hypertension as Captopril, given at its effective dose of 12.5–25 mg twice daily."[2]

In an open, controlled, parallel group, co-twin trial published in 2008 in *Phytotherapy Research,* researchers from Germany and Switzerland examined the effect of olive leaf extract on 40 identical (monozygotic) twins, between the ages of 18 and 60, with untreated suboptimal blood pressure—"exceeding 120 mmHg systolic or 80 mmHg diastolic at rest." The participants were given either capsules containing 500- or 1,000-mg doses of olive leaf extract or capsules containing placebos. The pairs of twins were assigned to different treatments. At the end of eight weeks, the researchers determined that olive leaf extract had antihypertensive properties. The researchers noted that "for the 1000 mg dose, these actions were substantial in subjects with borderline hypertension whereas, for the 500 mg dose, they were only detectable using the co-twin approach."[3]

Helps Prevent the Development of Atherosclerosis

In a study published in 2008 in the *European Journal of Nutrition,* researchers from China and Japan wanted to learn if olive leaf extract could be used to lower the incidence of atherosclerosis. They began by randomly placing 24 rabbits into one of three groups. The rabbits in the first group were fed standard rabbit food. They became the control group. The rabbits in the second group were fed a high-lipid diet. And, the rabbits in the third group were fed a high-lipid diet and olive leaf extract. At the end of the six-week trial, the researchers noted that "the administration of OLE [olive leaf extract] was able to decrease serum level of lipid and suppress the development of atherosclerosis." Furthermore, "the administration of OLE not only decreased the levels of blood lipid but also inhibited inflammatory response. The combined effect might account for the beneficial effects of OLE on preventing and reducing the development of atherosclerosis."[4]

Skin Protection Properties

In a study published in 2009 in *The Journal of Nutrition,* researchers from Japan investigated the skin protective properties of the oral administration of olive leaf extract in hairless mice exposed to chronic ultraviolet radiation. After 30 weeks, the researchers found that the olive leaf extract and its component, oleuropein, "significantly inhibited increases in skin thickness and reductions in skin elasticity." In addition, it reduced the numbers of skin cancers and growths. The researchers concluded that "the oral administration of an olive leaf extract and its component, oleuropein, prevents UVB-induced skin photoaging and carcinogenesis."[5]

Brain Protection Properties

In a study published in 2011 in *Phytomedicine: International Journal of Phytotherapy & Phytopharmacology,* researchers from Iran wanted to determine if olive leaf extract could help protect brain cells. The researchers began by dividing 72 rats into four groups of 18 each. One group, which served as the control, received only distilled water. The three other groups received varying amounts of olive leaf extract—50, 75, and 100 mg/kg/day, respectively. After 30 days, the rats were subjected to 60-minute arterial occlusions of their cerebral arteries, which induced strokes. The researchers found that the rats taking the higher amounts of olive leaf extract had less brain damage. The researchers concluded that olive leaf extract "may be cerebroprotective in a rat model of ischemia-reperfusion."[6]

Attenuates Symptoms of Metabolic Syndrome

In a study published in 2010 in *The Journal of Nutrition,* researchers from Australia tested the ability of olive leaf extract to diminish some of the symptoms associated with metabolic disorder, such as elevated amounts of abdominal fat. The researchers began by dividing 50 rats into four groups. The first group of 10 rats, which served as the control, were fed cornstarch; the second group of 10 rats were fed cornstarch and olive leaf extract; the third group of 20 rats were fed a high-carbohydrate, high-fat diet; and the fourth group of 10 rats were fed a high-carbohydrate, high-fat diet and olive leaf extract. The trial continued for 16 weeks. At that point, the rats fed the high-carbohydrate, high-fat diet developed signs of metabolic syndrome. On the other hand, when compared with rats on a high-carbohydrate, high-fat diet, rats on a high-carbohydrate high-fat diet and olive leaf extract diet "had improved or normalized cardiovascular, hepatic, and metabolic signs with the exception of elevated blood pressure." The researchers commented that their findings "demonstrate that treatment of diet-induced metabolic syndrome in rats with OLE [olive leaf extract] attenuated the metabolic, as well as structural and functional, changes in the heart and liver without decreasing blood pressure."[7]

Helps with Diabetes

In a study published in 2009 in *Phytotherapy Research,* researchers from Iran tested the ability of olive leaf extract to help normal and strepto-zotocin (STZ)-induced diabetic rats. The cohort consisted of 24 normal rats and 30 rats with diabetes. The rats were divided into several different groups. Some of the groups served as the controls; others were fed varying amounts of olive leaf alcohol extract. The rats in one group were treated with glibenclamide, a medication used for diabetes. The results were remarkable. The researchers found that the oral administration of olive leaf extract "produced significant hypoglycemic effects only in streptozotocin-induced diabetic rats and not in normal rats." Even more significant is the fact that the researchers found that olive leaf extract "is more effective in comparison with glibenclamide in attenuating the increased serum parameters resulting from damage of STZ-induced diabetic rats." And, they concluded that olive leaf extract "may be of use as an antidiabetic agent."[8]

Is Olive Leaf Extract Beneficial?

Though less well known than many other herbs, olive leaf extract appears to have a number of excellent properties. It may well be an herb that should be discussed with health care providers.

Notes

1. Erickson, Kim. September 2009. "All About Olive Leaf: Clear Up Acne-Prone Skin, Alleviate Eczema, and Benefit Your Heart in Multiple Ways with Olive Leaf Extract, a Potent Medicinal Herb." *Better Nutrition* 71(9): 30.
2. Susalit, E., N. Agus, I. Effendi, et al. February 2011. "Olive (*Olea europaea*) Leaf Extract effective in Patients with Stage-1 Hypertension: Comparison with Captopril." *Phytomedicine: International Journal of Phytotherapy & Phytopharmacology* 18(4): 251–258.
3. Perrinjaquet-Moccette, Tania, Andreas Busjahn, Caesar Schmidlin, et al. 2008. "Food Supplementation with an Olive (*Olea europaea* L.) Leaf Extract Reduces Blood Pressure in Borderline Hypertensive Monozygotic Twins." *Phytotherapy Research* 22: 1239–1242.

4. Wang, L., C. Geng, L. Jiang, et al. August 2008. "The Anti-Atherosclerotic Effect of Olive Leaf Extract Is Related to Suppressed Inflammatory Response in Rabbits with Experimental Atherosclerosis." *European Journal of Nutrition* 47(5): 235–243.

5. Kimura, Yoshiyuki, and Maho Sumiyoshi. November 2009. "Olive Leaf Extract and Its Main Component Oleuropein Prevent Chronic Ultraviolet B Radiation-Induced Skin damage and Carcinogenesis in Hairless Mice." *The Journal of Nutrition* 139(11): 2079–2086.

6. Mohagheghi, Fatemeh, Mohammad Reza Bigdeli, Bahram Rasoulian, et al. January 2011. "The Neuroprotective Effect of Olive Leaf Extract Is Related to Improved Blood–Brain Barrier Permeability and Brain Edema in Rat with Experimental Focal Cerebral Ischemia." *Phytomedicine: International Journal of Phytotherapy & Phytopharmacology* 18(2–3): 170–175.

7. Poudyal, H., F. Campbell, and L. Brown. May 2010. "Olive Leaf Extract Attenuates Cardiac, Hepatic, and Metabolic Changes in High Carbohydrate-, High Fat-Fed Rats." *The Journal of Nutrition* 140(5): 946–953.

8. Eidi, A., M. Eidi, and R. Darzi. March 2009. "Antidiabetic Effect of *Olea europaea* L. in Normal and Diabetic Rats." *Phytotherapy Research* 23(3): 347–350.

References and Resources

Magazines, Journals, and Newspapers
Eidi, A., M. Eidi, and R. Darzi. March 2009. "Antidiabetic Effect of *Olea europaea* L. in Normal and Diabetic Rata." *Phytotherapy Research* 23(3): 347–350.

Erickson, Kim. September 2009. "All About Olive Leaf: Clear Up Acne-Prone Skin, Alleviate Eczema Benefit Your Heart, in Multiple Ways with Olive Leaf Extract, a Potent Medicinal Herb." *Better Nutrition* 71(9): 30.

Kimura, Yoshiyuki, and Maho Sumiyoshi. November 2009. "Olive Leaf Extract and Its Main Component Oleuropein Prevent Chronic Ultraviolet C Radiation-Induced Skin Damage and Carcinogenesis in Hairless Mice." *The Journal of Nutrition* 139(11): 2079–2086.

Mohagheghi, Fatemeh, Mohammad Reza Bigdeli, Bahram Rasoulian, et al. January 2011. "The Neuroprotective Effect of Olive Leaf Extract Is Related to Improved Blood–Brain Barrier Permeability and Brain Edema in Rat with Experimental Focal Cerebral Ischemia." *Phytomedicine: International Journal of Phytotherapy & Phytopharmacology* 18(2–3): 170–175.

Perrinjaquet-Moccetti, Tania, Andreas Busjahn, Caesar Schmidlin, et al. 2008. "Food Supplementation with an Olive (*Olea europaea* L.) Leaf Extract Reduces Blood Pressure in Borderline Hypertensive Monozygotic Twins." *Phytotherapy Research* 22: 1239–1242.

Poudyal, H., F. Campbell, and L. Brown. May 2010. "Olive Leaf Extract Attenuates Cardiac, Hepatic, and Metabolic Changes in High Carbohydrate–High Fat-Fed Rats." *The Journal of Nutrition* 140(5): 946–953.

Susalit, E., N. Agus, I. Effendi, et al. February 2011. "Olive (*Olea europaea*) Leaf Extract Effective in Patients with Stage-1 Hypertension: Comparison with Captopril." *Phytomedicine: International Journal of Phytotherapy & Phytopharmacology* 18(4): 251–258.

Wang, L., C. Geng, L. Jiang, et al. August 2008. "The Anti-Atherosclerotic Effect of Olive Leaf Extract Is Related to Suppressed Inflammatory Response in Rabbits with Experimental Atherosclerosis." *European Journal of Nutrition* 47(5): 235–243.

Websites
Drugs.com. www.drugs.com.
Livestrong. www.livestrong.com.

Oregano ❦

Like many herbs, oregano has ancient roots. The Greeks and Romans considered oregano to be a symbol of happiness and joy. On their wedding days, Greek and Roman brides and grooms adorned their heads with laurels made from oregano. By the Middle Ages, the French were cultivating this herb. But, oregano did not make its way to the United States until the early 20th century.[1]

Today, oregano is grown primarily in Turkey. A member of the mint family, it flourishes in high altitudes and in hot, dry weather.[2] Oregano, also known as *Origanum vulgare,* has excellent amounts of vitamin K and very good amounts of manganese, iron, dietary fiber, and omega 3 fatty acids. It has good amounts of calcium and vitamins A and C. The volatile oils found in oregano, such as thymol and carvacrol, have antibacterial properties. Oregano contains phytonutrients that function as powerful antioxidants. But, what have the researchers learned?

Antibacterial, Antimicrobial, and Antifungal Agents
In a U.S. Department of Agriculture (USDA) study published in 2009 in the *Journal of Food Science,* researchers tested the ability—after 24 and 48 hours—of oregano, allspice, and garlic essential oils to inhibit the growth of three types of bacteria—*Escherichia coli, Salmonella enterica,* and *Listeria monocytogenes*—on edible films of apple

puree. The researchers learned that of the three essential oils, oregano had the strongest antimicrobial activity against these pathogens. Vapor tests of oregano essential oil determined that it diffused more efficiently through the air than through direct contact with the bacteria.[3]

In a study published in 2010 in the *Journal of Drugs in Dermatology,* researchers from Florida examined the types of microorganisms that oregano extract could inhibit and also attempted to determine the minimal amounts of oregano needed to facilitate such inhibition. During the course of the study, the researchers tested oregano extracts on at least 10 microorganisms including methicillin-resistant *Staphylococcus aureus* (MRSA), the well-known bacterium that is highly resistant to certain antibiotics. The researchers found that "an oregano-based ointment could effectively inhibit a wide range of microorganisms associated with skin infections." Apparently, the optimal amount of oregano in the ointments varied between 5% and 20%. Ointment containing more than 20% oregano caused "mild burning sensation comparable to the application of alcohol." When the researchers compared the oregano ointment to the triple-antibiotic products, a generic and Neosporin, the oregano ointment proved to be a more effective product. Additionally, the researchers found that the oregano ointment worked better than commercial antiseptic solutions, and "for complex infections involving multiple microorganisms, an oregano ointment may be a superior option."[4]

In an in vitro study published in 2009 in *Phytomedicine: International Journal of Phytotherapy & Phytopharmacology,* researchers from Bari, Italy noted that nystatin is the "a drug of choice" for treating fungal infections. However, because of its side effects, such as renal damage, it has the potential to cause serious problems. So, the researchers wondered if they combined nystatin with essential oils could medical providers reduce the levels of nystatin. The researchers combined nystatin with three essential oils made from *O. vulgare* (oregano), *Pelargonium graveolens* (rose geranium), and *Melaeuca alternifolia* (tea tree oil). Among the oils that were tested, oregano was found to be the most effective. The researchers commented that "nystatin essential oil combination administered against the Candida species [fungal infection] is likely to reduce the minimum efficient dose of nystatin." Moreover, "the combination of *O. vulgare* [oregano] oil and nystatin in the treatment of Candida is the best association . . . we have found in our experiments so far."[5]

Another study on the effectiveness of oregano against fungal infections was published in 2008 in the *Canadian Journal of Microbiology*. In this in vitro study, Brazilian researchers evaluated the usefulness of several plant essential oils against fungal infections. Of the essential oils tested, oregano was the most effective. The researchers suggested that it is the carvacrol, which is found in oregano and Mexican oregano extract at concentrations of 92% and 58.8%, respectively, that may be "the main compound responsible" for the antifungal activity.[6]

Enhancing Health

In a study published in 2009 in the *Journal of Medicinal Food,* researchers from Ireland examined the bioactive effects of oregano and sage in cooked beef patties. Could the addition of oregano improve meat quality and increase levels of antioxidants? The researchers found that the antioxidant potential of the oregano- or sage-enriched beef was "much greater" than the untreated beef patties. According to the researchers, "this suggests that these herbal extracts, as added ingredients in beef, exhibit antioxidant potential following digestion." The researchers see these herbs "as possible alternatives to synthetic antioxidants in meat products."[7]

Anti-Inflammatory

In a study published in 2008 in the *Proceedings of the National Academy of Sciences,* researchers from several countries determined that beta-caryophyllin (E-BCP), an active ingredient in oregano, has anti-inflammatory properties. The researchers administered small doses of E-BCP to mice with inflamed paws. In up to 70% of the cases, the symptoms improved. The researchers believe that the E-BCP in oregano may be useful for inflammatory illnesses such as Crohn's disease.[8]

Colon Cancer

In a trial published in 2009 in *Nutrition and Cancer,* researchers from Rome, Italy, studied the effects of oregano extract on certain types of colon cancer cells. The researchers found that the oregano extract stopped the growth of cancer cells "in a dose- and time-dependent manner." Oregano appeared to activate "both extrinsic and intrinsic apoptotic [cell death] pathways." Furthermore, "whole extract, instead of a specific component, can be responsible for the observed cytotoxic [toxic to cells] effects."[9]

In a study published in 2008 in the *Canadian Journal of Physiology & Pharmacology,* researchers from India investigated the effect of oregano on fecal bacterial enzymes in rats injected with a compound to induce colon cancer. The researchers determined that the rats fed oregano supplementation in the three different doses had lower levels of bacterial enzymes than those in the control group. Since these enzymes are strongly linked to the development of colon cancer, oregano seemed to reduce the risk of colon cancer.[10]

Useful for People with Diabetes

In a study published in 2004 in the *Journal of Ethnopharmacology,* researchers from Morocco investigated the effect of an aqueous extract of oregano on the blood glucose levels of normal rats and rats with induced diabetes. In the normal rats, single or multiple administrations of oregano slightly decreased the glucose levels. However, the same administration of oregano to the rats with diabetes resulted in significant reductions in blood glucose levels. This effect was independent of insulin.[11]

Is Oregano Beneficial?

Oregano appears to have a number of useful qualities. In fact, the antimicrobial qualities of oregano appear to be rather dramatic. Could oregano be a realistic option for someone dealing with a bacterial or fungal infection? Can oregano really help prevent colon cancer? Is it useful for people with diabetes? Although more research is needed, oregano may eventually be considered an extraordinarily beneficial herb.

Notes

1. The George Mateljan Foundation Website. www.whfoods.com.
2. Kane, Emily A. July 2007. "Control Candida with Oregano: Yeast Is a Normal Part of the Body, but If It Becomes Overgrown, It Can Create a Condition Called Candida. Learn How Oregano Can Help Restore Balance." *Better Nutrition* 69(7): 22–23.
3. Du, W. X., C. W. Olsen, R. J. Avena-Bustillos, et al. September 2009. "Antibacterial Effects of Allspice, Garlic, and Oregano Essential Oils in Tomato Films Determined by Overlay and Vapor-Phase Methods." *Journal of Food Science* 74(7): M390–M397.
4. Eng, William, and Robert Norman. April 2010. "Development of an Oregano-Based Ointment with Anti-Microbial Activity Including Activity against

Methicillin-Resistant *Staphlococcus aureus.*" *Journal of Drugs in Dermatology* 9(4): 377–380.

5. Rosato, Antonio, Cesare Vitali, Monica Piarulli, et al. October 2009. "In Vitro Synergic Efficacy of the Combination of Nystatin with the Essential Oils of *Origanum vulgare* and *Pelargonium graveolens* against Some Candida Species." *Phytomedicine: International Journal of Phytotherapy & Phytopharmacology* 16(10): 972–975.

6. Pozzatti, Patricia, Liliane Alves Scheid, Tatiana Borba Spader, et al. 2008. "In Vitro Activity of Essential Oils Extracted from Plants Used as Spices against Fluconazole-Resistant and Fluconazole-Susceptible *Candida* spp. [Species]." *Canadian Journal of Microbiology* 54(11): 950–956.

7. Ryan, E., S.A. Aherne, M.N. O'Grady, et al. August 2009. "Bioactivity of Herb-Enriched Beef Patties." *Journal of Medicinal Food* 12(4): 893–901.

8. Gertsch, Jürg, Marco Leonti, Stefan Raduner, et al. July 2008. "Beta-Caryophyllene Is a Dietary Cannabinoid." *Proceedings of the National Academy of Sciences* 105(26): 9099–9104.

9. Savini, Isabella, Rosaria Arnone, Maria Valeria, et al. May–June 2009. "*Origanum vulgare* Induces Apoptosis in Human Colon Cancer Caco$_2$." *Nutrition and Cancer* 61(3): 381–389.

10. Srihari, T., V. Balasubramaniyan, and N. Nalini. 2008. "Role of Oregano on Bacterial Enzymes in 1,2-Dimethylhydrazine-Induced Experimental Colon Carcinogenesis." *Canadian Journal of Physiology & Pharmacology* 86(10): 667–674.

11. Lemhadri, A., N.-A. Zeggwagh, M. Maghrani, et al. June 2004. "Anti-Hyperglycaemic Activity of the Aqueous Extract of *Origanum vulgare* Growing Wild in Tafilalet Region." *Journal of Ethnopharmacology* 92(2–3): 251–256.

References and Resources

Magazines, Journals, and Newspapers

Du, W.X., C.W. Olsen, R.J. Avena-Bustillos, et al. September 2009. "Antibacterial Effects of Allspice, Garlic, and Oregano Essential Oils in Tomato Films Determined by Overlay and Vapor-Phase Methods." *Journal of Food Science* 74(7): M390–M397.

Eng, William, and Robert Norman. April 2010. "Development of an Oregano-Based Ointment with Anti-Microbial Activity Including Activity against Methiciliin-Resistant *Staphlococcus aureus.*" *Journal of Drugs in Dermatology* 9(4): 377–380.

Gertsch, Jürg, Marco Leonti, Stefan Raduner, et al. July 2008. "Beta-Caryophyllene Is a Dietary Cannabinoid." *Proceedings of the National Academy of Sciences* 105(26): 9099–9104.

Kane, Emily. July 2007. "Control Candida with Oregano: Yeast Is a Normal Part of the Body, but If It Becomes Overgrown, It Can Create a Condition Called

Candida. Learn How Oregano Can Help Restore Balance." *Better Nutrition* 69(7): 22–23.

Lemhadri, A., N.-A. Zeggwagh, M. Maghrani, et al. June 2004. "Anti-Hyperglycaemic Activity of the Aqueous Extract in *Origanum vulgare* Growing Wild in Tafilalet Region." *Journal of Ethnopharmacology* 92(2–3): 251–256.

Pozzatti, Patricia, Liliane Alves Scheid, Tatiana Borba Spader, et al. 2008. "In Vitro Activity of Essential Oils Extracted from Plants Used as Spices against Fluconazole-Resistant and Fluconazole-Susceptible *Candida* Spp [Species]." *Canadian Journal of Microbiology* 54(11): 950–956.

Rosato, Antonio, Cesare Vitali, Monica Piarulli, et al. October 2009. "In Vitro Synergic Efficacy of the Combination of Nystatin with the Essential Oils of *Origanum vulgare* and *Pelargonium graveolens* against Some Candida Species." *Phytomedicine: International Journal of Phytotherapy & Phytopharmacology* 16(10): 972–975.

Ryan, E., S. A. Aherne, M. N. O'Grady, et al. August 2009. "Bioactivity of Herb-Enriched Beef Patties." *Journal of Medicinal Food* 12(4): 893–901.

Savini, Isabella, Rosaria Arnone, Maria Valeria, et al. May–June 2009. "*Origanum vulgare* Induces Apoptosis in Human Colon Cancer Caco$_2$ Cells." *Nutrition and Cancer* 61(3): 381–389.

Singletary, Keith. May–June 2010. "Oregano: Overview of the Literature on Health Benefits." *Nutrition Today* 45(3): 129–138.

Srihari, T., V. Balasubramaniyan, and N. Nalini. 2008. "Role of Oregano on Bacterial Enzymes in 1,2-Dimethylhydrazine-Induced Experimental Colon Carcinogenesis." *Canadian Journal of Physiology & Pharmacology* 86(10): 667–674.

Website

The George Mateljan Foundation. www.whfoods.com.

P

Peppermint and Peppermint Oil 🍃

Grown throughout Europe and North America, peppermint (*Mentha piper-ita*) is a perennial flowering member of the mint family. The medicinal use of peppermint may be traced to ancient Greece where it was considered helpful for digestive problems. Additionally, when inhaled, peppermint, which contains menthol, was thought to be therapeutic for upper respiratory symptoms and cough. Peppermint oil is made from the stem, leaves, and flowers. Today, it is probably best known as a treatment for the symptoms of irritable bowel syndrome (IBS), such as pain, bloating, diarrhea, consti-pation, and gas. These symptoms occur without any apparent mechanical, inflammatory, or biochemical explanation. But, peppermint may be effec-tive for other medical problems.[1] What have the researchers learned?

Irritable Bowel Syndrome

In a randomized, double-blind, placebo-controlled study that was published in 2010 in *Digestive Diseases and Sciences,* researchers from Tehran, Iran tested an enteric-coated, delayed-release capsule of peppermint oil (brand name Colpermin). (Why enteric-coated? The coating prevents the capsule from dissolving in the stomach, enabling it to remain intake until reaching the intestines.) For eight weeks, every day, 90 people with IBS took either three capsules of Colpermin or three placebos. The researchers found that "the severity of abdominal pain was . . . reduced significantly in the Colper-min groups as compared to controls." Moreover, "Colpermin significantly improved the quality of life." They concluded that "Colpermin is effective and safe as a therapeutic agent in patients with IBS suffering from abdomi-nal pain or discomfort."[2]

In a randomized, double-blind, placebo-controlled study published in 2007 in the journal *Digestive and Liver Disease,* Italian researchers investigated the use of peppermint oil (Mintoil) in 57 subjects who had normal lactose and lactulose breath tests and negative antibody screening for celiac disease. (Thus, the researchers eliminated anyone who had irritable bowel symptoms from another obvious source.) For four weeks, the subjects, who were between the ages of 18 and 89, took daily doses of either two enteric-coated peppermint capsules or two placebos. At the end of the fourth week, a remarkable 75% of the subjects who took peppermint oil capsules experienced at least a 50% reduction in their IBS symptoms. This compared to 38% of those taking placebos. Four weeks after the study ended, the difference was 54% to 11%, respectively. The researchers concluded that "a four week treatment with peppermint oil improves abdominal symptoms in patients with irritable bowel syndrome."[3]

In a study published in 2008 in the *British Medical Journal,* researchers from Canada and several sites in the United States reported on a meta-analysis that they conducted on the use of fiber, antispasmodics, and peppermint oil for treating IBS. Of these, four studies compared the use of peppermint oil to placebos in a total of 392 subjects. The researchers learned that 26% of the participants taking peppermint oil had persistent symptoms after treatment. This compared to 65% of those taking placebos. Of the three agents reviewed in this meta-analysis, peppermint oil was the most effective, and it had a low rate of adverse effects.[4]

Migraine Headaches

In a study published in 2010 in the *International Journal of Clinical Practice,* researchers from Shiraz, Iran, treated 35 patients, suffering from non-aura migraine attacks, with either a 10% ethanol solution of menthol (as drug), such as that found in peppermint, or a 0.5% ethanol solution of menthol (placebo). The liquids were applied to the forehead and temporal area. The 10% solution proved to be markedly better in the treatment of migraine-related symptoms, such as nausea and/or vomiting, and/or abnormal sensitivity to sounds and lights. The researchers wrote that "in the per-protocol population, there were significantly higher number of patients who experienced at least one pain free/pain relief after the application of menthol rather than the placebo."[5]

Infection Reduction

In a study published in 2009 in the *Journal of Cranio-Maxillofacial Surgery,* researchers from Germany, Australia, and the United Kingdom tested a number of different essential oils, including peppermint oil, for their ability to fight hospital-acquired infections such as Staphylococcus, Streptococcus, and Candida. Except for a few oils, all the essential oils, including peppermint oil, had "demonstrated efficacy against hospital-acquired isolates and reference strains." The researchers concluded that "essential oils represent a cheap and effective antiseptic topical treatment option even for antibiotic-resistant strains such as MRSA and antimycotic-resistant Candida species."[6]

A study on reducing levels of Candida was published in 2009 in *Mycopathologia.* Researchers from India investigated the ability of essential oils, including peppermint oil, to inhibit the growth of Candida. They found that 18 of the 30 essential oils that they tested had anti-Candida activity. Moreover, "four oils, eucalyptus, peppermint, ginger grass, and clove showed 80.87%, 74.16%, 40.46%, and 28.57% biofilm reduction respectively." The researchers noted that these essential oils had "substantial antifungal activity."[7]

In a study published in 2003 in *Phytomedicine: International Journal of Phytotherapy and Phytopharmacology,* German researchers conducted in vitro trials to determine if peppermint oil could inhibit the activity of type 1 and type 2 herpes simplex viruses. They found that "peppermint oil exhibited high levels of virucidal activity against HSV-1 and HSV-2 in viral suspension tests." In a truly stunning finding, the researchers noted that after three hours of incubation "of herpes simplex with peppermint oil an antiviral activity of about 99% could be demonstrated." Peppermint oil was also found to be active against strains of type 1 herpes simplex that are resistant to acyclovir, a drug prescribed for herpes infections. The researchers concluded that "peppermint oil might be suitable for topical therapeutic use a virucidal agent in recurrent herpes infection."[8]

Improved Alertness

In a study published in 2009 in the *North American Journal of Psychology,* researchers from West Virginia included 16 females and 9 males, with a mean age of 19.7 and a mean number of 3.4 years of driving experience, in a simulated drive. During this "drive," they received peppermint, cinnamon, or a nonodor control via an oxygen concentrator for 30 seconds every 15 minutes. As the trial was conducted, measures of cognitive performance, wakefulness, mood, and workload were assessed.

When compared to the subjects who received no odor, the subjects who received peppermint and cinnamon had increased ratings of alertness and decreased driving frustration. Peppermint was also associated with a decrease in anxiety. The researchers noted that "Given the numerous deleterious effects of fatigue and inattention on driving performance, and the number of personal injuries and deaths brought about by such conditions, any non-pharmacological aid that could counter-act such conditions would be rapidly accepted. These results should be of particular interest to automobile manufacturers, departments of transportation, long-haul trucking firms, and insurance companies."[9]

Is Peppermint Beneficial?

It certainly seems to have some noteworthy uses. But, the following caveats should be noted.

Caveats

Products containing peppermint should never be used on infants and small children, and they should never be given peppermint tea to drink. Peppermint has the potential to cause serious, life-threatening reactions.

Also, while peppermint may be effective for IBS, it should not be used by people who have gastroesophageal reflux disease (GERD), a medical problem in which stomach acids return to the esophagus, or a hiatal hernia. By relaxing the sphincter between the stomach and the esophagus, peppermint may increase the amount of reflux, thereby making an already challenging medical problem even more difficult.

Notes

1. Kligler, Benjamin, and Sapna Chaudhary. April 2007. "Peppermint Oil." *American Family Physician* 75(7): 1027–1030.
2. Merat, Shahin, Shadi Khalili, Pardise Mostajabi, et al. May 2010. "The Effect of Enteric-Coated, Delayed-Release Peppermint Oil on Irritable Bowel Syndrome." *Digestive Disease and Sciences* 55(5): 1385–1390.
3. Cappello, G., M. Spezzaferro, L. Grossi, et al. June 2007. "Peppermint Oil (Mintoil) in the Treatment of Irritable Bowel Syndrome: A Prospective Double

Blind Placebo-Controlled Randomized Trial." *Digestive and Liver Disease* 39(6): 530–536.

4. Ford, Alexander C., Nicholas J. Talley, Brennan M. R. Spiegel, et al. 2008. "Effect of Fibre, Antispasmodics, and Peppermint Oil in the Treatment of Irritable Bowel Syndrome: Systematic Review and Meta-Analysis." *British Medical Journal* 337: a2313.

5. Borhani Haghighi, A., S. Motazedian, R. Rezaii, et al. March 2010. "Cutaneous Application of Menthol 10% Solution as an Abortive Treatment of Migraine without Aura: A Randomised, Double-Blind, Placebo-Controlled, Crossed-Over Study." *International Journal of Clinical Practice* 64(4): 451–456.

6. Warnke, P. H., S. T. Becker, R. Podschun, et al. October 2009. "The Battle against Multi-Resistant Strains: Renaissance of Antimicrobial Essential Oils as a Promising Force to Fight Hospital-Acquired Infections." *Journal of Cranio-Maxillofacial Surgery* 37(7): 392–397.

7. Agarwal, V., P. Lal, and V. Pruthi. January 2008. "Prevention of Candida Albicans Biofilm by Plant Oils." *Mycopathologia* 165(1): 13–19.

8. Schuhmacher, A., J. Reichling, and P. Schnitzler. 2003. "Virucidal Effect of Peppermint Oil on the Enveloped Viruses Herpes Simplex Virus Type 1 and Type 2 *In Vitro*." *Phytomedicine: International Journal of Phytotherapy and Phytopharmacology* 10(6–7): 504–510.

9. Raudenbush, Bryan, Rebecca Grayhem, Tom Sears, and Ian Wilson. June 2009. "Effects of Peppermint and Cinnamon Odor Administration on Simulated Driving Alertness, Mood, and Workload." *North American Journal of Psychology* 11(2): 245+.

References and Resources

Magazines, Journals, and Newspapers

Agarwal, V., P. Lal, and V. Pruthi. January 2008. "Prevention of Candida Albicans Biofilm by Plant Oils." *Mycopathologia* 165(1): 13–19.

Borhani Haghighi, A., S. Motazedian, R. Rezaii, et al. March 2010. "Cutaneous Application of Menthol 10% Solution as an Abortive Treatment of Migraine without Aura: A Randomised, Double-Blind, Placebo-Controlled, Crossed-Over Study." *International Journal of Clinical Practice* 64(4): 451–456.

Cappello, G., M. Spezzaferro, L. Grossi, et al. June 2007. "Peppermint Oil (Mintoil) in the Treatment of Irritable Bowel Syndrome: A Prospective Double Blind Placebo-Controlled Randomized Trial." *Digestive and Liver Disease* 39(6): 530–536.

Ford, Alexander C., Nicolas J. Talley, Brennan M. R. Spiegel, et al. 2008. "Effect of Fibre, Antispasmodics, and Peppermint Oil in the Treatment of Irritable Bowel Syndrome: Systematic Review and Meta-Analysis." *British Medical Journal* 337: a2312.

Kligler, Benjamin, and Sapna Chaudhary. April 2007. "Peppermint Oil." *American Family Physician* 75(7): 1027–1030.

Merat, Shahin, Shadi Khalili, Pardise Mostajabi, et al. May 2010. "The Effect of Enteric-Coated, Delayed-Release Peppermint Oil on Irritable Bowel Syndrome." *Digestive Diseases and Sciences* 55(5): 1385–1390.

Raudenbush, Bryan, Rebecca Grayhem, Tom Sears, and Ian Wilson. June 2009. "Effects of Peppermint and Cinnamon Odor Administration on Simulated Driving Alertness, Mood, and Workload." *North American Journal of Psychology* 11(2): 245+.

Schuhmacher, A., J. Reichling, and P. Schnitzler. 2003. "Virucidal Effect of Peppermint Oil on the Enveloped Viruses Herpes Simplex Virus Type 1 and Type 2 *In Vitro.*" *Phytomedicine: International Journal of Phytotherapy and Phytopharmacology* 10(6–7): 504–510.

Warnke, P. H., S. T. Becker, R. Podschun, et al. October 2009. "The Battle against Multi-Resistant Strains: Renaissance of Antimicrobial Essential Oils as a Promising Force to Fight Hospital Acquired Infections." *Journal of Cranio-Maxillofacial Surgery* 37(7): 392–397.

Website
National Center for Complementary and Alternative Medicine. www.nccam.nih.gov.

Purple Coneflower 🌿

Scientifically known as *Echinacea purpurea,* purple coneflower has been used by Americans for hundreds of years. In the past, purple coneflower, which is generally referred to as echinacea, was thought to be a treatment for scarlet fever, syphilis, malaria, blood poisoning, and diphtheria. More recently, echinacea has been considered effective for infections, inflammation, pain, wounds, colds, cough, sore throats, and fevers. Many people regularly take purple coneflower to boost their immunity from everyday exposure to illnesses.[1] It is important to review what researchers have learned.

Prevention and Treatment of Colds
In an open, multicenter study published in 2006 in *Advances in Therapy,* researchers from Switzerland tested the tolerability and efficacy of echinacea among athletes. Why athletes? It has been well established that when athletes exceed their individual training thresholds, they may well experience immune suppression.

The cohort consisted of 80 men and women between the ages of 18 and 75. During their first visit, the participants were given 145 tablets of echinacea and told to take one in the morning and one in the evening for the next eight weeks. They were also provided with a journal, where they could record any cold symptoms. The researchers found that during the study period 71% of the subjects were free of cold symptoms. Twenty-six percent of the participants had one cold, and only 3% had two cold episodes. And, the treatment appeared to be effective. "About 75% of patients and investigators rate treatment efficacy during a common cold as 'very good' or 'good.' "[2]

Writing about this study, an article published in 2010 in *Holistic Nursing Practice* noted that echinacea supplementation is an effective method for dealing with the susceptibility of athletes to the common cold. "This study indicates a high tolerability for the standardized *E. purpurea* . . . and demonstrates its efficacy as a prophylactic and as a treatment for the common cold in athletes, a patient population at high risk."[3]

On the other hand, a randomized, controlled study published in 2010 in the *Annals of Internal Medicine* had different results. In this study, researchers from Wisconsin, United States, and Australia assigned 719 subjects, between the ages of 12 and 80, who were experiencing the first symptoms of the common cold, to one of four groups. The members of the first group took no pills; the members of the second group took placebos. Meanwhile, the members of the third group took blinded echinacea pills; and, the members of the fourth group took unblinded, open-label echinacea pills. The participants recorded their symptoms twice a day or as long as the cold continued—up to two weeks. Seven hundred and thirteen people, with a mean age of 33.7, completed the trial. The people taking echinacea experienced a 7- to 10-hour reduction of cold symptoms, which was not statistically significant.

The researchers concluded that "the pharmacologic activity of echinacea probably has only a small beneficial effect on persons with the common cold. . . . Any underlying benefit of echinacea was not large and was not demonstrated by our results." Still, the researchers acknowledged that some people may want to continue to use echinacea for their colds. "Individual choices about whether to use echinacea to treat the common cold should be guided by personal health values and preferences, as well as by the limited evidence available."[4]

Treatment for Acute Score Throats

In a multicenter, randomized, double-blind controlled trial published in 2009 in the *European Journal of Medical Research,* researchers from Switzerland and Germany assessed the efficacy of an echinacea/sage spray to that of a chlorhexidine/lidocaine (chemical antiseptic/pain killer) spray for the treatment of acute sore throats. Initially, the cohort consisted of 154 patients, at least 12 years old, who were dealing with an acute sore throat for no more than 72 hours. The patients received either a bottle of echinacea/sage or chlorhexidine/lidocaine. To conceal the identity of the active spray, the patients also received placebo spray that matched their active spray. They were told to spray their throat with two sprays from each bottle every two hours—up to 10 times per day. They were also instructed to continue this protocol for no more than five days or until they were symptom free. With the 133 people who completed the study, the researchers found that both sprays had similar results—they were about equally effective for treating sore throats. It is interesting to note that the majority of people in the chlorhexidine/lidocaine group thought they were using the echinacea/sage treatment. The researchers concluded that "the echinacea/sage spray demonstrated equivalent efficacy compared to the chlorhexidine/lidocaine treatment and was very well tolerated."[5]

Helps Treat Symptoms of Chronic
Obstructive Pulmonary Disease

In a single-center, randomized, double-blind, placebo-controlled trial published in 2011 in the *Journal of Clinical Pharmacy and Therapeutics,* researchers from Indonesia and Switzerland examined the ability of people with chronic obstructive pulmonary disease (COPD), who also have acute upper respiratory tract infections (URTI), to obtain a degree of a relief from a supplement that contains echinacea or a supplement that contains echinacea as well as zinc, selenium, and vitamin C. At the beginning of the trial, the cohort consisted of 120 people who were at least 40 years old. Upon enrollment, all participants received 500 mg ciprofloxacin, an antibiotic, for seven days. Then, for two weeks, the subjects took daily doses of either a placebo, 500 mg pure echinacea, or 500 mg echinacea and small amounts of zinc, selenium, and vitamin C. One hundred and eight subjects completed the trial.

The researchers found that "based on overall symptoms, exacerbations were significantly less severe and lasted significantly shorter under treatment with the combination of echinacea, selenium, zinc, and vitamin C as compared with placebo." The researchers noted that they were surprised to find "a statistically non-significant opposite trend . . . in the group given the same basic echinecea extract alone." The researchers concluded that the most likely explanation for their results was "a synergistic interaction between echinacea and the micronutrients."[6]

Useful for Benign Prostate Hyperplasia

In a study published in 2009 in *Phytotherapy Research,* researchers from Lithuania wanted to learn the effect echinacea would have on rats with experimentally induced benign prostate hyperplasia, or a condition in which the prostate gland is enlarged, a medical problem more often seen in older men. The researchers began by dividing rats into several groups. While some rats served as controls, other rats were treated with echinacea for either four or eight weeks. The results were notable. According to the researchers, the rats demonstrated significant reductions in prostate mass as well as a reversal of degenerative changes.[7]

Anxiety Relief

In a study published in 2010 in *Phytotherapy Research,* researchers from Hungary tested the ability of five different echinacea preparations to relieve anxiety in rats. And, they compared their results to the effectiveness of chlordiazepoxide, a prescription medication used for anxiety and agitation. Of the five echinacea preparations, three reduced anxiety-like behavior. Of these, only one preparation "robustly decreased anxiety in three different tests, with an effective dose-range that was comparable to that of chlordiazepoxide." Moreover, echinacea accomplished this goal without affecting locomotion. (Chlordiazepoxide is known for affecting locomotion.) The researchers noted that "from the point of view of safety, echinacea preparations are excellent candidates for the alternative treatment of anxiety." Furthermore, "the remarkable anxiolytic effects demonstrated . . . suggest that certain Echinacea preparations are excellent alternative anxiolytics from the point of view of efficacy as well."[8]

Is Echinacea Beneficial?

For years, echinacea has primarily been known as a treatment for colds. And, while it may or may not be useful for that common condition—or it may be useful for some people and not for others—research has also demonstrated that echinacea may well be an effective treatment for several other medical problems. It is a good idea to discuss echinacea with medical providers.

Notes

1. University of Maryland Medical Center Website. www.umm.edu.
2. Schoop, Roland, Samuel Büechi, and Andy Suter. September–October 2006. "Open, Multicenter Study to Evaluate the Tolerability and Efficacy of Echinaforce Forte Tablets in Athletes." *Advances in Therapy* 23(5): 823–833.
3. Ross, Stephanie Maxine. 2010. "A Standardized Echinacea Extract Demonstrates Efficacy in the Prevention and Treatment of Colds in Athletes." *Holistic Nursing Practice* 24(2): 107–109.
4. Barrett, B., R. Brown, D. Rakel, et al. December 2010. "Echinacea for Treating the Common Cold: A Randomized Trial." *Annals of Internal Medicine* 153(12): 769–777.
5. Schapowal, A., D. Berger, P. Klein, and A. Suter. September 2009. "Echinacea/Sage or Chlorhexidine/Lidocaine for Treating Acute Sore Throats: A Randomized Double-Blind Trial." *European Journal of Medical Research* 14(9): 406–412.
6. Isbaniah, F., W.H. Wiyono, F. Yunus, et al. October 2011. "*Echinacea purpurea* along with Zinc, Selenium and Vitamin C to Alleviate Exacerbations of Chronic Obstructive Pulmonary Disease: Results from a Randomized Controlled Trial." *Journal of Clinical Pharmacy and Therapeutics* 36(5), 568–576.
7. Skaudickas, D., A.J. Kondrotas, E. Kevelaitis, and P.R. Venskutonis. October 2009. "The Effect of *Echinacea purpurea* (L.) Moench Extract on Experimental Prostate Hyperplasia." *Phytotherapy Research* 23(10): 1474–1478.
8. Haller, J., J. Hohmann, and T.F. Freund. November 2010. "The Effect of Echinacea Preparations in Three Laboratory Tests of Anxiety: Comparison with Chlordiazepoxide." *Phytotherapy Research* 24(11): 1605–1613.

References and Resources

Magazines, Journals, and Newspapers

Barrett, Bruce, Roger Brown, Dave Rakel, et al. December 2010. "Echinacea for Treating the Common Cold: A Randomized Trial." *Annals of Internal Medicine* 153(12): 769–777.

Haller, J.J. Hohmann, and T.F. Freund. November 2010. "The Effect of Echinacea Preparations in Three Laboratory Tests of Anxiety: Comparison with Chlordiazepoxide." *Phytotherapy Research* 24(11): 1605–1613.

Isbaniah, F., W.H. Wiyoo, F. Yunus, et al. October 2011. "*Echinacea purpurea* along with Zinc, Selenium and Vitamin C to Alleviate Exacerbations of Chronic

Obstructive Pulmonary Disease: Results from a Randomized Controlled Trial." *Journal of Clinical Pharmacy and Therapeutics* 36(5): 568–576.

Ross, Stephanie Maxine. 2010. "A Standardized Echinacea Extract Demonstrates Efficacy in the Prevention and Treatment of Colds in Athletes." *Holistic Nursing Practice* 24(2): 107–109.

Schapowal, A., D. Berger, P. Klein, and A. Suter. September 2009. "Echinacea/ Sage of Chlorhexidine/Lidocaine for Treating Acute Sore Throats: A Randomized Double-Blind Trial." *European Journal of Medical Research* 14(9): 406–412.

Schoop, Roland, Samuel Büechi, and Andy Suter. September–October 2006. "Open, Multicenter Study to Evaluate the Tolerability and Efficacy of Echinaforce Forte Tablets in Athletes." *Advances in Therapy* 23(5): 823–833.

Skaudickas, D., A.J. Kondrotas, E. Kevelaitis, and P.R. Venskutonis. October 2009. "The Effect of *Echinacea purpurea* (L.) Moench Extract on Experimental Prostate Hyperplasia." *Phytotherapy Research* 23(10): 1474–1478.

Website

University of Maryland Medical Center. www.umm.edu.

R

Red Clover 🌿

Native to the Mediterranean regions, red clover, scientifically known as *Trifolium pretense,* is now available throughout the world. It contains isoflavones, which are plant-based chemicals that have estrogen-like properties. Over the years, red clover proponents have claimed that it has a host of like-enhancing properties. Some maintain that it reduces the number of hot flashes associated with menopause, supports cardiovascular and bone health, and fights cancer cells. Additionally, red clover is said to have anti-inflammatory properties and is, therefore, useful for skin conditions such as psoriasis and eczema.[1] But, what have the researchers learned?

Menopausal Symptoms

In a randomized, double-blind, placebo-controlled trial published in 2002 in *Maturitas,* researchers from the Netherlands enrolled 30 menopausal women who had more than five hot flashes per day. For the first four weeks, all the women took a placebo tablet. Then, for the next 12 weeks, the women were placed on either a placebo or a tablet containing 80 mg isoflavones from red clover. By the end of the study, the researchers observed that the women taking red clover had 44% fewer hot flashes than the women on the placebo, a finding that was statistically significant.[2]

A few years later, in 2005, another study on red clover was published in *Gynecological Endocrinology.* In this randomized, double-blind, placebo-controlled trial, researchers from Ecuador gave 60 subjects either a placebo or an 80-mg/day red clover isoflavone supplement for 90 days. After a 7-day washout period, the subjects took the alternate treatment for 90 days. The researchers found that when compared with the placebo, the menopausal symptoms of the 53 women who completed the study were "significantly decreased."[3]

In 2007, a meta-analysis of studies on the association between red clover supplementation and the incidence of hot flashes in menopausal women was published in *Phytomedicine: International Journal of Phytotherapy and Phytopharmacology*. Although 17 articles were retrieved, the U.K. researchers decided that only 5 should be included in the meta-analysis. The researchers concluded that red clover had a "marginally significant" ability to reduce the frequency of hot flashes.[4]

Different results were obtained in a randomized, double-blind study published in 2009 in *Menopause*. Illinois researchers compared treating 89 women with moderate to severe hot flashes (at least 35 hot flashes and night sweats per week) with black cohosh, red clover, placebo, and hormone therapy. After 12 months, the researchers found that all four groups experienced decreases in the numbers of hot flashes. Black cohosh decreased hot flashes by 34%; red clover decreased the flashes by 57%; placebo decreased them by 63%; and hormone therapy decreased them by 94%. The researchers noted that "the effect [of red clover and black cohosh] was no better than that observed in women using placebo." Thus, "the women taking red clover or black cohosh did not have reduced vasomotor symptoms [such as hot flashes] compared to the placebo group."[5]

Cardiovascular Health

In a study published in 2009 in *The Journal of Obstetrics and Gynecology Research,* Serbian researchers recruited 40 healthy postmenopausal women who were an average age of 56. The women were then divided into two groups. For the next 12 months, one group of 22 took red clover-derived isoflavones; the other group of 18 women took no red clover supplementation. The researchers found that the women taking red clover had significant reductions in total serum cholesterol, low-density lipoprotein (LDL or "bad" cholesterol), and levels of triglycerides. Moreover, levels of high-density lipoprotein (HDL or "good" cholesterol) were significantly increased. The researchers concluded that red clover supplementation had "favorable metabolic effects on serum lipids" in postmenopausal women.[6]

In a study published in 2007 in *Phytotherapy Research,* Iranian researchers investigated the effect of red clover on the development of atherosclerosis in 20 male rabbits with high levels of fat in their blood. The rabbits were divided into four groups of five. The rabbits in two of the groups ate a normal diet or a normal diet supplemented with red clover. Meanwhile, the rabbits in the two other groups received the same normal diet or normal diet with red clover, but both their diets were supplemented with 1% cholesterol. The researchers found that the dietary use of red clover in rats with high levels of blood fats significantly decreased levels of C-reactive protein, triglycerides, total cholesterol, and LDL "bad" cholesterol while it also increased levels of HDL "good" cholesterol. Likewise, "fatty streak formation was also significantly lower in aorta and left and right coronary arteries in the same animals due to use of dietary RC [red clover] supplementation." The researchers concluded that "dietary RC may reduce cardiovascular risk factors."[7]

Osteoporosis

In a double-blind, randomized, placebo-controlled study published in 2004 in *The American Journal of Clinical Nutrition,* U.K. researchers examined the effect of a daily dose of red clover supplementation in 177 women between the ages of 49 and 65. At the end of 12 months, the researchers found that the loss of lumbar spine bone mineral content and bone mineral density were significantly lower in the women taking red clover supplement than the women taking a placebo. They noted that "through attenuation of bone loss, isoflavones have a potentially protective effect on the lumbar spine in women."[8]

In a study published in 2007 in *Phytotherapy Research,* Italian researchers divided female rats into four groups. In a procedure known as an ovariectomy, the ovaries of the rats in three of the groups were removed. The rats in one group did not have the surgery. The rats that had the surgery experienced an immediate drop in their levels of estrogen. The reduced amounts of estrogen resulted in lowered levels of bone mineral content, femoral weight, femoral density, and other symptoms of osteoporosis. One week after the surgery, two groups of rats that had the surgery received daily red clover supplementation. For the next 14 weeks, one group received 20 mg/day and the other group received 40 mg/day. The researchers found that red clover "reduced bone loss induced by ovariectomy." Most likely, they wrote, red clover results in a reduction in "bone turnover via inhibition of bone resorption."[9]

Anxiety and Depression

In a study published in 2010 in *Maturitas,* Austrian researchers randomly assigned 109 postmenopausal women aged 40 or more to one of two groups.

For 90 days, the women in the first group received two daily capsules (80 mg) of red clover isoflavones, and the women in the second group took placebos. After a seven-day washout period, the women in the first group were given placebos, and the women in the second group took the same two capsules (80 mg) of red clover isoflavones every day. The second half of the study continued for 90 days. The researchers found that after taking the red clover, the women experienced significant reductions in anxiety and depression. They noted that "this effect was equivalent to a 76.9% reduction in the total HADS [Hospital Anxiety and Depression Scale] score (76% for anxiety and 78.3% for depression) and an 80.6% reduction in the total SDS [Self Rating Depression Scale] score."[10]

Is Red Clover Beneficial?

It is evident that red clover may well be beneficial, especially to postmenopausal women dealing with a variety of symptoms. And, thus far, studies have not found any negative side effects.

Notes

1. University of Maryland Medical Center Website. www.umm.edu.
2. van de Weijer, P. H., and R. Barentsen. July 2002. "Isoflavones from Red Clover (Promensil) Significantly Reduce Menopausal Hot Flush Symptoms Compared with Placebo." *Maturitas* 42(3): 187–193.
3. Hidalgo, L. A., P. A. Chedraui, N. Morocho, et al. November 2005. "The Effect of Red Clover Isoflavones on Menopausal Symptoms, Lipids and Vaginal Cytology in Menopausal Women: A Randomized, Double-Blind, Placebo-Controlled Study." *Gynecological Endocrinology* 21(5): 257–264.
4. Coon, Joanna Thompson, Max H. Pittler, and Edzard Ernst. February 2007. "*Trifolium pratense* Isoflavones in the Treatment of Menopausal Hot Flushes: A Systematic Review and Meta-Analysis." *Phytomedicine: International Journal of Phytotherapy and Phytopharmacology* 14(2–3): 153–159.
5. Geller, Stacie E., Lee P. Shulman, Richard B. van Breemen, et al. November–December 2009. "Safety and Efficacy of Black Cohosh and Red Clover for the Management of Vasomotor Symptoms: A Randomized Controlled Trial." *Menopause* 16(6): 1156–1166.
6. Terzic, M. M., J. Dotlic, S. Maricic, et al. December 2009. "Influence of Red Clover-Derived Isoflavones on Serum Lipid Profile in Postmenopausal Women." *The Journal of Obstetrics and Gynecology Research* 35(6): 1091–1095.
7. Asgary, S., J. Moshtaghian, G. Naderi, et al. August 2007. "Effects of Dietary Red Clover on Blood Factors and Cardiovascular Fatty Streak Formation in Hypercholesterolemic Rabbits." *Phytotherapy Research* 21(8): 768–770.

8. Atkinson, Charlotte, Juliet E. Compston, Nicholas E. Day, et al. February 2004. "The Effects of Phytoestrogen Isoflavones on Bone Density in Women: A Double-Blind, Randomized, Placebo-Controlled Trial." *The American Journal of Clinical Nutrition* 79(2): 326–333.

9. Occhiuto, F., R. D. Pasquale, G. Guglielmo, et al. February 2007. "Effects of Phytoestrogenic Isoflavones from Red Clover (*Trifolium pratense* L.) on Experimental Osteoporosis." *Phytotherapy Research* 21(2): 130–134.

10. Lipovac, M., P. Chedraui, C. Gruenhut, et al. March 2010. "Improvement of Postmenopausal Depressive and Anxiety Symptoms after Treatment with Isoflavones Derived from Red Clover Extracts." *Maturitas* 65(3): 258–261.

References and Resources

Magazines, Journals, and Newspapers

Asgary, S., J. Moshtaghian, G. Naderi, et al. August 2007. "Effects of Dietary Red Clover on Blood Factors and Cardiovascular Streak Formation in Hypercholesterolemic Rabbits." *Phytotherapy Research* 21(8): 768–770.

Atkinson, Charlotte, Juliet E. Compston, Nicholas E. Day, et al. February 2004. "The Effects of Phytoestrogen Isoflavones on Bone Density in Women: A Double-Blind Randomized, Placebo-Controlled Trial." *The American Journal of Clinical Nutrition* 79(2): 326–333.

Baumann, Leslie S. April 2005. "Red Clover." *Skin & Allergy News* 36(4): 14.

Coon, Joanna Thompson, Max H. Pittler., and Edzard Ernst. February 2007. "*Trifolium pratense* Isoflavones in the Treatment of Menopausal Hot Flushes: A Systematic Review and Meta-Analysis." *Phytomedicine: International Journal of Phytotherapy and Phytopharmacology* 14(2–3): 153–159.

Geller, Stacie E., Lee P. Shulman, Richard B. van Breemen, et al. November–December 2009. "Safety and Efficacy of Black Cohosh and Red Clover for the Management of Vasomotor Symptoms: A Randomized Controlled Trial." *Menopause* 16(6): 1156–1166.

Hidalgo, L. A., P. A. Chedraui, N. Morocho, et al. November 2005. "The Effect of Red Clover Isoflavones on Menopausal Symptoms, Lipids and Vaginal Cytology in Menopausal Women: A Randomized, Double-Blind, Placebo-Controlled Study." *Gynecological Endocrinology* 21(5): 257–264.

Lipovac, M., P. Chedraui, C. Gruenhut, et al. March 2010. "Improvement of Postmenopausal Depressive and Anxiety Symptoms after Treatment with Isoflavones Derived from Red Clover Extracts." *Maturitas* 65(3): 258–261.

Occhiuto, F., R. D. Pasquale, G. Guglielmo, et al. February 2007. "Effects of Phytoestrogenic Isoflavones from Red Clover (*Trifolium pratense* L.) on Experimental Osteoporosis." *Phytotherapy Research* 21(2): 130–134.

Terzic, M. M., J. Dotlic, S. Maricic, et al. December 2009. "Influence of Red Clover-Derived Isoflavones on Serum Lipid Profile in Postmenopausal Women." *The Journal of Obstetrics and Gynecology Research* 35(6): 1091–1095.

van de Weijer, P. H., and R. Barentsen. July 2002. "Isoflavones from Red Clover (Promensil) Significantly Reduce Menopausal Hot Flush Symptoms Compared with Placebo." *Maturitas* 42(3): 187–193.

Website
University of Maryland Medical Center. www.umm.edu.

Rhodiola 🌿

Also known as golden root, arctic root, and roseroot, rhodiola is a perennial plant with yellow flowers that has grown since ancient times in the high alpine and arctic regions of the Northern Hemisphere. Despite the challenging climatic conditions, it thrived.

Nevertheless, until the past decade, rhodiola, scientifically known as *Rhodiola rosea,* was not well known in North America. But, it was considered an excellent medicinal herb in other parts of the world. Eastern Europeans and Asians, especially Russians and Scandinavians, have long believed that the plant's rhizome or flashy underground stem was useful for a wide variety of conditions. These include fatigue, depression, headaches, altitude sickness, colds, influenza, gastrointestinal upset, and infections.[1] But what have the researchers determined?

Depression

In a double-blind, randomized, placebo-controlled Swedish study published in 2007 in the *Nordic Journal of Psychiatry,* researchers examined the use of a standardized extract of rhodiola on 89 subjects between the ages of 18 and 70. All the subjects, who had been diagnosed with significant levels of clinical depression by two different standard psychiatric measurements, were randomly assigned to one of three groups. The members of the first group received two tablets once daily (340 mg/day) of a rhodiola root extract known as SHR-5; the members of the second group received two tablets twice daily (680 mg/day) of the same extract. The subjects in the third group took two placebo tablets, which were identical in appearance to the other tablets, once per day.

At the end of six weeks, both the groups that took rhodiola had significant reductions in depression. The members of the placebo group did not show any meaningful change in depressive symptoms. Moreover, the researchers found that the members of the groups on rhodiola had improvements in insomnia, emotional instability, and levels of somatization (physical symptoms caused by psychological problems). The subjects taking the placebo did not have any significant changes in these health concerns. Additionally, the subjects on the higher dose of rhodiola had significant increases in their levels of self-esteem. Those on the lower dose and the placebo did not have changes in their levels of self-esteem. None of the subjects reported any serious side effects. The researchers concluded that "the standardized extract SHR-5 shows anti-depressive potency in patients with mild to moderate depression when administered in dosages of either 340 or 680 mg/day over a six-week period."[2]

Generalized Anxiety Disorder

In a pilot study published in 2008 in *The Journal of Alternative and Complementary Medicine,* researchers from the University of California, Los Angeles, recruited 10 participants, between the ages of 34 and 55, from the UCLA Anxiety Disorders program. For 10 weeks, all the participants, who had been diagnosed with generalized anxiety disorder, received daily doses of 340 mg rhodiola. By the end of the study, the participants had significant reductions in anxiety. Side effects tended to be mild; dizziness and dry mouth were the most common. The researchers noted that the improvement in symptoms was similar to what may be obtained in clinical trials.[3]

Stress-Related Fatigue

In a study published in 2009 in *Planta Medica,* researchers from Uppsala University in Sweden investigated the use of rhodiola for the treatment of stress-induced fatigue in 60 men and women between the ages of 20 and 55. The subjects were divided into two groups of 30. One group received four daily tablets of SHR-5 extract (a total of 576 mg extract/day); the other group received four daily placebo tablets.

At the end of one month, the members of both groups reported better levels of attention and less fatigue. However, the improvement was most dramatic among those taking rhodiola. In addition, the members of the rhodiola group had lower levels of cortisol in the blood. Higher levels of serum cortisol increase muscle fatigue. The researchers concluded that the rhodiola had an "antifatigue" effect that enhanced "mental performance, particularly the ability to concentrate." The rhodiola also lowered "cortisol response to awakening stress in burnout patients with fatigue syndrome."[4]

Anti-Aging

In a study published in 2007 in *Rejuvenation Research,* researchers from the University of California, Irvine, examined the effects of rhodiola supplementation on the lifespan of fruit flies (*Drosophilia melanogaster*). The researchers divided their fruit flies into two groups. The fruit flies in one group received 30 mg/mL rhodiola supplementation every other day; the fruit flies in the other group served as the control. The researchers found that "when comparing the distribution of deaths between rhodiola-supplemented and control flies, rhodiola-fed flies exhibited decelerated aging."[5]

Symptom Improvement in People with Physical and Cognitive Deficiencies

In a 12-week drug monitoring study published in 2007 in *Advances in Therapy,* researchers from Hamburg, Germany, evaluated the "efficiency and safety" of rhodiola and vitamins and minerals for 120 adults (83 women and 37 men between the ages of 50 and 89) with physical and cognitive deficiencies. The subjects were divided into two groups of 60. The participants in group 1 took two capsules after breakfast; the participants in group 2 took one capsule after breakfast and a second capsule after lunch. During the study, there were three medical evaluations—at baseline, after 6 weeks, and after 12 weeks. The researchers determined that the men and women in both groups experienced "a statistically highly significant improvement . . . in physical and cognitive deficiencies." However, the "improvements in group 1 were more pronounced than in group 2," which meant that it was probably better to take both capsules together after breakfast. During the study, the rhodiola, vitamins, and minerals did not result in any adverse effects.[6]

Mental Alertness

In a randomized, double-blind, placebo-controlled, parallel group study published in 2003 in *Phytomedicine: International Journal of Phytotherapy and Phytopharmacology,* researchers from Russia and Sweden attempted to quantify the effect of a single dose of rhodiola (SHR-5) on the "capacity for mental work against a background of fatigue and stress."

Since the researchers also wanted to learn if there were varying responses to the different doses, they gave one group of subjects the "standard mean dose" of 370 mg and the other group received a dose that was 555 mg, a 50% increase. A third group served as the control.

The subjects consisted of 161 male military cadets between the ages of 19 and 21 who were stressed and sleep deprived. Researchers found that the cadets in both treated groups had significant improvements in fatigue. There appeared to be "no significant difference between the two dosage groups."[7]

Enhancing Exercise

In a double-blind study that was published in 2008 in the *International Journal of Sport Nutrition and Exercise Metabolism,* Polish researchers assigned 11 members of the Polish Rowing Team to a group that received 100 mg of rhodiola extract twice daily for four weeks. During this same time period, an additional 11 members of the same team took placebos. The researchers found that the rowers taking rhodiola had an increased amount of free radical-fighting antioxidants in their blood, but the rhodiola appeared to have no effect "on oxidative damage induced by exhaustive exercise."[8]

Is Rhodiola Beneficial?

While rhodiola has some clear benefits, it may have side effects. These include stomach upset, drowsiness, dizziness, and insomnia.

Moreover, it has become evident that some people should avoid rhodiola. Rhodiola should not be taken by women who are pregnant or are trying to become pregnant. Researchers do not know if rhodiola may harm a growing fetus. Because of its ability to stimulate, rhodiola should not be used without the approval and supervision of a healthcare provider by people with a bipolar diagnosis, depression, or other mental health issues. Rhodiola has the potential to trigger a manic phase. And, women dealing with breast cancer with estrogen receptor positive tumors and are on antiestrogenic medication must not consume any rhodiola. It may well interfere with the treatment.

Notes

1. The Herb Companion Website. www.herbcompanion.com.
2. Darbinyan, V., G. Aslanyan, E. Amroyan, et al. 2007. "Clinical Trial of *Rhodiola rosea* L. Extract SHR-5 in the Treatment of Mild to Moderate Depression." *Nordic Journal of Psychiatry* 61(5): 343–348.

3. Bystritsky, A., L. Kerwin, and J. D. Feusner. March 2008. "A Pilot Study of *Rhodiola rosea* (Rhodax) for Generalized Anxiety Disorder (GAD)." *The Journal of Alternative and Complementary Medicine* 14(2): 175–180.

4. Olsson, E. M., B. von Schéele, and A. G. Panossian. February 2009. "A Randomised, Double-Blind, Placebo-Controlled, Parallel-Group Study of the Standardised Extract SHR-5 of the Roots of *Rhodiola rosea* in the Treatment of Subjects with Stress-Related Fatigue." *Planta Medica* 75(2): 105–112.

5. Jefari, Mahtab, Jeffrey S. Felgner, Irvin I. Bussel, et al. December 2007. "Rhodiola: A Promising Anti-Aging Chinese Herb." *Rejuvenation Research* 10(4): 587–602.

6. Fintelmann, Volker, and Joerg Gruenwald. July 2007. "Efficacy and Tolerability of a *Rhodiola rosea* Extract in Adults with Physical and Cognitive Deficiencies." *Advances in Therapy* 24(4): 929–939.

7. Shevtsov, V. A., B. I. Zholus, V. I. Shervarly, et al. 2003. "A Randomized Trial of Two Different Doses of a SHR-5 *Rhodiola rosea* Extract versus Placebo and Control of Capacity for Mental Work." *Phytomedicine: International Journal of Phytotherapy and Phytopharmacology* 10(2–3): 95–105.

8. Skarpanska-Stejnborn, Anna, Lucja Pilaczynska-Szczesniak, Piotr Basta, and Ewa Deskur-Smielecka. April 2009. "The Influence of Supplementation with *Rhodiola rosea* L. Extract on Selected Redox Parameters in Professional Rowers." *International Journal of Sport Nutrition and Exercise Metabolism* 19(2): 186–199.

References and Resources

Magazines, Journals, and Newspapers

Bystritsky, A., L. Kerwin, and J. D. Feusner. March 2008. "A Pilot Study of *Rhodiola rosea* (Rhodax) for Generalized Anxiety Disorder." *The Journal of Alternative and Complementary Medicine* 14(2): 175–180.

Darbinyan, V., G. Aslanyan, E. Amroyan, et al. 2007. "Clinical Trial of *Rhodiola rosea* L. Extract SHR-5 in the Treatment of Mild to Moderate Depression." *Nordic Journal of Psychiatry* 61(5): 343–348.

Fintelmann, Volker, and Joerg Gruenwald. July 2007. "Efficacy and Tolerability of a *Rhodiola Rosea* Extract in Adults with Physical and Cognitive Deficiencies." *Advances in Therapy* 24(4): 929–939.

Jafari, Mahtab, Jeffrey S. Felgner, Irvin I. Bussel, et al. December 2007. "Rhodiola: A Promising Anti-Aging Chinese Herb." *Rejuvenation Research* 10(4): 587–602.

Olsson, E. M., B. von Schéele, and A. G. Panossian. February 2009. "A Randomised, Double-Blind, Placebo-Controlled, Parallel-Group Study of the Standardized Extract SHR-5 of the Roots of *Rhodiola Rosea* in the Treatment of Subjects with Stress-Related Fatigue." *Planta Medica* 75(2): 105–112.

Shevtsov, V. A., B. I. Zholus, V. I. Shervarly, et al. 2003. "A Randomized Trial of Two Different Doses of SHR-5 *Rhodiola rosea* Extract versus Placebo and Control of Capacity for Mental Work." *Phytomedicine: International Journal of Phytotherapy and Phytopharmacology* 10(2–3): 95–105.

Skarpanska-Stejnborn, Anna, Lucja Pilaczynska-Szczeniak, Piotr Basta, and Ewa Deskur-Smielecka. April 2009. "The Influence of Supplementation with *Rhodiola rosea* L. Extract on Selected Redox Parameters in Professional Rowers." *International Journal of Sport Nutrition and Exercise Metabolism* 19(2): 186–199.

Websites
American Botanical Council. www.herbalgram.org.
The Herb Companion. www.herbcompanion.com.

Rosemary 🌿

Scientifically known as *Rosmarinus officinalis,* rosemary has been traditionally thought to be useful for a wide variety of health concerns. These include improving memory, relieving muscle pain and spasms, stimulating the growth of hair, and supporting the circulatory and nervous system. Rosemary is also believed to be useful for increasing the flow of urine and treating indigestion.[1] But, it is important to review what researchers have learned.

Useful for Preventing Thrombosis (Blood Clots)
In a study published in 2008 in *Thrombosis Research,* researchers from Japan investigated how the long-term use of rosemary and common thyme affected the platelets, thrombus formation, and bleeding times in mice fed a high-fat, Western-style diet. For 12 weeks, the diets of the mice included either 5% or 0.5% of rosemary or 5% of common thyme. The researchers found that both the rosemary and common thyme "significantly suppressed the rate of thrombus formation." And, unlike antiplatelet agents, which often cause bleeding, "rosemary and common thyme did not prolong but rather shortened (statistically not significantly) the bleeding time."[2]

Anti-Aging Protection

In a study published in 2009 in *Experimental Gerontology,* researchers from Madrid, Spain, wanted to learn if supplementing the diets of elderly rats (20 months old) with rosemary extract would reduce their levels of oxidative stress. The researchers began by dividing their 30 rats into three groups of 10 rats. The rats in the first group received no rosemary; the rats in the second group received a 0.2% concentration of rosemary; and, the rats in the third group received 0.02% concentration of rosemary. After 12 weeks, the rats were sacrificed, and the researchers collected tissue samples from their hearts and brains. The researchers found that the rosemary supplement had protective effects on both these organs. They concluded that "rosemary extract could be incorporated . . . [into] the diet as a nutritional supplement, to augment the body's defenses against oxidative stress."[3]

Improves Cognition

In an often mentioned study that was published in 2003 in the *International Journal of Neuroscience,* researchers from the United Kingdom divided 144 young adults into three groups. One group sat in cubicles with rosemary aroma; another group sat in cubicles with lavender aroma. The third group, whose members served as controls, sat in cubicles with no aroma. During the study, the subjects were given a number of tests. The researchers found that "rosemary produced a significant enhancement of performance for overall quality of memory and secondary memory factors."[4]

Supports Cardiovascular Health

In a study published in 2011 in *Phytotherapy Research,* researchers from Slovenia wondered if rosemary supplementation in younger, healthier people could decrease their risk of atherosclerosis. The cohort consisted of 7 men and 12 women, with a mean age of 34.3. Eight of the subjects were smokers, and three had a family history of symptomatic atherosclerosis. During the study, the subjects took rosemary extract for 21 days. The researchers found that rosemary increased circulation by dilating the subjects' arteries. In addition, rosemary was found to have antioxidant properties that reduce the risk of atherosclerosis.[5]

Antidepressant Properties

In a study published in 2009 in *Progress in Neuro-Psychopharmacology and Biological Psychiatry,* researchers from Brazil used two behavioral models—forced swimming test and tail suspension test—to induce depressive symptoms in mice. To determine if rosemary could reduce some of these symptoms, they treated some of the mice with rosemary extract. Other mice, which were not treated, served as controls. The researchers learned that rosemary "produces a specific antidepressant-like effect in animal models." Furthermore, "the effect of the acute or repeated administration of this extract was similar to the action produced by the classical antidepressant fluoxetine [Prozac]."[6]

Anti-Anxiety Properties

In a study published in 2009 in *Holistic Nursing Practice,* researchers from Florida examined the use of rosemary and lavender aromatherapy to reduce test-taking anxiety of 40 students in the master's program in advanced nursing practice. To complete the program, the students were required to pass four examinations with a grade of at least 80%. In order to have control data, there was no aromatherapy with the first test. Both before and during the second test, students breathed lavender aromatherapy; before and during the third test, they breathed rosemary aromatherapy. The researchers found no differences in pre- and post test anxiety during the first test. However, during the second and third tests, there were significant decreases in test anxiety. During the discussions following each exam, the students noted that they preferred rosemary aromatherapy; they indicated that lavender aromatherapy made them too relaxed.[7]

Anti-Cancer Properties

In a study published in 2010 in *Plant Foods for Human Nutrition,* researchers from Turkey obtained rosemary from three different locations in Turkey. They then applied these extracts to various types of cancer cells and leukemia (blood cancer) cells. The researchers found that rosemary inhibited cancer cell proliferation and killed most cancer cells. However, it had little effect on leukemia cells. The researchers concluded that "rosemary extract is a potential candidate to be included in the anti-cancer diet with pre-determined doses avoiding toxicity."[8]

Anti-Fungal Properties

In a study published in 2010 in the *Brazilian Journal of Biology*, researchers from Brazil analyzed the anti-fungal properties of rosemary and several other medicinal herbs. The researchers found that rosemary had "strong activity" against fungus; the addition of rosemary extract killed most fungal spores. Why is it important to identify additional anti-fungal agents? According to the researchers, "because of the increasing development of drug resistance to human pathogens and the appearance of undesirable effects of certain anti-fungal agents, the search for new antimicrobial agents is of great concern today."[9]

May Be of Use in the Treatment of Parkinson's Disease

While the cause of Parkinson's disease is unclear, it is known that Parkinson's disease involves dopamine-producing cells deep within the brain. Sometimes these cells degrade, causing unwanted body movements. In a study published in 2010 in *Cellular and Molecular Neurobiology*, researchers from Korea investigated the ability of rosemary to protect dopamine-producing cells. The researchers began by exposing human dopamine cells with hydrogen peroxide. This created an experimental model of Parkinson's disease. When they exposed human dopamine cells to hydrogen peroxide and rosemary extract, the damage was prevented. While acknowledging that more research on the use of rosemary for Parkinson's disease is needed, the researchers noted that their findings "may offer a new therapeutic strategy in treating Parkinson's disease."[10]

Not Very Useful for Oral Pathogens

In a study published in 2010 in *Zeitschrift fur Naturforschung*, researchers from Brazil tested constituents in rosemary essential oil against a number of different microorganisms that have the potential to cause dental cavities (caries) in humans. Unfortunately, the researchers found that "essential oil displayed low activity against the selected microorganisms." And, they concluded that rosemary essential oil "as well as its major compounds were not active against some important oral pathogens."[11]

Is Rosemary Beneficial?

It is evident that rosemary has a number of different benefits. For most people, it is probably a useful addition to the diet.

Notes

1. University of Maryland Medical Center Website. www.umm.edu.
2. Naemura, A., M. Ura, T. Yamashita, et al. 2008. "Long-Term Intake of Rosemary and Common Thyme Herbs Inhibits Experimental Thrombosis without Prolongation of Bleeding Time." *Thrombosis Research* 122(4): 517–522.
3. Posadas, S. J., V. Caz, C. Largo, et al. June–July 2009. "Protective Effect of Supercritical Fluid Rosemary Extract, *Rosmarinus officinalis*, on Antioxidants of Major Organs of Aged Rats." *Experimental Gerontology* 44(6–7): 383–389.
4. Moss, M., J. Cook, K. Wesnes, and P. Duckett. January 2003. "Aromas of Rosemary and Lavender Essential Oils Differentially Affect Cognition and Mood in Health Adults." *International Journal of Neuroscience* 113(1): 15–38.
5. Sinkovic, A., D. Suran, L. Lokar, et al. March 2011. "Rosemary Extracts Improve Flow-Mediated Dilation of the Brachial Artery and Plasma PAI-1 Activity in Healthy Young Volunteers." *Phytotherapy Research* 25(3): 402–407.
6. Machado, D. G., L. E. Bettio, M. P. Cunha, et al. June 2009. "Antidepressant-Like Effect of the Extract of *Rosmarinus officinalis* in Mice: Involvement of the Monoaminergic System." *Progress in Neuro-Psychopharmacology and Biological Psychiatry* 33(4): 642–650.
7. McCaffrey, R., D. J. Thomas, and A. O. Kinzelman. March–April 2009. "The Effects of Lavender and Rosemary Essential Oils on Test-Taking Anxiety among Graduate Nursing Students." *Holistic Nursing Practice* 23(2): 88–93.
8. Yesil-Celiktas, O., C. Sevimli, E. Bedir, and F. Vardar-Sukan. June 2010. "Inhibitory Effects of Rosemary Extracts, Carnosic Acid and Rosmarinic Acid, on the Growth of Various Human Cancer Cell Line." *Plant Foods for Human Nutrition* 65(2): 158–163.
9. Höfling, J. F., P. C. Anibal, G. A. Obando-Pereda, et al. 2010. "Antimicrobial Potential of Some Plant Extracts against *Candida* Species." *Brazilian Journal of Biology* 70(4): 1065–1068.
10. Park, Se-Eun, Seung Kim, Kumar Sapkota, and Sung-Jun Kim. 2010. "Neuroprotective Effect of *Rosmarinus officinalis* Extract on Human Dopaminergic Cell Line, SH-SY5Y." *Cellular and Molecular Neurobiology* 30: 759–767.
11. Bernardes, W. A., R. Lucarini, M.G. Tozatti, et al. September–October 2010. "Antibacterial Activity of the Essential Oil from *Rosmarinus officinalis* and Its Major Components against Oral Pathogens." *Zeitschrift für Naturforschung A* [*A Journal of Physical Sciences*] 65c(9–10): 588–593.

References and Resources

Magazines, Journals, and Newspapers

Bernardes, W. A., R. Lucariri, M.G. Tozatti, et al. September–October 2010. "Antibacterial Activity of the Essential Oil from *Rosmarinus officinalis* and Its

Major Components against Oral Pathogens." *Zeitschrift für Naturforschung A [A Journal of Physical Sciences]* 65c (9–10): 588–593.

Höfling, J. F., P. C. Anibal, G. A. Obando-Pereda, et al. 2010. "Antimicrobial Potential of Some Plant Extracts against *Candida* Species." *Brazilian Journal of Biology* 70(4): 1065–1068.

Machado, D. G., L. E. Bettio, M. P. Cunha, et al. June 2009. "Antidepressant-Like Effect of the Extract of *Rosmarinus officinalis* in Mice: Involvement of the Monoaminergic System." *Progress in Neuro-Psychopharmacology and Biological Psychiatry* 33(4): 642–650.

McCaffrey, E., D. J. Thomas, and A. O. Kinzelman. March–April 2009. "The Effects of Lavender and Rosemary Essential Oils on Test-Taking Anxiety among Graduate Nursing Students." *Holistic Nursing Practice* 23(2): 88–93.

Moss, M., J. Cook, K. Wesnes, and P. Duckett. January 2003. "Aromas of Rosemary and Lavender Essential Oils Differentially Affect Cognition and Mood in Healthy Adults." *International Journal of Neuroscience* 113(1): 15–38.

Naemura, A., M. Ura, T. Yamashita, et al. 2008. "Long-Term Intake of Rosemary and Common Thyme Herbs Inhibits Experimental Thrombosis without Prolongation of Bleeding Time." *Thrombosis Research* 122(4): 517–522.

Park, Se-Eun, Seung Kim, Kumar Sapkota, and Sung-Jun Kim. 2010. "Neuroprotective Effect of *Rosmarinus officinalis* Extract on Human Dopaminergic Cell Lines, SH-SY5Y." *Cellular and Molecular Neurobiology* 30: 759–767.

Posadas, S. J., V. Caz, C. Largo, et al. June–July 2009. "Protective Effect of Supercritical Fluid Rosemary Extract, *Rosmarinus officinalis*, on Antioxidants of Major Organs of Aged Rats." *Experimental Gerontology* 44(6–7): 383–389.

Sinkovic, A., D. Suran, L. Lokar, et al. March 2011. "Rosemary Extracts Improve Flow-Mediated Dilation of the Brachial Artery and Plasma PAI-1 Activity in Healthy Young Volunteers." *Phytotherapy Research* 25(3): 402–407.

Yesil-Celiktas, O., C. Sevimli, E. Bedir, and F. Vardar-Sukan. June 2010. "Inhibitory Effects of Rosemary Extracts, Carnosic Acid and Rosmarinic Acid, on the Growth of Various Human Cancer Cell Lines." *Plant Foods for Human Nutrition* 65(2): 158–153.

Website

University of Maryland Medical Center. www.umm.edu.

S

Saffron 🌿

While herbs are generally modestly priced, saffron, used since ancient times, is expensive. In fact, saffron, which is native to southwest Asia and primarily grown today in France, Spain, Sicily, and Iran, is the most costly of all plant products on the market. There are primarily two reasons for the high price. People who farm saffron, which is scientifically known as *Crocus sativus,* obtain very little product for the amount of acreage and labor required. Farmers need an astonishing three acres of flowers to produce a single pound of saffron. And, the harvesting of saffron is time-consuming and back-breaking.[1]

Over the years, saffron has been said to be useful for a wide variety of medical problems. These include coughs, whooping cough, gastrointestinal upset, jaundice, insomnia, menstrual pain, menopause, impotence, infertility, anemia, enlarged liver, depression, and chronic diarrhea.[2] Can one herb really be useful for so many dissimilar medical concerns? It is interesting to review what the researchers have learned.

Skin Cancer

In a study published in 2010 in *Acta Histochemica,* researchers from Washington DC and India tested the ability of saffron to kill skin cancer cells. They began by dividing mice into five groups: carcinogen (cancer) control (CC), normal control, saffron-treated A, saffron treated B, and saffron treated C. Then, the researchers used a chemical to induce skin cancer on the backs of mice in groups A, B, C, and CC. Acetone was placed on the back of the mice in the normal control group. Three groups of mice also received oral infusion of saffron. The mice in group

A received oral infusion before the procedure, and the mice in group C received it after the procedure to induce skin cancer. The mice in group B received saffron both before and after the procedure. The researchers noted that the mice in group B clearly benefited from the saffron. They wrote that "Standard histological [microscopic] examination of the skin demonstrated a beneficial action of saffron in mice where saffron treatments were given both before and after the induction of skin carcinogenesis [development of cancer]."[3]

Pancreatic Cancer

In a study published in 2009 in *Molecular Cancer Therapeutics,* researchers from several locations in Kansas conducted in vitro and in vivo trials on the ability of crocetin, a carotenoid compound derived from saffron, to kill pancreatic cancer cells. During their in vitro work, the researchers found that "pancreatic cancer cells . . . [were] significantly inhibited by crocetin treatment." During their in vivo work, the researchers injected highly aggressive pancreatic cancer cells into the legs of mice. After they observed palpable tumors, crocetin was administered orally. The crocetin was found to result in significant "regression in tumor growth." The researchers concluded that "crocetin has a significant antitumorigenic effect in both in vitro and in vivo on pancreatic cancer."[4]

Wound Healing

In a study published in 2008 in *The Keio Journal of Medicine,* researchers from Iran investigated the use of pollen of saffron extract cream to treat second-degree burns in rats. Forty-eight rats that sustained burns from hot water were divided into four groups; each group had 12 rats. One group received no topical treatment for the burns; that group served as the control. The rats in a second group were treated with a base cream that had no healing agent. The wounds of the rats in a third group were treated with a 1% silver sulfadiazine cream, a wound-healing cream. And, the wounds of the last group of rats were treated with a 20% saffron cream. The treatments, which were scheduled twice daily, began 24 hours after the administration of the wounds. By the 25th day, "the wound size of the saffron group was significantly smaller than other groups." As a result, the researchers added, "the results of this study raise the possibility of potential efficacy of saffron in accelerating wound healing in burn injuries."[5]

Weight Control

In a randomized, placebo-controlled, double-blind trial published in 2010 in *Nutrition Research,* French researchers attempted to determine if Satiereal, an extract of saffron, could help mildly overweight women reduce their snacking and achieve increased rates of satiety, thereby contributing to weight loss. The cohort consisted of 60 women "homogenous for age, body weight, and snacking frequency." For eight weeks, 31 women took a Satiereal capsule twice daily; 29 women took a matching placebo. At the end of the trial, the researchers found that "the mean snacking frequency was significantly decreased in the Satiereal group as compared with the placebo group." The researchers noted that their findings "indicate that Satiereal consumption produces a reduction of snacking and creates a satiating effect that could contribute to body weight loss." Moreover, "the combination of an adequate diet with Satiereal supplementation might help subjects engaged in a weight loss program in achieving their objective."[6]

Cardiovascular Health

In a study published in 2010 in *Applied Biochemistry and Biotechnology,* researchers from India evaluated the ability of saffron and crocin, another of its active components, to lower serum lipid levels and increase antioxidants in hyperlipidemic rats (rats with high-lipid levels). The researchers fed rats either a diet with a normal amount of fat or a high amount of fat. Then, for five consecutive days, the rats were divided into groups and fed varying amounts of saffron or crocin. The researchers found that both saffron and crocin reduced levels of triglycerides and total cholesterol and increased amounts of antioxidants. Still, "the saffron was found to be superior to crocin indicating the involvement of other potential constituents of saffron apart from crocin. For its synergistic behavior of quenching the free radicals and ameliorating the damages of hyperlipidemia."[7]

In a study published in 2010 in *Phytotherapy Research,* researchers from Iran used saffron, and its components crocin and safranal, to lower high blood pressure levels in rats with elevated levels. The researchers found that the saffron, crocin, and safranal reduced the levels of blood pressure in a dose-dependent manner. The researchers concluded that saffron lowers blood pressure; safranal seems to have stronger blood pressure lowering properties than crocin.[8]

Alzheimer's Disease

In a double-blind study published in 2010 in the *Journal of Clinical Pharmacy and Therapeutics,* researchers from Iran assessed the ability of saffron to play a role in the treatment of mild to moderate Alzheimer's disease. The cohort consisted of 46 patients with "probable" Alzheimer's disease. Patients were randomly assigned to take 15 mg of saffron or a placebo, twice daily. At the end of 16 weeks, the researchers observed that "saffron produced a significantly better outcome on cognitive function than placebo." And, there did not appear to be any negative side effects. "There were no significant differences in the two groups in terms of observed adverse events."[9]

Age-Related Macular Degeneration

In a study published in 2010 in *Investigative Ophthalmology & Visual Science,* researchers from Italy evaluated the ability of short-term supplementation with saffron to aid those dealing with early age-related macular degeneration (AMD). The cohort consisted of 25 people. They were randomly assigned to oral saffron 20 mg/day or placebo supplementation. The initial trial continued for three months. Then, for the next three months, those who had taken saffron took the placebo, and those who had taken the placebo took saffron. The researchers found that those taking saffron had some improvement in the electrical responses in the retina. They noted that their findings "provide important clues that nutritional carotenoids may impact AMD [age-related macular degeneration] in novel and unexpected ways, possibly beyond their antioxidant properties."[10]

Is Saffron Beneficial?

Clearly, more research is needed on saffron. But, the available research is impressive. It may well be an herb that should be discussed with medical providers. At the least, most people should probably consume more.

Notes

1. Medicinal Herb Info Website. www.medicinalherbinfo.org.
2. Medicinal Herb Info Website. www.medicinalherbinfo.org.
3. Das, lla, Sukta Das, and Tapas Saha. July 2010. "Saffron Suppresses Oxidative Stress in DMBA-Induced Skin Carcinoma: A Histopathological Study." *Acta Histochemica* 112(4): 317–327.

4. Dhar, A., S. Mehta, G. Dhar, et al. February 2009. "Crocetin Inhibits Pancreatic Cancer Cell Proliferation and Tumor Progression in a Xenograft Mouse Model." *Molecular Cancer Therapeutics* 8(2): 315–323.

5. Khorasani, G., S.J. Hosseinimehr, P. Zamani, et al. December 2008. "The Effect of Saffron (*Crocus sativus*) Extract for Healing of Second-Degree Burn Wounds in Rats." *The Keio Journal of Medicine* 57(4): 190–195.

6. Gout, B., C. Bourges, and S. Paineau-Dubreuil. May 2010. "Satiereal, a *Crocus sativus* L Extract, Reduces Snacking and Increases Satiety in a Randomized Placebo-Controlled Study of Mildly Overweight, Healthy Women." *Nutrition Research* 30(5): 305–313.

7. Asdaq, S.M., and M.N. Inamdar. September 2010. "Potential of *Crocus sativus* (Saffron) and Its Constituent, Crocin, as Hypolipidemic and Antioxidant in Rats." *Applied Biochemistry and Biotechnology* 162(2): 358–372.

8. Imenshahidi, Mohsen, Hossein Hosseinzadeh, and Yaser Javadpour. July 2010. "Hypotensive Effect of Aqueous Saffron Extract (*Crocus sativus* L.) and Its Constituents, Safranal and Crocin, in Normotensive and Hypertensive Rats." *Phytotherapy Research* 24(7): 990–994.

9. Akhondzadeh, S., M.S. Sabet, M.H. Harirchian, et al. October 2010. "Saffron in the Treatment of Patients with Mild to Moderate Alzheimer's Disease: A 16-Week, Randomized and Placebo-Controlled Trial." *Journal of Clinical Pharmacy and Therapeutics* 35(5): 581–588.

10. Falsini, B., M. Piccardi, A. Minnella, et al. December 2010. "Influence of Saffron Supplementation on Retinal Flicker Sensitivity in Early Age-Related Macular Degeneration." *Investigative Ophthalmology & Visual Science* 51(12): 6118–6124.

References and Resources

Magazines, Journals, and Newspapers

Akhondzadeh, S., M.S. Sabet, M.H. Harirchian, et al. October 2010. "Saffron in the Treatment of Patients with Mild to Moderate Alzheimer's Disease: A 16-Week, Randomized and Placebo-Controlled Trial." *Journal of Clinical Pharmacy and Therapeutics* 35(5): 581–588.

Asdaq, S.M., and M.N. Inamdar. September 2010. "Potential of *Crocus sativus* (Saffron) and Its Constituent, Crocin, as Hypolipidemic and Antioxidant in Rats." *Applied Biochemistry and Biotechnology* 162(2): 358–372.

Das, lla, Sukta Das, and Tapas Saha. July 2010. "Saffron Suppresses Oxidative Stress in DMBA-Induced Skin Carcinoma: A Histopathological Study." *Acta Histochemica* 112(4): 317–327.

Dhar, A., S. Mehta, G. Dhar, et al. February 2009. "Crocetin Inhibits Pancreatic Cancer Cell Proliferation and Tumor Progression in a Xenograft Mouse Model." *Molecular Cancer Therapeutics* 8(2): 315–323.

Falsini, B., M. Piccardi, A. Minnella, et al. December 2010. "Influence of Saffron Supplementation on Retinal Flicker Sensitivity in Early Age-Related Macular Degeneration." *Investigative Ophthalmology & Visual Science* 51(12): 6118–6124.

Gout, B., C. Bourges, and S. Paineau-Dubreuil. May 2010. "Satiereal, a *Crocus sativus* L. Extract, Reduces Snacking and Increases Satiety in a Randomized Placebo-Controlled Study of Mildly Overweight, Healthy Women." *Nutrition Research* 30(5): 305–313.

Imenshahidi, Mohsen, Hossein Hosseinzadeh, and Yaser Javadpour. July 2010. "Hypotensive Effect of Aqueous Saffron Extract (*Crocus sativus* L.) and Its Constituents, Safranal and Crocin, in Normotensive and Hypertensive Rats." *Phytotherapy Research* 24(7): 990–994.

Khorasani, G., S.J. Hosseinimehr, P. Zamani, et al. December 2008. "The Effect of Saffron (*Crocus sativus*) Extract for Healing of Second-Degree Burn Wounds in Rats." *The Keio Journal of Medicine* 57(4): 190–195.

Website
Medicinal Herb Info. www.medicinalherbinfo.org.

Sage 🐏

Like many other medicinal herbs, sage, which is native to countries near the Mediterranean Sea, has truly ancient roots. The Greeks and Romans held sage in high esteem for its ability to heal medical problems, and they used it as a preservative for meat; the ancient Romans even designed a special ceremony for gathering sage.[1]

By the 14th century, Europeans were using sage to protect against witchcraft. And, in the 17th century, the Chinese allegedly traded the Dutch three cases of tea leaves for every one case of sage leaves. In 2001, sage was named "Herb of the Year" by the International Herb Association.[2]

Today, sage, scientifically known as *Salvia officinalis,* is probably best known as a memory enhancer. But, sage is also believed to have antioxidant and anti-inflammatory properties. It is important to review what the researchers have learned.

Improvements in Memory and Mood
In a randomized, placebo-controlled, double-blind, five-period crossover study published in 2008 in *Psychopharmacology,* researchers from the

United Kingdom and Australia investigated the acute effects of sage on the cognitive performance of 20 healthy volunteers. All the participants were over the age of 65, and they had a mean age of 72.95. On separate occasions, the volunteers received four "active" doses of sage extract—167, 333, 666, and 1,332 mg—and a placebo. Between each visit, there were seven-day washout periods. While people on the placebo experienced "the characteristic performance decline over the day," those taking the 333-mg dose had "significant enhancement of secondary memory performance at all testing times." Participants on the other doses also showed improvement, but to a lesser extent. Furthermore, the researchers observed that there "were significant improvements to accuracy of attention following the 333 mg dose."[3]

In a double-blind, placebo-controlled, balanced crossover study published in 2011 in *Journal of Psychopharmacology,* researchers from the United Kingdom and Australia assessed the effects of a single dose of sage extract on cognitive performance and mood. Researchers gave 36 healthy participants capsules containing extract of two very similar types of sage or a placebo. Seven days later, the procedure was repeated. The researchers found that "oral consumption [of sage] led to improved performance of secondary memory and attention tasks . . . and reduced mental fatigue and increased alertness."[4]

And, in a study that was published in 2010 in *Human Psychopharmacology: Clinical and Experimental,* U.K. researchers tested whether the aromas of two similar types of sage would affect the cognition and mood of 135 healthy volunteers. Forty-five participants were in each sage group. An additional 45 people were in the control group; they were not exposed to aromas. The researchers found that when compared to the members of the control group, the members of the *Salvia officinalis* aroma group had significant improvements in memory. And, when compared to the control group, both sage groups had significant improvements in mood. The researchers concluded that their two types of sage "reproduced some but not all of the effects found following oral herb administration."[5]

Alzheimer's Disease

In a four-month, parallel group, placebo-controlled trial published in 2003 in the *Journal of Clinical Pharmacy and Therapeutics,* researchers from Iran attempted to determine if sage extract would be useful for people dealing with mild to moderate Alzheimer's disease. The cohort consisted of 42 people between the ages of 65 and 80. At the end of the trial, the researchers found that the people taking sage extract had a significantly "better outcome on cognitive functions than [those taking the] placebo." The two groups did not appear to have any differences in observed side effects "except agitation that appears to be more frequent in the placebo group."[6]

Antibacterial

In a study published in 2010 in *Phytotherapy Research*, researchers from Australia analyzed the antibacterial activities of 21 herbal extracts and four essential oils against *Helicobacter pylori*, a bacterium that causes ulcers, and *Campylobacter jejuni*, a bacterium that causes a potentially severe gastrointestinal illness. Sage was one of four herbs that demonstrated the highest antibacterial activity against *H. pylori* and among the six herbs that had the most antibacterial activity against *C. jejuni*. Still, the researchers acknowledged that "the herbal extracts have a much lower efficacy than the marketed antibiotics," so they "can only be seen as an adjunct treatment."[7]

Disinfectant Properties

In a study published in 2009 in *Food and Chemical Toxicology*, researchers from Tunisia examined the disinfectant properties of sage essential oils. During their various types of testing, the researchers found that the sage essential oils had "strong bacterial and fungicidal effects." They concluded that sage essential oils "showed a potent vapour activity against a panel of bacteria, yeasts, and fungi." According to the researchers, sage is an "eco-friendly disinfectant" that may be used "to manage airborne microbes."[8]

Skin Redness and Rashes

In a prospective, randomized, double-blind, placebo-controlled trial published in 2007 in *Planta Medica*, researchers from Freilburg, Germany, examined the anti-inflammatory properties of sage extract. They began by irradiating test areas on the backs of 40 healthy volunteers. The test areas were then treated with 2% sage extract in an ointment. Control areas were treated with either 1% hydrocortisone or 0.1% betamethasone (steroids creams used for skin conditions). The researchers found that after 48 hours sage extract "significantly reduced the ultraviolet-induced erythema [skin condition characterized by redness or rash], to a similar extent as hydrocortisone." According to the researchers, their findings "suggest that SE [sage extract] might be useful in the topical treatment of inflammatory skin conditions."[9]

Cardiovascular Health

In a nonrandomized, crossover study published in 2009 in the *International Journal of Molecular Sciences,* researchers from Braga, Portugal investigated whether drinking 300 mL of sage tea two times a day for four weeks would improve diabetes parameters and associated complications in six women between the ages of 40 and 50. While the researchers observed no effects of sage on the blood glucose levels in the women, drinking sage tea did improve the women's lipid profile (lowered total cholesterol and gradually increased HDL—"good" cholesterol) and increased their intake of antioxidants. Though the researchers commented that their study found that sage did not affect the regulation of glucose in healthy women, their findings nevertheless demonstrated that drinking sage tea was safe, and their work may "pave the way for sage's effects to be tested in diabetic patients."[10] Still, it is important to add that the number of participants in this research was very small. It is hard to propose any definitive conclusion with so few study subjects.

Acute Sore Throat

In a study published in 2009 in the *European Journal of Medical Research,* researchers from Switzerland compared the efficacy of treating an acute sore throat with a spray containing the two herbs echinacea and sage or a spray containing chlorhexidine and lidocaine, an antiseptic antibacterial agent and a local anesthetic that works by stopping nerves from sending pain signals. Each spray had a corresponding placebo. The cohort consisted of 154 patients who had a sore throat for not more than 72 hours prior to inclusion in the study. By the time the results were evaluated, the cohort was down to 143 people. The researchers found that both sprays were similarly effective and were well tolerated by the participants.[11]

Is Sage Beneficial?

Sage appears to have a number of benefits. It may well be an herb that many people should discuss with their medical providers.

Notes

1. The George Mateljan Foundation Website. www.whfoods.com.
2. The George Mateljan Foundation Website. www.whfoods.com.
3. Scholey, A. B., N. T. Tidesley, C. G. Ballard, et al. May 2008. "An Extract of Salvia (Sage) with Anticholinesterase Properties Improves Memory and Attention in Healthy Older Volunteers." *Psychopharmacology* 198(1): 127–139.
4. Kennedy, D. O., F. L. Dodd, B. C. Robertson, et al. August 2011. "Monoterpenoid Extract of Sage (*Salvia lavandulaefolia*) with Cholinesterase Inhibiting Properties Improves Cognitive Performance and Mood in Healthy Adults." *Journal of Psychopharmacology* 25(8): 1088–1100.
5. Moss, L., M. Rouse, K. A. Wesnes, and M. Moss. July 2010. "Differential Effects of the Aromas of *Salvia* Species on Memory and Mood." *Human Psychopharmacology: Clinical and Experimental* 25(5): 388–396.
6. Akhondzadeh, S., M. Noroozian, M. Mohammadi, et al. February 2003. "*Salvia officinalis* Extract in the Treatment of Patients with Mild to Moderate Alzheimer's Disease: A Double Blind, Randomized and Placebo-Controlled Trial." *Journal of Clinical Pharmacy and Therapeutics* 28(1): 53–59.
7. Cwikla, C., K. Schmidt, A. Matthias, et al. May 2010. "Investigations into the Antibacterial Activities of Phytotherapeutics against *Helicobacter pylori* and *Campylobacter jejuni*." *Phytotherapy Research* 24(5): 649–656.
8. Bouaziz, M., T. Yangui, S. Sayadi, and A. Dhouib. November 2009. "Disinfectant Properties of Essential Oils from *Salvia officinalis* L. Cultivated in Tunisia." *Food and Chemical Toxicology* 47(11): 2755–2760.
9. Reuter, J., A. Jocher, S. Hornstein, et al. September 2007. "Sage Extract Rich in Phenolic Diterpenes Inhibits Ultraviolet-Induced Erythema In Vivo." *Planta Medica* 73(11): 1190–1191.
10. Sá, C. M., A. A. Ramos, M. F. Azevedo, et al. September 2009. "Sage Tea Drinking Improves Lipid Profile and Antioxidant Defences in Humans." *International Journal of Molecular Sciences* 10(9): 3937–3950.
11. Schapowal, A., D. Berger, P. Klein, and A. Suter. September 2009. "Echinacea/Sage or Chlorhexidine/Lidocaine for Treating Acute Sore Throats: A Randomized Double-Blind Trial." *European Journal of Medical Research* 14(9): 406–412.

References and Resources

Magazines, Journals, and Newspapers

Akhondzadeh, S., M. Noroozian, M. Mohammadi, et al. February 2003. "*Salvia officinalis* Extract in the Treatment of Patients with Mild to Moderate Alzheimer's Disease: A Double Blind, Randomized and Placebo-Controlled Trial." *Journal of Clinical Pharmacy and Therapeutics* 28(1): 53–59.

Bouaziz, M., T. Yangui, S. Sayadi, and A. Dhouib. November 2009. "Disinfectant Properties of Essential Oils from *Salvia officinalis* L. Cultivated in Tunisia." *Food and Chemical Toxicology* 47(11): 2755–2760.

Cwikla, C., K. Schmidt, A. Matthias, et al. May 2010. "Investigations into the Antibacterial Activities of Phytotherapeutics against *Helicobacter pylori* and *Campylobacter jejuni*." *Phytotherapy Research* 24(5): 649–656.

Kennedy, D.O., F.L. Dodd, B.C. Robertson, et al. August 2011. "Monoterpenoid Extract of Sage (*Salvia lavandulaefolia*) with Cholinesterase Inhibiting Properties Improves Cognitive Performance and Mood in Healthy Adults." *Journal of Psychopharmacology* 25(8): 1088–1100.

Moss, L., M. Rouse, K.A. Wesnes, and M. Moss. July 2010. "Differential Effects of the Aromas of *Salvia* Species on Memory and Mood." *Human Psychopharmacology: Clinical and experimental* 25(5): 388–396.

Reuter, J., A. Jocher, S. Hornstein, et al. September 2007. "Sage Extract Rich in Phenolic Diterpenes Inhibits Ultraviolet-Induced Erythema In Vivo." *Planta Medica* 73(11): 1190–1191.

Sá, C.M., A.A. Ramos, M.F. Azevedo, et al. September 2009. "Sage Tea Drinking Improves Lipid Profile and Antioxidant Defences in Humans." *International Journal of Molecular Sciences* 10(9): 3937–3950.

Schapowal, A., D. Berger, P. Klein, and A. Suter. September 2009. "Echinacea/Sage or Chlorhexidine/Lidocaine for Treating Acute Sore Throats: A Randomized Double-Blind Trial." *European Journal of Medical Research* 14(9): 406–412.

Scholey, A.B., N.T. Tidesley, C.G. Ballard, et al. May 2008. "An Extract of Salvia (Sage) with Anticholinesterase Properties Improves Memory and Attention in Healthy Older Volunteers." *Psychopharmacology* 198(1): 127–139.

Website
The George Mateljan Foundation. www.whfoods.com.

Sea Buckthorn 🌿

Scientifically known as *Hippophae rhamnoides,* sea buckthorn, which may also be written as seabuckthorn, is believed to be useful for a wide variety of medical concerns. While generally considered to be an effective treatment for skin problems, such as wounds, burns, lesions, eczema, and sun damage, sea buckthorn has also been used for digestive and respiratory disorders and cardiovascular health. A 2010 article in *Better Nutrition* summarized the benefits of this herb. According to the article, sea buckthorn is a powerful "nutrient-packed shrub" that contains carotenoids, tocopherals, sterols, vitamins B1, B2, B5, B6, C, folate, flavonoids, and fatty acids, such as omega-3, omega-6, omega-7, and omega-9. It even has high concentrations of palmitoleic acid—"a fatty acid naturally found in sebum—the oil that lubricates the skin." To many, sea buckthorn is "the Swiss Army knife of supplements." It may be found in a wide range of products such as "body oils, creams, soaps and shampoos, juices, jams, candies, elixirs, wine and beer."[1] Still, it is important to examine what researchers have learned.

Wound Healing

In a study published in 2009 in *Food and Chemical Toxicology,* researchers from India applied two different doses of sea buckthorn seed oil to burn wounds on rats for a period of seven days. As a control, they had rats with burns that they did not treat. The researchers found that the sea buckthorn seed oil "augmented the wound healing process." And, they concluded that sea buckthorn seed oil "possesses significant wound healing activity and has no associated toxicity or side effects."[2]

In a study published a year earlier, in 2008, in *Wound Repair and Regeneration,* some of the same researchers from India examined the use of an herbal formulation containing sea buckthorn, aloe vera, and tumeric to treat the wounds of rats with and without diabetes. The researchers found that the herbal formation "showed potent wound healing activity in both normal . . . [and] diabetic rats."[3] If this finding proves to be applicable to humans, it may have life-enhancing effects for people with diabetes who frequently have wound-healing problems.

Cardiovascular Health

In a randomized, double-blind trial published in 2009 in the *European Journal of Nutrition,* researchers from Finland examined the effect that a low dose of sea buckthorn berries had on circulating lipid markers (associated with cardiovascular disease) as well as concentrations of flavonol in the blood. For three months, the members of the cohort, which consisted of 229 healthy participants, consumed 28 g/day of sea buckthorn berry or placebo. When compared to those consuming placebos, the researchers found that "the consumption of SBB [sea buckthorn berry] increased the plasma concentration of the flavonols quercetin and isorhamnetin significantly." However, there was no significant change in the concentration of the flavonol kaempferol, and sea buckthorn berries did not alter lipid markers or triglyceride levels.[4]

In a study published in 2008 in the *Journal of Ethnopharmacology,* researchers from China and Denmark investigated the antihypertensive role of sea buckthorn in rats fed large amounts of sucrose. The researchers began by dividing rats into two groups. The first group consisted of 11 rats; they were fed a normal rat diet. The second group of 55 rats, which were all fed high-sucrose diets, was divided into five groups, each containing 11 rats. One group of rats was the "model control." A second group was placed on the antihypertensive medication irbesartan. The final three groups were fed different doses of sea buckthorn. The researchers found that hypertension (high blood pressure), hyperinsulinmia (excess levels of insulin circulating in the blood), dyslipidemia (abnormal amounts of lipids in the blood), and activated angiotensin (hormone released by kidneys that increases blood pressure) triggered by the high sucrose diet were able to be "ameliorated or modulated" by intake of sea buckthorn. The best results were obtained with a dose of 150 mg/kg/day.[5]

In a study published in 2009 in *Clinical Hemorheology and Microcirculation,* researchers from Japan fed hypertensive, stroke-prone rats regular rat food supplemented with sea buckthorn dry fruits for 60 days. The control rats were fed regular rat food without the sea buckthorn supplement. The researchers found that the rats fed the supplemented food had significant decreases in "mean arterial blood pressure, heart rate, total plasma cholesterol, triglycerides, and glycated hemoglobin." Moreover, "there was a trend for an increase in the total capillary density." The researchers concluded that sea buckthorn fruit "improved the metabolic processes accompanied by reduction of hypertensive stress on the ventricular microvessels."[6]

In a study published in 2009 in *Sichuan Da Xue Xue Bao Yi Xue Ban* (*Journal of Sichuan University: Medical Science Edition*), researchers based in China attempted to understand the role that sea buckthorn may play in treating spontaneously hypertensive rats. The researchers divided 12-week-old spontaneously hypertensive rats into three groups. One group of rats was treated with sea buckthorn; a second group was treated with Enalapril, a high blood pressure medication; and a third group was treated with hydrochlorothiazide, a diuretic that is often used to lower blood pressure. There were also two control groups. At the end of 12 weeks, the researchers found that the systolic blood pressure levels of the rats on sea buckthorn were significantly lower. They were similar to the levels seen in rats treated with both Enalapril and hydrochlorothiazide.[7]

Cardiovascular Disease and Type 2 Diabetes

In a study published in 2010 in the *Journal of Food Biochemistry,* researchers from China investigated the antihyperglycemic activity of sea buckthorn seed residues in 10 rats without type 2 diabetes, 10 rats with type 2 diabetes, and 10 rats with type 2 diabetes that were fed a daily dose of sea buckthorn seed residues for 10 weeks. The researchers found that the administrations of the sea buckthorn seed residues "lowered body weight, serum glucose, total cholesterol and low-density lipoprotein cholesterol levels in diabetic rats" while it also "significantly increased insulin sensitivity."[8]

Sea Buckthorn and the Health of Children with Type 1 Diabetes

In a study published in 2008 in *Acta Physiologica Hungarica,* researchers from Romania examined whether a supplement containing sea buckthorn and blueberry would improve some of the health problems faced by children with type 1 diabetes. During their trial, the researchers treated 30 children who had type 1 diabetes with the supplement for a period of two months. The researchers found that the supplement positively addressed a few problems. For example, they noted that after treatment, the children had significantly higher levels of c-peptide concentrations in their bodies. That meant that the children were producing higher amounts of insulin. At the same time, their levels of glycated hemoglobin were significantly reduced. So, the sugar levels in their bodies were lower. The researchers concluded that "treatment with this dietary supplement has a beneficial effect in the treatment of type 1 diabetic children, and it should be considered as a phytotherapeutic product in the fight against diabetes mellitus."[9]

Is Sea Buckthorn Beneficial?

Though it would be useful to have more research on sea buckthorn, it clearly has a number of obvious benefits. Most significantly, from the research reviewed in this entry, it seems effective for skin problems and improving cardiovascular health.

Notes

1. Erickson, Kim. January 2010. "Secrets of Sea Buckthorn: Learn Why This Natural Supplement Is Great for Skin, Heart Health, and More." *Better Nutrition* 72(1): 26.

2. Upadhyay, N. K., R. Kumar, S. K. Mandotra, et al. June 2009. "Safety and Healing Efficacy of Sea Buckthorn (*Hippophae rhamnoides* L.) Seed Oil on Burn Wounds in Rats." *Food and Chemical Toxicology* 47(6): 1146–1153.
3. Gupta, A., N. K. Upadhyay, R. C. Sawhney, and R. Kumar. November–December 2008. "A Poly-Herbal Formulation Accelerates Normal and Impaired Diabetic Wound Healing." *Wound Repair and Regeneration* 16(6): 784–790.
4. Larmo, P. S., B. Yang, S. A. Hurme, et al. August 2009. "Effect of a Low Dose of Sea Buckthorn Berries on Circulating Concentrations of Cholesterol, Triacyglycerols, and Flavonols in Health Adults." *European Journal of Nutrition* 48(5): 277–282.
5. Pang, X., J. Zhao, W. Zhang, et al. May 2008. "Antihypertensive Effect of Total Flavones Extracted from Seed Residues of *Hippophae rhamnoides* L. in Sucrose-Fed Rats." *Journal of Ethnopharmacology* 117(2): 325–331.
6. Koyama, T., A. Taka, and H. Togashi. 2009. "Effects of a Herbal Medicine, *Hippophae rhamnoides*, on Cardiovascular Functions and Coronary Microvessels in the Spontaneously Hypertensive Stroke-Prone Rat." *Clinical Hemorheology and Microcirculation* 41(1): 17–26.
7. He, J., Y. Chen, H. Y. Xiao, et al. May 2009. "Effect of Total Flavonoids of *Hippophae rhamnoides* L. on the Expression of MCP-1 in Aorta of Spontaneously Hypertensive Rats." *Sichuan Da Xue Xue Bao Yi Xue Ban* [*Journal of Sichuan University: Medical Science Edition*] 40(3): 481–485.
8. Zhang, Wen, Jingjing Zhao, Xinglei Zhu, et al. August 2010. "Antihyperglycemic Effect of Aqueous Extract of Sea Buckthorn (*Hippophae rhamnoides* L.) Seed Residues in Streptozotocin-Treated and High Fat-Diet-Fed Rats." *Journal of Food Biochemistry* 34(4): 856–868.
9. Nemes-Nagy, E., T. Szocs-Molnár, T. Dunca, et al. December 2008. "Effects of Dietary Supplement Containing Blueberry and Sea Buckthorn Concentrate on Antioxidant Capacity in Type 1 Diabetic Children." *Acta Physiologica Hungarica* 95(4): 383–393.

References and Resources

Magazines, Journals, and Newspapers

Erickson, Kim. January 2010. "Secrets of Sea Buckthorn: Learn Why This Natural Supplement Is Great for Skin, Heart Health, and More." *Better Nutrition* 72(1): 26.

Gupta, A., N. K. Upadhyay, R. C. Sawhney, and R. Kumar. November–December 2008. "A Poly-Herbal Formulation Accelerates Normal and Impaired Diabetic Wound Healing." *Wound Repair and Regeneration* 16(6): 784–790.

He, J., Y. Chen, H. Y. Xiao, et al. May 2009. "Effect of Total Flavonoids of *Hippophae rhamnoides* L. on the Expression of MCP-1 in Aorta of Spontaneously Hypertensive Rats." *Sichuan Da Xue Xue Bao Yi Xue Ban* [*Journal of Sichuan University: Medical Science Edition*] 40(3): 481–485.

Koyama, T., A. Taka, and H. Togashi. 2009. "Effects of a Herbal Medicine, *Hippophae rhamnoides*, on Cardiovascular Functions and Coronary Microvessels in the Spontaneously Hypertensive Stroke-Prone Rat." *Clinical Hemorheology and Microcirculation* 41(1): 17–26.

Larmo, P. S., B. Yang, S. A. Hurme, et al. August 2009. "Effect of a Low Dose of Sea Buckthorn Berries on Circulating Concentrations of Cholesterol, Triacylglycerols, and Flavonols in Health Adults." *European Journal of Nutrition* 48(5): 277–282.

Nemes-Nagy, E., T. Szocs-Molnár, I. Dunca, et al. December 2008. "Effect of Dietary Supplement Containing Blueberry and Sea Buckthorn Concentrate on Antioxidant Capacity in Type 1 Diabetic Children." *Acta Physiologica Hungarica* 95(4): 383–393.

Pang, X., J. Zhao, W. Zhang, et al. May 2008. "Antihypertensive Effect of Total Flavones Extracted from Seed Residues of *Hippophae rhamnoides* L. in Sucrose-Fed Rats." *Journal of Ethnopharmacology* 117(2): 325–331.

Upadhyay, N. K., R. Kumar, S. K. Mandotra, et al. June 2009. "Safety and Healing Efficacy of Sea buckthorn (*Hippophae rhamnoides* L.) Seed Oil on Burn Wounds in Rats." *Food and Chemical Toxicology* 47(6): 1146–1153.

Zhang, Wen, Jingjing Zhao, Xinglei Zhu, et al. August 2010. "Antihyperglycemic Effect of Aqueous Extract of Sea Buckthorn (*Hippophae rhamnoides* L.) Seed Residues in Streptozotocin-Treated and High Fat-Diet-Fed Rats." *Journal of Food Biochemistry* 34(4): 856–868.

Websites

American Botanical Council. www.cms.herbalgram.org.

Sea Buckthorn Research. www.seabuckthornresearch.com.

St. John's Wort 🌿

Scientifically known as *Hypericum perforatum,* St. John's wort is probably one of the world's most recognizable herbs. It is also extremely controversial. While St. John's wort is praised by many for bringing relief to people suffering from complex medical problems such as depression, fatigue, anxiety, insomnia, and loss of appetite, it is also criticized for interfering with or compromising the integrity of other medications. Additionally, it is possible that taking St. John's wort supplementation may create a health problem such as mania in someone who is depressed and psychosis in someone who is dealing with a diagnosis of schizophrenia.[1] It is important to review what researchers have learned.

Depression and Anxiety

In a randomized, double-blind, placebo-controlled study published in 2009 in *Human Psychopharmacology: Clinical and Experimental,* researchers from Australia examined whether people suffering from a major depressive disorder and anxiety could benefit from treatment with St. John's wort and kava, an herb that is sometimes used for anxiety. While there were 114 initial volunteers, only 28 adults (21 women and 7 men between the ages of 18 and 64) fulfilled the criteria of the study. For example, the subjects could not currently be taking St. John's wort or kava. The trial included a two-week placebo period followed by two controlled phases of four weeks each. During the first controlled phase, St. John's wort and kava had "a significant effect on depression." However, during the second controlled phase, these results were not replicated. The researchers concluded that "the combination of SJW [St. John's wort] and Kava demonstrated efficacy in reducing depression within one of two controlled phases of doubled-blind RCT [randomized controlled trial] on people with MDD [major depressive disorder] and comorbid anxiety."[2]

A 2009 article in *Evidence-Based Mental Health* summarized a British researcher's meta-analysis of studies on the use of St. John's wort for depression. Twenty-nine double-blind studies ($n = 5489$) met the criteria required for inclusion. Of these, 18 compared St. John's wort with a placebo and 17 compared St. John's wort to standard antidepressants. In 19 studies, the subjects had mild to moderate depression; in 9 studies, the subjects had moderate to severe depression. The researcher found that St. John's wort "extracts are more effective than placebo in people with major depression," and "they are similarly effective to standard antidepressants but with fewer side effects."[3]

In an eight-week, double-blind, placebo-controlled, randomized trial published in 2010 in the *Journal of Psychiatric Research,* researchers from Germany and New Jersey tested the effect that St. John's wort had on people dealing with symptoms of atypical depression, such as hyperphagia (overeating) and hypersomnia (excessive daytime sleepiness). The cohort consisted of 100 subjects with mild atypical depression and 100 subjects with moderate atypical depression. The subjects took either a daily dose of 600 mg of St. John wort extract or a placebo. Although the researchers found that there was no clear benefit to subjects with mild atypical depression, subjects with moderate atypical depression experienced "a highly significant benefit."[4]

Premenstrual Syndrome

In a randomized, double-blind, placebo-controlled crossover study that was conducted at the Institute of Psychological Sciences at the University of Leeds in the United Kingdom and was published in 2010 in *CNS Drugs,* researchers tested the ability of St. John's wort to relieve symptoms from premenstrual syndrome. The cohort consisted of 36 women between the ages of 18 and 45 who had regular menstrual cycles and mild premenstrual syndrome symptoms, such as anxiety, depression, aggression, and impulsivity. After all the women had a "two-cycle placebo run-in phase," they were randomly assigned to take either St. John's wort (900 mg/day) or a placebo for two months. At the end of that time, there was a placebo-treated washout cycle, which was followed by two months on the alternate supplement. The researchers found that the women with premenstrual syndrome symptoms obtained more relief from a daily dose of St. John's wort than a daily dose of a placebo.[5]

Hot Flashes

In a study published in 2010 in *Menopause,* researchers from Iran tested the ability of St. John's wort to control hot flashes in 100 women with an average age of 50.4. For eight weeks, 50 women took 20 drops of St. John's wort three times each day; the other 50 women took a placebo of distilled water. Forty-five women in the treatment group and 43 in the placebo group completed the study. In the women taking St. John's wort, the number of hot flashes began to decline during the first four weeks. But, there was a greater decline during the last four weeks. The women taking the placebo did not show any significant decrease in hot flashes during the first four weeks. But, they had some improvement during the second month, though not as great as those on the herb. The researchers concluded that "there was a significant difference between the two study groups during intervention, and women who received St. John's wort felt more comfortable than did those who were on placebo."[6]

Smoking Cessation

In a randomized, placebo-controlled, clinical trial published in 2010 in *The Journal of Alternative and Complementary Medicine,* researchers from the Mayo Clinic College of Medicine in Rochester, Minnesota investigated the use of St. John's wort for assistance with smoking cessation. A total of 118 subjects were randomly assigned to take one of two different doses of St. John's wort or a matching placebo tablet three times per day. This was combined with a behavioral intervention. The trial continued for 12 weeks. The researchers found that St. John's wort did not assist with smoking cessation and "has little role in the treatment of tobacco dependence."[7]

Irritable Bowel Syndrome

In a randomized, double-blind, placebo-controlled study published in 2010 in *The American Journal of Gastroenterology,* Mayo Clinic researchers from Rochester, Minnesota and Jacksonville, Florida tested St. John's wort for the treatment of irritable bowel syndrome. The cohort consisted of 70 subjects with a mean age of 42. For 12 weeks, the subjects received either 450-mg tablets twice daily or a placebo. At the end of the trial, the subjects taking the placebo reported more improvement in their irritable bowel symptoms than those on St. John's wort. The researchers concluded that St. John's wort "seems to be less effective than placebo."[8]

Is St. John's Wort Beneficial?

St. John's wort may well be beneficial for certain medical concerns. But, it is important to know that there are researchers who caution that it should not be used with certain medications. For example, in an article published in 2010 in *Pharmacological Research,* a researcher from Milan, Italy said that there are a number of different herbs, including St. John's wort, that have the potential to interact with medications, which may "lead to toxicity or loss of therapeutic efficacy." According to the researcher, "in order to assess this risk, it is important to consider all potential mechanisms of pharmacokinetic interference."[9] Moreover, a 2010 article in the *Journal of Psychosocial Nursing and Mental Health Services* noted that "a systematic review of available literature provided very weak evidence for the safety of the use of St. John's wort during pregnancy and lactation."[10] And, a 2010 article in *Heart Advisor* advised people with cardiovascular diseases to discuss herbal use with their physicians. Specifically, it mentioned that St. John's wort may interact with certain medications that stop abnormal rhythms of the heart.[11]

Notes

1. MedlinePlus Website. www.medlineplus.gov.
2. Sarris, J., D. J. Kavanagh, G. Deed, and K. M. Bone. January 2009. "St. John's Wort and Kava in Treating Major Depressive Disorder with Comorbid Anxiety: A Randomised Double-Blind Placebo-Controlled Pilot Trial." *Human Psychopharmacology: Clinical and Experimental* 24(1): 41–48.
3. Ernst, Edzard. 2009. "St. John's Wort Superior to Placebo and Similar to Antidepressants for Major Depression but with Fewer Side Effects." *Evidence-Based Mental Health* 12:78.
4. Mannel, Marcus, Ulrike Kuhn, Ulrich Schmidt, et al. September 2010. "St. John's Wort LI160 for the Treatment of Depression with Atypical Features—A Double-Blind, Randomized, and Placebo-Controlled Trial." *Journal of Psychiatric Research* 44(12): 760–767.
5. Canning, Sarah, Mitch Waterman, Nic Orsi, et al. March 2010. "The Efficacy of *Hypericum perforatum* (St. John's Wort) for the Treatment of Premenstrual Syndrome: A Randomized, Double-Blind, Placebo-Controlled Trial." *CNS Drugs* 24(3): 207–225.
6. Abdali, K., M. Khajehei, and H. R. Tabatabaee. March 2010. "Effect of St. John's Wort on Severity, Frequency, and Duration of Hot Flashes in Premenopausal, Perimenopausal, and Postmenopausal Women: A Randomized, Double-Blind, Placebo-Controlled Study." *Menopause* 17(2): 326–331.
7. Sood, A., J. O. Ebbert, K. Prasad, et al. July 2010. "Randomized Clinical Trial of St. John's Wort for Smoking Cessation." *The Journal of Alternative and Complementary Medicine* 16(7): 761–767.
8. Saito, Yuri A., Enrique Ray, Ann E. Almazar-Elder, et al. January 2010. "A Randomized, Double-Blind, Placebo-Controlled Trial of St. John's Wort for Treating Irritable Bowel Syndrome." *The American Journal of Gastroenterology* 105: 170–177.
9. Colalto, Cristiano. September 2010. "Herbal Interactions on Absorption of Drugs: Mechanisms of Action and Clinical Risk Assessment." *Pharmacological Research* 62(3): 207–227.
10. Gossler, S. M. November 2010. "Use of Complementary and Alternative Therapies during Pregnancy, Postpartum, and Lactation." *Journal of Psychosocial Nursing and Mental Health Services* 48(11): 30–36.
11. "Share Your Herbal Supplement Use with Your Doctor: Research Shows That Some Popular Supplements May Be Dangerous for People with Cardiovascular Diseases." April 2010. *Heart Advisor* 13(4): 6–7.

References and Resources

Magazines, Journals, and Newspapers

Abdali, K., M. Khajehei, and H. R. Tabatabaee. March 2010. "Effect of St. John's Wort on Severity, Frequency, and Duration of Hot Flashes in Premenopausal, Perimenopausal, and Postmenopausal Women: A Randomized, Double-Blind, Placebo-Controlled Study." *Menopause* 17(2): 326–331.

Canning, Sarah, Mitch Waterman, Nic Orsi, et al. March 2010. "The Efficacy of *Hypericum perforatum* (St. John's Wort) for the Treatment of Premenstrual Syndrome: A Randomized, Double-Blind, Placebo-Controlled Trial." *CNS Drugs* 24(3): 207–225.

Colalto, Cristiano. September 2010. "Herbal Interactions on Absorption of Drugs: Mechanisms of Action and Clinical Risk Assessment." *Pharmacological Research* 62(3): 207–227.

Ernst, Edzard. 2009. "St. John's Wort Superior to Placebo and Similar to Antidepressants for Major Depression but with Fewer Side Effects." *Evidence-Based Mental Health* 12: 78.

Gossler, S. M. November 2010. "Use of Complementary and Alternative Therapies during Pregnancy, Postpartum, and Lactation." *Journal of Psychosocial Nursing and Mental Health Services* 48(11): 30–36.

Mannel, Marcus, Ulrike Kuhn, Ulrich Schmidt, et al. September 2010. "St. John's Wort Extract LI160 for the Treatment of Depression with Atypical Features—a Double-Blind Randomized and Placebo-Controlled Trial." *Journal of Psychiatric Research* 44(12): 760–767.

Saito, Yuri A., Enrique Ray, Ann E. Almazar-Elder, et al. January 2010. "A Randomized, Double-Blind, Placebo-Controlled Trial of St. John's Wort for Treating Irritable Bowel Syndrome." *The American Journal of Gastroenterology* 105: 170–177.

Sarris, J., D. J. Kavanagh, G. Deed, and K. M. Bone. January 2009. "St. John's Wort and Kava in Treating Major Depression Disorder with Comorbid Anxiety: A Randomised Double-Blind Placebo-Controlled Pilot Trial." *Human Psychopharmacology: Clinical and Experimental* 24(1): 41–48.

"Share Your Herbal Supplement Use with Your Doctor: Research Shows that Some Popular Supplements May be Dangerous for People with Cardiovascular Diseases." April 2010. *Heart Advisor* 13(4): 6–7.

Sood, A., J. O. Ebbert, K. Prasad, et al. July 2010. "Randomized Clinical Trial of St. John's Wort for Smoking Cessation." *The Journal of Alternative and Complementary Medicine* 16(7): 761–767.

Website

MedlinePlus. www.medlineplus.gov.

Stinging Nettle 🌿

Used medicinally for hundreds of years, stinging nettle has fine hairs on its leaves and stems. These fine hairs contain chemicals that are released when they come into contact with skin. Normally, this is quite uncomfortable. However, when stinging nettle is placed on a painful part of the body, it reduces the discomfort. According to scientists, stinging nettle lowers the levels of inflammatory chemicals in the body and interferes with the way the body transmits pain signals.[1]

But, stinging nettle, scientifically known as *Urtica dioica,* has also been used for a host of other medical problems. These include painful muscles and joints, eczema, arthritis, gout, anemia, urinary tract infections, enlarged prostate (benign prostatic hyperplasia), hay fever (allergic rhinitis), sprains and strains, tendonitis, and insect bites.[2] Is stinging nettle really effective for all these conditions? It is important to review what researchers have learned.

Benign Prostatic Hyperplasia

In a prospective, randomized, double-blind, placebo-controlled, crossover study published in 2005 in the *Journal of Herbal Pharmacotherapy,* a researcher from Iran evaluated the ability of stinging nettle to help relieve the lower urinary track symptoms associated with an enlarged prostate, such as problems with the flow of urine. The researcher began by dividing the cohort of 620 men into two groups. For six months, one group received stinging nettle and the other took a placebo. Then, the groups switched. The men who had taken stinging nettle were placed on a placebo, and those who had taken a placebo were given stinging nettle.

Ninety percent of the men completed the study. In general, when the men took stinging nettle, they saw improvements in symptoms. When they discontinued the herb, the symptoms returned. "At 18-month follow-up, only patients who continued therapy had a favorable treatment variables value." The researcher concluded that stinging nettle had "beneficial effects in the treatment of symptomatic BPH [benign prostatic hyperplasia]."[3]

Lowers Severity of Urinary Tract Symptoms

In a study published in 2010 in *Urologia,* Italian researchers investigated whether a combination of three herbs—stinging nettle, saw palmetto, and

an herb from the bark of the cluster pine tree (*Pinus pinaster*)—could reduce the incidence of lower urinary tract symptoms. During the years 2007
and 2008, 320 men were treated with a combination of these herbs. All
the men received these supplements for as little as 30 days or as long as a
year. Some patients were also placed on antibiotics or alpha-blockers. The
researchers noted that "a marked reduction of LUTS [lower urinary tract
symptoms] was observed in 85% of evaluable cases, especially with regard
to pain and irritative symptoms."[4]

Prostatitis

In a prospective, randomized study published in 2009 in the *International
Journal of Antimicrobial Agents,* researchers from France evaluated the
therapeutic effect of stinging nettle and other herbs on men with chronic
bacterial prostatitis (infection of the prostate gland) who are treated with
prulifloxacin (an antibiotic). The cohort consisted of 143 men with chronic
bacterial prostatitis. Everyone received prulifloxacin 600 mg daily for
14 days. While 37 men were treated only with the antibiotic, 106 men
were also treated with stinging nettle, saw palmetto (herb often used for
prostate problems), curcumin (source of the spice turmeric), and quercetin
(an antioxidant). The results were truly remarkable. One month after the
treatment, 89.6% of those who received the antibiotics and the herbs had
not experienced a recurrence of their prostatitis symptoms. On the other
hand, only 27% of those who only had antibiotic therapy were recurrence-
free. The addition of the herbal extracts significantly improved the clinical
efficacy of the antibiotics.[5]

Osteoarthritis

In a study published in 2009 in *Alternative Therapies in Health and Medicine,* researchers from San Jose, California, recruited 23 patients with
confirmed osteoarthritis. For two weeks, these subjects applied a cream
containing stinging nettle twice each day to the affected areas. The patients reported improved functioning and reduced pain. Only two people
noted side effects—transient tingling and mild discomfort. According to
the researchers, "many of the enrolled subjects requested continuance
of the treatment after the study was over." The researchers concluded
that "If stinging nettle effectively relieves pain, then that is valuable in
its own right." Additionally, "managing pain relief itself may slow or

reverse pathophysiology by allowing for regular exercise, thereby increasing protective muscular strength and improving biomechanics."[6]

In another study published in 2009 in *Arthritis Research & Therapy,* researchers from France tested the ability of Phytalgic, a food supplement that contained stinging nettle, fish oil, vitamin E, and zinc, to relieve the pain associated with osteoarthritis of the hip or knee. This randomized, double-blind, parallel-group, three-month clinical trial had a cohort of 81 people with osteoarthritis who regularly took nonsteroidal anti-inflammatory medications (NSAIDs) or analgesics to help cope with their pain. The participants, who had an average age of 57 years, were divided into two groups. One group of 41 took three capsules per day of Phytalgic; the other group of 40 took three similarly appearing placebos each day. The researchers found that the people taking the supplements experienced a significant reduction—greater than 50%—in the amount of pain medication they used. They concluded that they had demonstrated that "three capsules a day over three months of this nutraceutical compound might decrease disease scores in patients with osteoarthritis of the knee and/or hip, and reduce their use of analgesics and NSAIDs."[7]

Allergic Rhinitis

In an article published in 2009 in *Phytotherapy Research,* researchers based in Florida examined the in vitro properties of stinging nettle extract. They found that stinging nettle extract has multiple anti-inflammatory activities, and it inhibited "several key inflammatory events that cause the symptoms of seasonal allergies [allergic rhinitis]." The researchers noted that their results "provide, for the first time, a mechanistic understanding of the role of nettle extracts in reducing allergic and other inflammatory responses in vitro."[8]

Cardiovascular Health

In a study published in 2009 in *Zhong Xi Yi Jie He Xue Bao* (*Journal of Chinese Integrative Medicine*), researchers from Iran examined the role that stinging nettle may play in lowering cholesterol levels in rats. For four weeks, male rats were fed a high-cholesterol diet and either 100 or 300 mg/kg of stinging nettle extract or 10 mg/kg of lovastatin, a cholesterol-lowering medication. The researchers found that both doses of stinging nettle "significantly reduced the levels of total cholesterol (TC) and low-density lipoprotein-cholesterol (LDL-C)."[9]

Improvements in Health and Memory

In a study published in 2009 in *The Journal of Nutritional Biochemistry,* researchers from Hungary, Finland, and Korea reviewed the effect of stinging nettle and exercise on rats with injection-induced brain lesions. The lesions had caused a deterioration in behaviors and learning abilities. The researchers found that stinging nettle "has an effective antioxidant role . . . and could also promote learning performance in the brain." They concluded that their findings "revealed that natural, physiological factors such as nutrition and regular exercise could play an important role in brain health."[10]

Is Stinging Nettle Beneficial?

Stinging appears to have a number of benefits. However, a brief article in a 2008 issue of the *European Journal of Emergency Medicine* should be noted. Medical providers described a 78-year-old man with diabetes who became hypoglycemic after taking a supplement containing four herbs, including stinging nettle. The authors of the article commented that "patients with multiple comorbidities may well take a nonprescribed medication, including herbal remedies, with deleterious effects."[11]

Notes

1. University of Maryland Medical Center Website. www.umm.edu.
2. University of Maryland Medical Center Website. www.umm.edu.
3. Safarinejad, M.R. 2005. "*Urtica dioica* for Treatment of Benign Prostatic Hyperplasia: A Prospective, Randomized, Double-Blind, Placebo-Controlled Crossover Study." *Journal of Herbal Pharmacotherapy* 5(4): 1–11.
4. Pavone, C., D. Abbadessa, M.L. Tarantino, et al. September 2010. "Associating *Serenoa repens, Urtica dioica,* and *Pinus pinaster.* Safety and Efficacy in the Treatment of Lower Urinary Tract Symptoms. Prospective Study on 320 Patients." *Urologia* 77(1): 43–51.
5. Cai, T., S. Mazzoli, A. Bechi, et al. June 2009. "*Serenoa repens* Associated with *Urtica dioica* (ProstaMEV) and Curcumin and Quercitin (FlogMEV) Extracts Are Able to Improve the Efficacy of Prulifloxacin in Bacterial Prostatitis Patients: Results from a Prospective Randomised Study." *International Journal of Antimicrobial Agents* 33(6): 549–553.

6. Rayburn, K., E. Fleischbein, J. Song, et al. July–August 2009. "Stinging Nettle Cream for Osteoarthritis." *Alternative Therapies in Health and Medicine*
15(4): 60–61.

7. Jacquet, A., P. O. Girodet, A. Pariente, et al. 2009. "Phytalgic, a Food Supplement, vs. Placebo in Patients with Osteoarthritis of the Knee or Hip: A Randomised Double-Blind Placebo-Controlled Clinical Trial. *Arthritis Research
& Therapy* 11(6): R192.

8. Roschek, B. Jr., R. C. Fink, M. McMichael, and R. S. Alberte. July 2009.
"Nettle Extract (*Urtica dioica*)Affects Key Receptors and Enzymes Associated with Allergic Rhinitis." *Phytotherapy Research* 23(7): 920–926.

9. Nassiri-Asl, M., F. Zamansolt, E. Abbasi, et al. May 2009. "Effects of *Urtica
dioica* on Lipid Profile in Hypercholesterolemic Rats." *Zhong Xi Yi Jie He Xue
Bao* [*Journal of Chinese Integrative Medicine*] 7(5): 428–433.

10. Toldy, Anna, Mustafa Atalay, Krisztián Stadler, et al. December 2009.
"The Beneficial Effects of Nettle Supplementation and Exercise on Brain
Lesion and Memory in Rat." *The Journal of Nutritional Biochemistry*
20(12): 974–981.

11. Edgcumbe, D. P., and D. McAuley. August 2008. "Hypoglycaemia Related
to Ingestion of a Herbal Remedy." *European Journal of Emergency Medicine*
15(4): 236–237.

References and Resources

Magazines, Journals, and Newspapers

Cai, T., S. Mazzoli, A. Bechi, et al. June 2009. "*Serenoa repens* Associated with
Urtica dioica (ProstaMEV) and Curcumin and Quercitin (FlogMEV) Extracts
Are Able to Improve the Efficacy of Prulifloxacin in Bacterial Prostatitis Patients: Results from a Prospective Randomised Study." *International Journal
of Antimicrobial Agents* 33(6): 549–553.

Edgcumbe, D. P., and D. McAuley. "Hypoglycaemia Related to Ingestion
of a Herbal Remedy." *European Journal of Emergency Medicine* 15(4):
236–237.

Jacquet, A., P. O. Girodet, A. Pariente, et al. 2009. "Phytalgic, a Food Supplement,
vs. Placebo in Patients with Osteoarthritis of the Knee or Hip: A Randomised,
Double-Blind Placebo-Controlled Clinical Trial." *Arthritis Research & Therapy* 11(6): R192.

Nassiri-Asl, M., F. Zamansolt, E. Abbasi, et al. May 2009. "Effects of *Urtica dioica* Extract on Lipid Profile in Hypercholesterolemic Rats." *Zhong Xi Yi Jie He
Xue Bao* [*Journal of Chinese Integrative Medicine*] 7(5): 428–433.

Pavone, C., D. Abbadessa, M. L. Tarantino, et al. September 2010. "Associating
Serenoa repens, Urtica dioica, and *Pinus pinaster.* Safety ad Efficacy in the
Treatment of Lower Urinary Tract Symptoms. Prospective Study on 320 Pa-
tients." *Urologia* 77(1): 43–51.

Rayburn, K., E. Fleischbein, J. Song, et al. July–August 2009. "Stinging Nettle Cream for Osteoarthritis." *Alternative Therapies in Health and Medicine* 15(4): 60–61.

Roschek, B. Jr., R. C. Fink, M. McMichael, and R. S. Alberte. July 2009. "Nettle Extract (*Urtica dioica*) Affects Key Receptors and Enzymes Associated with Allergic Rhinitis." *Phytotherapy Research* 23(7): 920–926.

Safarinejad, M. R. 2005. "*Urtica dioica* for Treatment of Benign Prostatic Hyperplasia: A Prospective, Randomized, Double-Blind, Placebo-Controlled, Crossover Study." *Journal of Herbal Pharmacology* 5(4): 1–11.

Toldy, Anna, Mustafa Atalay, Krisztián Stadler, et al. December 2009. "The Beneficial Effects of Nettle Supplementation and Exercise on Brain Lesion and Memory in Rat." *The Journal of Nutritional Biochemistry* 20(12): 974–981.

Website
University of Maryland Medical Center. www.umm.edu.

Sweet Basil 🌿

A truly ancient herb, sweet basil, scientifically known as *Ocimum basilicum,* was initially grown in India, Asia, and Africa. In the ancient civilizations, it was acclaimed; in fact, the word basil may be traced to the Greek word *basilikohn,* which means "royal." Today, sweet basil is ubiquitous. It is grown throughout the world and is sold in a wide variety of venues ranging from local farmers' markets to giant supermarkets. People who use sweet basil often grow it in their homes.

Sweet basil contains excellent amounts of vitamin K and very good amounts of iron, calcium, and vitamin A. It also has good amounts of dietary fiber, manganese, magnesium, vitamin C, and potassium. Sweet basil is well-known for its antimicrobial and antibacterial properties, and basil is said to support the cardiovascular system.[1] But, what have the researchers learned?

Antimicrobial and Antibacterial

In a food study published in 2010 in *Bioscience, Biotechnology, and Biochemistry,* researchers from Thailand investigated the antimicrobial activity of nine essential oils—sweet basil, cinnamon, clove, fingerroot, garlic, lemongrass, oregano, thyme, and tumeric—against six strains of *Salmonella enteritidis*. (*S. enteritidis* is a bacterium that infects the ovaries of seemingly healthy hens. It contaminates the eggs before the shells are formed.) The findings were quite remarkable. Sweet basil oil was found to have "the strongest antimicrobial activity against all the tested bacteria." As a result, the researchers concluded that "based on its antimicrobial activity against *S. enteritidis* both *in vitro* and in a food model and acceptance by consumers when applied in food, basil oil is a candidate for a food preservative."[2]

In an in vitro study published in 2008 in the *African Journal of Traditional, Complementary and Alternative Medicines,* researchers from Turkey examined the antimicrobial actions of chloroform, acetone, and two different concentrations of methanol extracts of sweet basil against 10 bacteria and 4 strains of yeast. While the chloroform and acetone had no effect, the extracts of sweet basil "showed antimicrobial activity against the test microorganisms and caused the degradation of cell walls of sensitive bacteria."[3]

In a study published in 2009 in the *Journal of Applied Sciences,* researchers from Malaysia and Sudan evaluated the antibacterial activity of essential oils made from five types of ornamental basil and one type of basil that grows in the wild. The researchers tested these different basil essential oils on three types of bacteria—*Escherichia coli, Staphylococcus aureus,* and *Salmonella typhimurium* (a type of bacterium that causes typhoid fever that is uncommon in the United States). The researchers learned that "the essential oils of all six basil types showed strong [dose-dependent] antibacterial activity against" the bacteria tested. As a result, they concluded that "basil essential oil has potential clinical or food applications as an antibacterial agent."[4]

In an in vitro study published in 2009 in the *Journal of Biological Sciences,* Iranian researchers attempted to learn if sweet basil inhibited the growth of *Helicobacter pylori,* a bacterium that may cause gastritis, peptic ulcers, and gastric cancer. The researchers noted that *H. pylori* is a "difficult infection to eradicate," and it is becoming increasingly resistant to antibiotics. By the end of the study, all 45 clinical isolates of *H. pylori* were inhibited by the extract of sweet basil. However, when they tested the antibiotic amoxicillin against the bacteria, the researchers found that it "was significantly more [effective] than each of [the] fractions of sweet basil."

Nevertheless, the researchers noted that "sweet basil is recommended for food preparation and as an alternative to synthetic compounds to improve flavor and taste." As far as an alternative treatment for *H. pylori* is concerned, "further studies are necessary."[5]

In a study published in 2009 in the *Pakistan Journal of Pharmaceutical Sciences,* researchers from Nigeria obtained oral swabs from 18 male and female dental patients in Benin City, Nigeria. The patients had been diagnosed with a variety of dental ailments—dental caries, periodontitis, aveola abscess, gingivitis, and propritis. Using those swabs, the researchers were able to isolate 29 different organisms. Then, the researchers treated the bacteria with different concentrations of two types of basil—sweet basil and African basil. To varying degrees, the two types of basil were found to inhibit bacteria growth. But, African basil appeared to be more "active" than sweet basil.[6]

In a study published in 2008 in the *Journal of Food Protection,* researchers from Ireland evaluated the antimicrobial activity of 11 different plant essential oils against food-borne pathogens and spoilage bacteria that may be found in ready-to-eat vegetables. Each essential oil contained either basil, caraway, funnel, lemon balm, marjoram, nutmeg, oregano, parsley, rosemary, sage, or thyme. The essential oils were tested on eight different types of bacteria. The essential oils of basil and marjoram proved to be particularly effective against four types of bacteria—*Bacillus cereus, Enterobacter aerogenes, E. coli,* and *Salmonella.*[7]

Overall Health

In an in vitro study published in 2010 in *Plant Foods for Human Nutrition,* researchers from Ireland wanted to determine the amount of carotenoids found in a number of different herbs. Why carotenoids? They are a class of yellow to red pigments found in many foods that have been associated with health benefits such as reduced risk of age-related macular degeneration, some cancers, and cardiovascular disease. During the investigation, the researchers determined the carotenoid content of sweet basil, coriander, dill, mint, parsley, rosemary, sage, and tarragon. When compared to the other herbs, basil contained the highest levels of the carotenoids beta-carotene, lutein, and zeaxanthin. The researchers noted that "basil and coriander were superior in carotenoid content and bioaccessibility."[8]

Cardiovascular Support

In a study published in 2006 in *Phytotherapy Research,* researchers from Morocco and Italy evaluated the ability of sweet basil to lower lipid levels in rats. At the beginning of the trial, the researchers used a medication to induce high levels of cholesterol in rats. Then, the rats were divided into three groups. One group was treated with a cholesterol-lowering medication; a second group had sweet basil added to the diet; and a third group had no interventions. When compared to the control rats and the rats on medication after 24 hours, the rats with sweet basil in their diets had markedly lower levels of cholesterol. There was also evidence that sweet basil had strong antioxidant properties.[9]

In a study published in 2009 in the *Journal of Ethnopharmacology,* researchers from Morocco divided rats into three groups. One group was fed the standard diet; the second group was fed a diet that was high in cholesterol; and a third group was fed a high-cholesterol diet and basil extract. The researchers found that the addition of sweet basil appeared to ease some of the problems associated with a high-cholesterol diet. For example, the sweet basil reduced the aggregation of platelets, thereby lowering the risk of a heart attack. The researchers concluded that use of sweet basil "as [a] medicinal plant could be beneficial for [the] cardiovascular system."[10]

Is Sweet Basil Beneficial?

Though there is clearly a need for more well-designed research studies on sweet basil, it appears to be a beneficial addition to the diet.

Notes

1. The George Mateljan Foundation Website. www.whfoods.com.
2. Rattanachaikunsopon, Pongsak, and Parichat Phumkhachorn. June 2010. "Antimicrobial Activity of Basil (*Ocimum basilicum*) Oil against *Salmonella enteritidis* In Vitro and in Food." *Bioscience, Biotechnology, and Biochemistry* 74(6): 1200–1204.
3. Kaya, Ilhan, Nazife Yiğit, and Mehlika Benli. June 2008. "Antimicrobial Activity of Various Extracts of *Ocimum basilicum* L. and Observation of the Inhibition Effect of Bacterial Cells by Use of Scanning Electron Microscopy." *African Journal of Traditional, Complementary and Alternative Medicines* 5(4): 363–369.
4. Nour, A. H., S. A. Ekhussein, N. A. Osman, et al. 2009. "Antibacterial Activity of the Essential Oils of Sudanese Accessions of Basil (*Ocimum basilicum* L.)." *Journal of Applied Sciences* 9: 4161–4167.

5. Moghaddam, M. N., M. A. Khajeh-Karamoddin, and M. Ramezani. 2009. "*In Vitro* Anti-Bacterial Activity of Sweet Basil Fractions against *Helicobacter pylori.*" *Journal of Biological Sciences* 9: 276–279.

6. Ahonkhai, I., A. Ba, O. Edogun, and U. Mu. October 2009. "Antimicrobial Activities of the Volatile Oils of *Ocimum bacilicum* L. and *Ocimum gratissimum* L. (Lamiaceae) against Some Aerobic Dental Isolates." *Pakistan Journal of Pharmaceutical Sciences* 22(4): 405–409.

7. Gutierrez, J., G. Rodriguez, C. Barry-Ryan, and P. Bourke. September 2008. "Efficacy of Plant Essential Oils against Foodborne Pathogens and Spoilage Bacteria Associated with Ready-to-Eat Vegetables: Antimicrobial and Sensory Screening." *Journal of Food Protection* 71(9): 1846–1854.

8. Daly, Trevor, Marvin A. Jiwan, Nora M. O'Brien, and S. Aisling Aherne. June 2010. "Carotenoid Content of Commonly Consumed Herbs and Assessment of Their Bioaccessibility Using an *In Vitro* Digestion Model." *Plant Foods for Human Nutrition* 65(2): 164–169.

9. Amrani, Souliman, Hicham Hamafi, Nour El Houda Bouanani, et al. December 2006. "Hypolipidaemic Activity of Aqueous *Ocimum basilicum* Extract in Acute Hyperlipidaemia Induced by Triton WR-1339 in Rats and Its Antioxidant Property." *Phytotherapy Research* 20(12): 1040–1045.

10. Amrani, S., H. Harnafi, D. Gadi, et al. August 2009. "Vasorelaxant and Anti-Platelet Effects of Aqueous *Ocimum basilicum* Extract." *Journal of Ethnopharmacology* 125(1): 157–162.

References and Resources

Magazines, Journals, and Newspapers

Ahonkhai, I., A. Ba, O. Edogun, and U. Mu. October 2009. "Antimicrobial Activities of the Volatile Oils of *Ocimum bacilicum* L. and *Ocimum gratissimum* L. (Lamiaceae) against Some Aerobic Dental Isolates." *Pakistan Journal of Pharmaceutical Sciences* 22(4): 405–409.

Amrani, S., H. Harnafi, D. Gadi, et al. August 2009. "Vasorelaxant and Anti-Platelet Aggregation Effects of Aqueous *Ocimum basilicum* Extract." *Journal of Ethnopharmacology* 125(1): 157–162.

Amrani, Souliman, Hicham Hamafi, Nour El Houda Bouanani, et al. December 2006. "Hypolipidaemic Activity of Aqueous *Ocimum basilicum* Extract in Acute Hyperlipidaemic Induced by Triton WR-1339 in Rats and Its Antioxidant Property." *Phytotherapy Research* 20(12): 1040–1045.

Daly, Trevor, Marvin A. Jiwan, Nora M. O'Brien, and S. Aisling Aherne. June 2010. "Carotenoid Content of Commonly Consumed Herbs and Assessment of their Bioaccessibility Using an *In Vitro* Digestion Model." *Plant Foods for Human Nutrition* 65(2): 164–169.

Gutierrez, J., G. Rodriguez, C. Barry-Ryan, and P. Bourke. September 2008. "Efficacy of Plant Essential Oils against Foodborne Pathogens and Spoilage

Bacteria Associated with Ready-to-Eat Vegetables: Antimicrobial and Sensory Screening." *Journal of Food Protection* 71(9): 1846–1854.

Kaya, Ilhan, Nazife Yiğit, and Mehlika Benli. June 2008. "Antimicrobial Activity of Various Extracts of *Ocimum basilicum* L. and Observation of the Inhibition Effects on Bacterial Cells by Use of Scanning Electron Microscopy." *African Journal of Traditional, Complementary and Alternative Medicines* 5(4): 363–369.

Moghaddam, M. N., M. A. Khajeh-Karamoddin, and M. Ramezani. 2009. "*In Vitro* Anti-Bacterial Activity of Sweet Basil Fractions against *Helicobacter pylori*." *Journal of Biological Sciences* 9: 276–279.

Nour, A. H., S. A. Elhussein, N. A. Osman, et al. 2009. "Antibacterial Activity of the Essential Oils of Sudanese Accessions of Basil (*Ocimum basilicum* L.)." *Journal of Applied Sciences* 9: 4161—4167.

Rattanachaikunsopon, Pongsak, and Parichat Phumkhachorn. June 2010. "Antimicrobial Activity of Basil (*Ocimum basilicum*) Oil against *Salmonella enteritidis* In Vitro and in Food." *Bioscience, Biotechnology, and Biochemistry* 74(6): 1200–1204.

Website

The George Mateljan Foundation. www.whfoods.com.

T

Thyme 🌿

Since ancient times, thyme, scientifically known as *Thymus vulgaris,* has been valued for its culinary, aromatic, and medicinal properties. The ancient Greeks burned thyme in their temples; the ancient Egyptians used it to preserve the bodies of their dead pharaohs. By the 16th century, thyme was also considered a topical antiseptic and mouthwash. Native to Asia, south Europe, and the Mediterranean region, thyme is also grown in North America.[1]

Thyme has excellent amounts of vitamin K, iron, and manganese. It has very good amounts of calcium and good amounts of dietary fiber.[2] But, what have the researchers learned?

Anti-Inflammatory Properties

In a study published in 2009 in *Biochemical Pharmacology,* researchers from Korea and the Agricultural Research Service, Western Human Nutrition Center at the University of California, Davis investigated six compounds in plants, including a compound known as luteolin. Luteolin is found in thyme, as well as celery, green peppers, and chamomile tea. Of the six compounds studied, the researchers determined that luteolin had the strongest ability to target an enzyme known as TBK1 and inhibit the enzyme's ability to activate a specific biochemical signal. In so doing, luteolin reduced the possibility that the signal will form gene products that trigger inflammation. Inflammation in the body has been associated with many chronic health problems such as cancer, cardiovascular disease, and insulin resistance.[3]

In a more recent study published in 2010 in the *Journal of Lipid Research,* researchers from Japan determined that six essential oils—thyme, clove, rose, fennel, bergamot, and eucalyptus—suppress the inflammatory COX-2 enzyme. Apparently, it does this in a way that is similar to resveratrol, the chemical in red wine that is associated with health benefits. According to the researchers, carvacrol, which is found in thyme, is the chemical that causes this suppressive activity. Of the six essential oils tested, thyme oil was the most active. It reduced COX-2 levels by almost 75%. But, the researchers then went an extra step. They used pure carvacrol extracts in their tests. When they did, COX-2 levels decreased by more than 80%.[4]

Antifungal and Antibacterial Agents

In a study published in 2009 in *Molecules,* researchers from Serbia and the Netherlands examined the antifungal properties of four essential oils, including thyme essential oil, on 17 different pathogens. Like the other essential oils, thyme essential oil was found "to show very strong antifungal activities." Interestingly, bifonazole, a commercial fungicide, which was used as the control, "had much lower antifungal activity than the oils and components investigated." The researchers commented that all four essential oils, including thyme essential oil, have "great antifungal potential and could be used as natural preservatives and fungicides."[5]

According to research presented at the spring 2010 meeting of the Society for General Microbiology, some essential oils, such as the essential oil of thyme, have the potential to protect against drug-resistant hospital "superbugs." The researchers, from the Technological Educational Institute of Ionian Islands in Greece, evaluated the antimicrobial abilities of eight plant essential oils. By far the most effective, thyme eliminated almost all the bacteria within 60 minutes. And, thyme was useful against some of the most drug-resistant bacteria, such as meticillin-resistant *Staphylococcus aureus* (MRSA).[6]

In a study published in 2008 in the *Journal of Antimicrobial Chemotherapy,* researchers from the College of Pharmacy at Oregon State University noted that *Staphylococcus aureus* has become "responsible for an increasing number of skin infections." So, they evaluated the ability of three different over-the-counter topical antibacterial wound care products to kill four different isolates of *S. aureus*—USA300–1, USA300–2, USA300–3, and USA400. One of the wound care products, an ointment-gel named Staphaseptic, contained benzethonium chloride, tea tree oil, and white thyme oil. The researchers determined that all three products "demonstrated variable activity against the four strains tested." However, Staphaseptic was quicker and far more effective in killing *S. aureus* than the other two products. In fact, it reduced the number of all four strains of tested bacteria by a factor of 1,000. Moreover, Staphaseptic continued to kill bacteria for 24 hours.[7]

Kills Bacteria and Cancer Cells

In a study published in 2010 in *Molecules,* researchers from China and Germany tested the ability of 10 different essential oils, including thyme essential oil, to kill *Propionibacterium acnes,* a type of bacterium responsible for acne and other skin problems, and three different types of human cancer cells. The researchers found that thyme, cinnamon, and rose essential oils "exhibited the best antibacterial activities towards *P. acnes*." Thyme essential oil was the most effective against the cancer cells. The researchers concluded that "the potential of essential oils for the treatment of acne and cancer merits further exploration in the future."[8]

Respiratory Infections

In a study published in 2007 in *Phytotherapy Research,* Italian researchers examined the antibacterial effects of 13 essential oils, including thyme essential oil, on respiratory tract pathogens. Thyme, cinnamon, and clove exhibited the strongest action against the pathogens, even against multiresistant strains. The researchers concluded that "thyme can be considered a potential antimicrobial against for the treatment of some tract respiratory infections in man."[9]

Acute Bronchitis

In a prospective, double-blind, placebo-controlled trial published in 2007 in *Arzneimittelforschung,* a German researcher assessed the efficacy and tolerability of a combination of thyme and primrose root for the treatment of acute bronchitis with a productive cough. The cohort included 361 outpatients. Of these, 183 patients were given 11 days of the herbal treatment (one tablet three times per day) and 178 were given a placebo. The researcher found that "the mean reduction in coughing fits on days 7 and 9 relative to baseline . . . was 67.1% under thyme–primrose combination compared to 51.3% under placebo." In addition, improvement occurred about two days earlier in the thyme–primrose group. The researcher concluded that "Oral treatment of acute bronchitis with thyme–primrose combination for about 11 days was superior to placebo in terms of efficacy. The treatment was safe and well tolerated."[10]

Metastatic Breast Cancer

In a study published in 2010 in *Phytomedicine: International Journal of Phytotherapy and Phytopharmacology,* a researcher from Hyderabad, India acknowledged that carvacrol (previously noted to be found in high amounts in thyme) has been associated with antitumor effects. The researcher, who focused on identifying the mechanism of carvacrol-induced cell death in human metastatic breast cells—MDA-MB 231—learned that carvacrol causes "morphological changes such as cell shrinkage" that cause apoptosis or cell death. The researcher commented that these findings "demonstrated the antiproliferative effects of carvacrol in metastatic breast cancer, MDA-MB 231." Consequently, "carvacrol could be a potent anti-tumor molecule against metatastic breast cancer cells."[11]

Reduce Clot Formation

In a study published in 2008 in *Thrombosis Research,* researchers from Japan investigated the effects of the long-term intake of thyme and rosemary on platelets, thrombus formation, and bleeding time. For 12 weeks, researchers fed mice a Western-style high-fat diet that also contained thyme or rosemary. They found that the mice that ate a diet consisting of 5% thyme had significantly lower rates of clot and platelet formation. This was accomplished without increasing the risk of bleeding issues, a problem associated with synthetic blood-thinning medications.[12]

Is Thyme Beneficial?

Thyme certainly appears to have a number of beneficial qualities. And, it is exceedingly hard to find any negative aspects of this herb. Perhaps, future research will yield even more information about all the ways that thyme supports a healthy lifestyle.

Notes

1. The George Mateljan Foundation Website. www.whfoods.com.
2. The George Mateljan Foundation Website. www.whfoods.com.

3. Kyung Lee, Jun, So Young Kim, Yoon Sun Kim, et al. April 2009. "Suppression of the TRIF-Dependent Signaling Pathway of Toll-Like Receptors by Luteolin." *Biochemical Pharmacology* 77(8): 1391–1400.
4. Hotta, M., R. Nakata, M. Katsukawa, et al. January 2010. "Carvacrol, a Component of Thyme Oil, Activates PPARalpha and Gamma and Suppresses COX-2 Expression." *Journal of Lipid Research* 51(1): 132–139.
5. Soković, M.D., J. Vukojević, P.D. Marin, et al. January 2009. "Chemical Composition of Essential Oils of Thymus and Mentha Species and Their Antifungal Activities." *Molecules* 14(1): 238–249.
6. Society for General Microbiology Website. http://www.sgm.ac.uk/.
7. Bearden, David T., George P. Allen, and J. Mark Christensen. October 2008. "Comparative *In Vitro* Activities of Topical Wound Care Products against Community-Associated Methicillin-Resistant *Staphylococcus aureus.*" *Journal of Antimicrobial Chemotherapy* 62(4): 769–772.
8. Zu, Y., H. Yu, L. Liang, et al. April 2010. "Activities of Ten Essential Oils Towards *Propionibacterium acnes* and PC-3, A-549 and MCF-7 Cancer Cells." *Molecules* 15(5): 3200–3210.
9. Fabio, A., C. Cermelli, G. Fabio, et al. April 2007. "Screening of the Antibacterial Effects of a Variety of Essential Oils on Microorganisms Responsible for Respiratory Infections." *Phytotherapy Research* 21(4): 374–377.
10. Kemmerich, B. 2007. "Evaluation of Efficacy of Tolerability of a Fixed Combination of Dry Extracts of Thyme Herb and Primrose Root in Adults Suffering from Acute Bronchitis with Productive Cough. A Prospective, Double-Blind, Placebo-Controlled Multicentre Clinical Trial." *Arzneimittelforschung/Drug Research* 5(9): 607–615.
11. Arunasree, K.M. July 2010. "Anti-Proliferative Effects of Carvacrol on a Human Metastatic Breast Cancer Line, MDA-MB 231." *Phytomedicine: International Journal of Phytotherapy and Phytopharmacology* 17(8): 581–588.
12. Naemura, Aki, Mayumi Ura, Tsutomu Yamashita, et al. 2008. "Long-Term Intake of Rosemary and Common Thyme Herbs Inhibits Experimental Thrombosis without Prolongation of Bleeding Time." *Thrombosis Research* 111(4): 517–522.

References and Resources

Magazines, Journals, and Newspapers

Arunasree, K.M. July 2010. "Anti-Proliferative Effects of Carvacrol on a Human Metastatic Breast cancer Cell Line, MDA-MB 231." *Phytomedicine: International Journal of Phytotherapy and Phytopharmacology* 17(8): 581–588.

Bearden, David T., George P. Allen, and J. Mark Christensen. October 2008. "Comparative *In Vitro* Activities of Topical Wound Care Products against Community-Associated Methicillin-Resistant *Staphylococcus aureus.*" *Journal of Antimicrobial Chemotherapy* 62(4): 769–772.

Fabio, A., C. Cermelli, G. Fabio, et al. April 2007. "Screening of the Antibacterial Effects of a Variety of Essential Oils on Microorganisms Responsible for Respiratory Infections." *Phytotherapy Research* 21(4): 374–377.

Hotta, M., R. Nakata, M. Katsukawa, et al. January 2010. "Carvacrol, a Component of Thyme Oil, Activates PPARalpha and Gamma and Suppresses COX-2 Expression." *Journal of Lipid Research* 51(1): 132–139.

Kemmerich, B. 2007. "Evaluation of Efficacy and Tolerability of a Fixed Combination of Dry Extracts of Thyme Herb and Primrose Root in Adults Suffering from Acute Bronchitis with Productive Cough. A Prospective Double-Blind, Placebo-Controlled Multicentre Clinical Trial." *Arzneimittelforschung/Drug Research* 57(9): 607–615.

Kyung Lee, Jun, So Young Kim, Yoon Sun Kim, et al. April 2009. "Suppression of the TRIF-Dependent Signaling Pathway of Toll-Like Receptors by Luteolin." *Biochemical Pharmacology* 77(8): 1391–1400.

Naemura, Aki, Mayumi Ura, Tsutomu Yamashita, et al. 2008. "Long-Term Intake of Rosemary and Common Thyme Herbs Inhibits Experimental Thrombosis without Prolongation of Bleeding Time." *Thrombosis Research* 122(4): 517–522.

Soković, M.D., J. Vukojević, P.D. Marin, et al. January 2009. "Chemical Composition of Essential Oils of Thymus and Mentha Species and Their Antifungal Activities." *Molecules* 14(1): 238–249.

Zu, Y., H. Yu, L. Liang, et al. April 2010. "Activities of Ten Essential Oils Towards *Propionibacterium Acnes* and PC-3, A-549 and MCF-7 Cancer Cells." *Molecules* 15(5): 3200–3210.

Websites
The George Mateljan Foundation. www.whfoods.com.

Society for General Microbiology. http://www.sgm.ac.uk/.

Turmeric 🌿

For centuries, turmeric has been an integral part of both traditional Chinese medicine and Ayurveda, the ancient Hindu science of health and medicine. A key component of curry, turmeric, scientifically known as *Curcuma longa,* contains curcumin, which has antioxidant and anti-inflammatory properties. Turmeric is believed to be useful for a wide variety of medical problems. But, what have the researchers learned?

Breast Cancer

In a laboratory study published in 2010 in *Breast Cancer Research and Treatment,* researchers from Michigan applied a solution of curcumin and piperine, which is found in black pepper, to cultures of breast cancer stem cells. The researchers used the equivalent of about 20 times the potency of curcumin and piperine that might be consumed in a diet. Apparently, piperine enhanced the effects of curcumin, and curcumin and piperine decreased the numbers of stem cells, while they had no effect on the normal process of cell development. The researchers commented that curcumin and piperine "could be potential cancer preventive agents."[1]

Esophageal Cancer

In a study published in 2009 in the *British Journal of Cancer,* researchers based at the Cork Cancer Research Centre in Ireland treated esophageal cancer cells with curcumin. Within 24 hours, the curcumin was killing cancer cells, and the cells were digesting themselves. Furthermore, the researchers determined that curcumin killed cells by provoking lethal cell death signals. The researchers noted that curcumin "represents a promising anticancer agent for prevention and treatment" of esophageal cancer.[2]

Pancreatic Cancer

In a study published in 2008 in *Clinical Cancer Research,* researchers from Texas and New Jersey examined the use of 8 g/day of curcumin supplementation on 25 patients with advanced pancreatic cancer. None of the patients was on any form of chemotherapy. The researchers noted that the curcumin temporarily stopped the progression of pancreatic cancer in two patients—one for 8 months and the other for 2.5 years. It also reduced the size of a tumor in another patient by 73%. Unfortunately, the tumor quickly grew back. The patients had no negative side effects from the curcumin.[3]

Prostate Cancer

In a study published in 2006 in *Cancer Research,* researchers from Rutgers, the State University of New Jersey, injected mice with curcumin and/or phenethyl isothiocyanate (PEITC), a naturally occurring substance found in vegetables such as broccoli and kale. The next day, they injected the mice with human prostate cancer cells. Then, for four weeks, the mice were injected with curcumin or PEITC three times per week. The researchers found that both the curcumin and PEITC significantly slowed the growth of cancerous tumors; when both curcumin and PEITC were used, the results were even better. The researchers also investigated the use of curcumin and/or PEITC on mice with well-established tumors. Separately, neither curcumin nor PEITC had an effect. However, when used together, they significantly reduced tumor growth.[4]

Alzheimer's Disease

In a study published in 2009 in the *Journal of Alzheimer's Disease,* California researchers tested their hypothesis that combining a type of vitamin D with curcumin may help stimulate the immune system to clear amyloid beta from the brain. Amyloid beta forms the plaques in the brains of people with Alzheimer's disease. The researchers began by taking blood samples from nine people with Alzheimer's disease, one person with mild cognitive impairment, and three healthy control subjects. They then isolated monocyte cells, which transformed themselves into macrophages. Macrophages, in turn, travel throughout the body and consume waste products, such as amyloid beta. The researchers incubated the macrophages with amyloid beta, vitamin D3, and natural or synthetic curcumin, and they found that curcuminoids (synthetic curcumin) and vitamin D prompted the immune system to clear the brain of amyloid beta. Future research on more people may help to determine if vitamin D and natural or synthetic curcumin, separately or in combination, may be useful for Alzheimer's disease.[5]

Diabesity (Diabetes Caused by Overweight or Obesity)

In a study published in 2008 in *Endocrinology,* researchers from Columbia University in New York City tested high doses of dietary curcumin in two different mouse models of obesity and type 2 diabetes—high-fat-diet-fed male mice and leptin-deficient obese female mice. Lean wild-type mice that were fed low-fat diets served as controls. (Leptin is a hormone that has a central role in fat metabolism.)

The researchers found that turmeric-treated mice had a reduced risk for developing type 2 diabetes. Moreover, when compared to controls, obese mice that were fed turmeric had lower levels of inflammation in fat tissue and the liver. The researchers concluded that the antioxidant and anti-inflammatory properties of turmeric reduced the incidence of insulin resistance and type 2 diabetes. "Orally ingested curcumin reverses many of the inflammatory and metabolic derangements associated with obesity and improves glycemic control in mouse models of type 2 diabetes." They added that their studies "revealed that high doses of oral curcumin safely treat diabetes in several mouse models of obesity-associated diabetes." Additionally, even when the mice had a normal or higher than normal calorie intake, the researchers observed that curcumin was associated with a small but significant decline in body weight and fat content. The researchers commented that "curcumin holds potential as an adjuvant treatment for diabesity complications."[6]

Reduce Fat Tissue

In a study published in 2009 in *The Journal of Nutrition,* Boston researchers divided 18 mice into three groups of 6. For 12 weeks, the mice in the control group were fed a diet consisting of 4% fat; the mice in the second group were fed a diet containing 22% fat; and the mice in the third group were fed a 22% fat diet, but they were also fed curcumin. The researchers found that the mice fed high-fat diet and curcumin had reductions in body-weight gain and total body fat. Similar reductions were not seen in the mice fed only the high-fat diet. Likewise, the mice fed the curcumin had less blood vessel growth in fat tissue, and they had lower levels of blood glucose, triglycerides, fatty acids, cholesterol, and liver fats. The researchers noted that their findings indicate "that dietary curcumin may have a potential benefit in preventing obesity."[7]

Knee Osteoarthritis

In a randomized, controlled study published in 2009 in *The Journal of Alternative and Complementary Medicine,* Thai researchers treated 107 patients with primary knee osteoarthritis with either 800-mg/day ibuprofen or 2-g/day turmeric. Fifty-two received turmeric and 55 took ibuprofen. At the end of six weeks, the subjects in the two groups were compared. The researchers found that the turmeric was as effective and safe for the pain associated with knee osteoarthritis as the ibuprofen.[8]

Cardiovascular Health

In a study published in 2008 in *The Journal of Clinical Investigation,* researchers from Kyoto, Japan, induced high blood pressure in one group of rats by overly salting their food. In a second group of rats, they performed surgery to mimic a heart attack. Normally, the rats in both groups would proceed to have heart failure. However, by feeding the rats curcumin, that inevitability was prevented. "In both models, curcumin prevented deterioration of systolic function and heart failure." The researchers concluded that "the nontoxic dietary compound curcumin may provide a novel therapeutic strategy for heart failure in humans."[9]

Is Turmeric Beneficial?

It certainly appears that turmeric should have greater recognition for its many benefits. But, some people should not use turmeric without a discussion with their medical provider. Since turmeric may affect the ability of blood to clot, people taking blood thinners, even aspirin, must be cautious. And, turmeric may interfere with the actions of drugs that reduce stomach acids and drugs for diabetes that lower blood sugar.

Notes

1. Kakarala, Madhuri, Dean E. Brenner, Hasan Korkaya, et al. 2010. "Targeting Breast Stem Cells with the Cancer Preventive Compounds Curcumin and Piperine." *Breast Cancer Research and Treatment* 122(3): 777–785.
2. O'Sullivan-Coyne, G., G.C. O'Sullivan, T.R. O'Donovan, et al. 2009. "Curcumin Induces Apoptosis-Independent Death in Oesophageal Cancer Cells." *British Journal of Cancer* 101: 1585–1595.
3. Dhillon, Navneet, Bharat B. Aggarwal, Robert A. Newman, et al. July 2008. "Phase II Trial of Curcumin in Patients with Advanced Pancreatic Cancer." *Clinical Cancer Research* 14(14): 4491–4499.
4. Khor, Tin Oo, Young-Sam Keum, Wen Lin, et al. January 2006. "Combined Inhibitory Effects of Curcumin and Phenethyl Isothiocyanate on the Growth of Human PC-3 Prostate Xenografts in Immunodeficient Mice." *Cancer Research* 66: 613–621.
5. Masoumi, A., B. Goldenson, S. Ghirmai, et al. July 2009. "1alpha,25-dihydroxyvitamin D3 Interacts with Curcuminoids to Stimulate Amyloid-Beta Clearance by Macrophages of Alzheimer's Disease Patients." *Journal of Alzheimer's Disease* 17(3): 703–717.
6. Weisberg, S.P., R. Leibel, and D.V. Tortoriello. July 2008. "Dietary Curcumin Significantly Improves Obesity-Associated Inflammation and Diabetes in Mouse Models of Diabesity." *Endocrinology* 149(7): 3549–3558.
7. Ejaz, A., D. Wu, P. Kwan, and M. Meydani. May 2009. "Curcumin Inhibits Adipogenesis in 3T3-L1 Adipocytes and Angiogenesis and Obesity in C57/BL Mice." *The Journal of Nutrition* 139(5): 919–925.
8. Kuptniratsaikul, Vilai, Sunee Thanakhumtorn, Pornsiri Chinswangwatanakul, et al. August 2009. "Efficacy and Safety of *Curcuma domestica* Extracts in Patients with Knee Osteoarthritis." *The Journal of Alternative and Complementary Medicine* 15(8): 891–897.

9. Morimoto, Tatsuya, Yoichi Sunagawa, Teruhisa Kawamura, et al. March 2008. "The Dietary Compound Curcumin Inhibits p300 Histone Acetyltransferase Activity and Prevents Heart Failure in Rats." *The Journal of Clinical Investigation* 118(3): 868–878.

References and Resources

Magazines, Journals, and Newspapers

Dhillon, Navneet, Bharat B. Aggarwal, Robert A. Newman, et al. July 2008. "Phase II Trial of Curcumin in Patients with Advanced Pancreatic Cancer." *Clinical Cancer Research* 14(14): 4491–4499.

Ejaz, A., D. Wu, P. Kwan, and M. Meydani. May 2009. "Curcumin Inhibits Adipogenesis in 3T3-L1 Adipocytes and Angiogenesis and Obesity in C57/BL Mice." *The Journal of Nutrition* 139(5): 919–925.

Kakarala, Madhuri, Dean E. Brenner, Hasan Korkaya, et al. 2010. "Targeting Breast Stem Cells with the Cancer Preventive Compounds Curcumin and Piperine." *Breast Cancer Research and Treatment* 122(3): 777–785.

Khor, Tin Oo, Young-Sam Keum, Wen Lin, et al. January 2006. "Combined Inhibitory Effects of Curcumin and Phenethyl Isothiocyanate on the Growth of Human PC-3 Prostate Xenografts in Immunodeficient Mice." *Cancer Research* 66: 613–621.

Kuptniratsaikul, Vilai, Sunee Thanakhumtorn, Pornsiri Chinswangwatanakul, et al. August 2009. "Efficacy and Safety of *Curcuma domestica* Extracts in Patients with Knee Osteoarthritis." *The Journal of Alternative and Complementary Medicine* 15(8): 891–897.

Masoumi, A., B. Goldenson, S. Ghirmai, et al. July 2009. "1alpha,25-dihydroxyvitamin D3 Interacts with Curcumoids to Stimulate Amyloid-Beta Clearance by Macrophages of Alzheimer's Disease in Patients." *Journal of Alzheimer's Disease* 17(3): 703–717.

Morimoto, Tatsuya, Yoichi Sunagawa, Teruhisa Kawamura, et al. March 2008. "The Dietary Compound Curcumin Inhibits p300 Histone Acetyltransferase Activity and Prevents Heart Failure in Rats." *The Journal of Clinical Investigation* 118(3): 868–878.

O'Sullivan-Coyne, G., G. C. O'Sullivan, T. R. O'Donovan, et al. 2009. "Curcumin Induces Apoptosis-Independent Death in Oesophageal Cancer Cells." *British Journal of Cancer* 101: 1585–1595.

Weisberg, S. P., R. Leibel, and D. V. Tortoriello. July 2008. "Dietary Curcumin Significantly Improves Obesity-Associated Inflammation and Diabetes in Mouse Models of Diabesity." *Endocrinology* 149(7): 3549–3558.

Website

The University of Texas—MD Anderson Cancer Center. www.mdanderson.org.

V

Valerian 🦌

Scientifically known as *Valeriana officinalis,* valerian has been used as a medicinal herb since ancient times. It is known that Hippocrates described using valerian in the 2nd century, and Galen prescribed valerian for insomnia. (Hippocrates and Galen were ancient Greek physicians. Hippocrates is often considered the Father of Medicine.) By the 16th century, valerian was thought to be effective against nervousness, trembling, headaches, and heart palpitations. However, by the mid-19th century, valerian was no longer considered a valuable herb. In fact, it was thought to cause a number of health problems. Then, during World War II, valerian reemerged in England to assist people forced to deal with the stress of the air raids. Today, valerian is said to be useful for insomnia, anxiety, gastrointestinal spasms and distress, epileptic seizures, and attention deficit hyperactivity disorder.[1] Still, it is important to review the results of some of the scientific research on valerian.

Sleep Problems

Although valerian is probably best known as a sleep aid, research studies on the usefulness for this medical concern offer mixed results. For example, in a study published in 2007 in *PLoS ONE,* researchers from Norway recruited via television and the Internet more than 400 people between the ages of 18 and 75 who had insomnia. The study began by asking the participants to complete a two-week sleep diary. Then, they were provided with valerian or placebo tablets to take for two weeks. Neither the participants nor the investigators knew which tablets they took. While the researchers found that the people taking valerian experienced some improvements in sleep over those on placebos, the differences were not statistically significant. When other factors were examined, such as night awakenings, the valerian group also had better outcomes. But, the benefits were only minimal. The researchers concluded that "valerian appears to be safe, but with modest beneficial effects at most on insomnia compared to placebo."[2]

In a prospective, tripled-blinded, randomized, placebo-controlled, parallel design trial published in 2009 in *Alternative Therapies in Health and Medicine,* researchers from Philadelphia, Pennsylvania wanted to determine if valerian would help people with restless legs syndrome (RLS) sleep better and obtain relief from their symptoms. The trial began with 48 participants. For eight weeks, half of them took 800 mg of valerian and the other half took a placebo. Thirty-seven participants, between the ages of 36 and 65, completed the trial. Interestingly, "both groups reported improvement in RLS symptoms severity and sleep." Moreover, the researchers found that valerian improved the quality of sleep and reduced RLS severity in people whose RLS symptoms kept them up at night and made them sleepy the following day.[3]

In a report published in 2010 in *Sleep Medicine,* researchers from Spain outlined their meta-analyses of 18 well-designed, randomized, placebo-controlled clinical trials of valerian. Still, their findings were far from remarkable. They noted that "valerian would be effective for subjective improvement of insomnia, although its effectiveness has not been demonstrated with quantitative or objective measures." At the same time, the researchers wrote that valerian "can be considered for some patients given its safety." However, they suggested that researchers focus their future investigations on "other more promising treatments."[4]

In a randomized, placebo-controlled, double-blind trial published in 2011 in *The Journal of Supportive Oncology,* researchers from several locations in the United States attempted to learn if valerian could help people undergoing cancer treatments obtain improved sleep. The researchers noted that sleep disturbances are not uncommon in people dealing with cancer therapies. The participants received either 450-mg valerian or a placebo, and they were instructed to take their supplementation orally one hour before bedtime for the next eight weeks. Although the researchers began with 227 participants, in the end data were available on 119 people—62 taking valerian and 57 taking the placebo. The researchers found that the valerian did not improve sleep. Still, participants on valerian found that they had less fatigue.[5]

In a randomized, double-blind, crossover, controlled study published in 2009 in *Sleep Medicine,* researchers from Seattle, Washington attempted to learn if valerian could assist older women who suffered from insomnia. The cohort consisted of 16 women with a mean age of 69.4. For two weeks, the women took either 300 mg of concentrated valerian extract or a placebo about 30 minutes before going to bed. The researchers wrote that they found "no statistically significant differences between valerian and placebo after a single dose or after two weeks of night dosing on any measure of sleep latency [the amount of time it takes to fall asleep], wake after sleep onset (WASO), sleep efficiency, and self-rated sleep quality." They concluded that "valerian did not improve sleep in this sample of older women with insomnia."[6]

Reduction in Anxiety

In a study published in 2010 in *Phytomedicine: International Journal of Phytotherapy & Phytopharmacology,* researchers from Oregon and Washington attempted to determine if valerian would be useful for those dealing with anxiety. They began by randomly dividing 50 female rats into five groups of 10 rats. The rats in the first group, which were administered ethanol, served as the control. The second group of rats had diazepam, an anti-anxiety medication. The rats in the third group were treated with valerian root exact. The rats in the fourth group had valerenic acid (the active constituent in valerian). And, the final group was treated with a solution of valerenic acid and gamma-aminobutyric acid (GABA), a neurotransmitter found in the brain. The rats were then placed in a maze. The researchers' findings were certainly notable. They wrote that "there was a significant reduction in anxious behavior when valerian extract or valerenic acid exposed subjects were compared to the ethanol control group." Furthermore, the researchers suggested that "valerian may be an effective alternative to the traditional" anti-anxiety medications that may have side effects such as nausea, tremor, and addiction.[7]

Anticonvulsant Properties

In a study published in 2010 in the *Journal of Ethnopharmacology,* researchers from Iran examined the effect of valerian extracts on an experimental model of temporal lobe epilepsy in rats. After inducing epilepsy in the rats, the rats were administered three different dosages of aqueous extract of valerian (200, 500, and 800 mg/kg). The convulsive activity was measured using electrodes place in a structure in the deep portion of the temporal lobe area of the brain. The researchers found that the administration of aqueous extract of valerian had an anticonvulsant effect. On the other hand, the administration of petroleum ether extracts of valerian (50 and 100 mg/kg) had a seizure-inducing effect.[8]

Is Valerian Beneficial?

From a review of the many websites that sell valerian, it is evident that it is a very popular herb. But, the research does not appear to offer strong support for such a widespread use. One cannot help but wonder if large numbers of people are benefiting from valerian because they simply believe that it is working, which is known as the placebo effect.

It is important to mention that some people have become ill when their intake of valerian has interfered with their prescribed medication. For example, a letter to the editor in a 2009 issue of *Phytotherapy Research* described a 40-year-old man who was taking lorazepam for generalized anxiety disorder and dream disorders. After self-medicating with valerian and passionflower, he developed movement disorders and drowsiness. When the herbs were discontinued, the man's symptoms resolved.[9]

Notes

1. National Institutes of Health, Office of Dietary Supplements. December 2007. "Questions and Answers about Valerian for Insomnia and Other Sleep Disorders." *Pamphlets by: National Institutes of Health, Office of Dietary Supplements.*
2. Oxman, A. D., S. Flottorp, K. Håvelsrud, et al. October 2007. "A Television, Web-Based Randomised Trial of an Herbal Remedy (Valerian) for Insomnia." *PLoS ONE* 2(10): e1040.
3. Cuellar, Norma G. and Sarah J. Ratcliffe. March–April 2009. "Does Valerian Improve Sleepiness and Symptoms Severity in People with Restless Legs Syndrome? *Alternative Therapies in Health and Medicine* 15(2): 22–28.
4. Fernández San Martin, M. I., R. Masa-Font, L. Palacios-Soler, et al. June 2010. "Effectiveness of Valerian on Insomnia: A Meta-Analysis of Randomized Placebo-Controlled Trials." *Sleep Medicine* 11(6): 505–511.
5. Barton, D. L., P. J. Atherton, B. A. Bauer, et al. January–February 2011. "The Use of *Valeriana officinalis* (Valerian) in Improving Sleep in Patients Who Are Undergoing Treatment for Cancer: A Phase III Randomized, Placebo-Controlled, Double-Blind Study." *The Journal of Supportive Oncology* 9(1): 24–31.

6. Taibi, Diana M., Michael V. Vitiello, Suzanne Barsness, et al. March 2009. "A Randomized Clinical Trial of Valerian Fails to Improve Self-Reported, Polysomnographic, and Actigraphic Sleep in Older Women with Insomnia." *Sleep Medicine* 10(3): 319–328.

7. Murphy, K., Z. J. Kubin, J. N. Shepherd, and R. H. Ettinger. July 2010. "*Valeriana officinalis* Root Extracts Have Potent Anxiolytic Effects in Laboratory Rats." *Phytomedicine: International Journal of Phytotherapy & Phytopharmacology* 17(8–9): 674–678.

8. Rezvani, Mohammad Ebrahim, Ali Roohbakhsh, Mohammad Allahtavakoli, and Ali Shamsizadeh. February 2010. "Anticonvulsant Effect of Aqueous Extract of *Valeriana officinalis* in Amygdala-Kindled Rats: Possible Involvement of Adenosine." *Journal of Ethnopharmacology* 127(2): 313–318.

9. Carrasco, Maria Consuelo, José Ramón Vallejo, Manuel Pardo-de-Santayana, et al. December 2009. "Interactions of *Valeriana officinalis* L. and *Passiflora incarnate* L. in a Patient Treated with Lorazepam." *Phytotherapy Research* 23(12): 1795–1796.

References and Resources

Magazines, Journals, and Newspapers

Barton, D. L., P. J. Atherton, B. A. Bauer, et al. January–February 2011. "The Use of *Valeriana officinalis* (Valerian) in Improving Sleep in Patients Who Are Undergoing Treatment for Cancer: A Phase III Randomized, Placebo-Controlled, Double-Blind Study." *The Journal of Supportive Oncology* 9(1): 24–31.

Carrasco, Maria Consuelo, José Ramón Vallejo, Manuel Pardo-de-Santayana, et al. December 2009, "Interactions of *Valeriana officinalis* L. and *Passiflora incarnate* L. in a Patient Treated with Lorazepam." *Phytotherapy Research* 23(12): 1795–1796.

Cuellar, Norma G. and Sarah J. Ratcliffe. March–April 2009. "Does Valerian Improve Sleepiness and Symptoms Severity in People with Restless Legs Syndrome? *Alternative Therapies in Health and Medicine* 15(2): 22–28.

Fernández San Martin, M. I., R. Masa-Font, L. Palacios-Soler, et al. June 2010. "Effectiveness of Valerian on Insomnia: A Meta-Analysis of Randomized Placebo-Controlled Trials." *Sleep Medicine* 11(6): 505–511.

Murphy, K., Z. J. Kubin, J. N. Shepherd, and R. H. Ettinger. July 2010. "*Valeriana officinalis* Root Extracts Have Potent Anxiolytic Effects in Laboratory Rats." *Phytomedicine: International Journal of Phytotherapy & Phytopharmacology* 17(8–9): 674–678.

National Institutes of Health, Office of Dietary Supplements. December 2007. "Questions and Answers about Valerian for Insomnia and Other Sleep Disorders." *Pamphlets by: National Institutes of Health, Office of Dietary Supplements.*

Oxman, A. D., S. Flottorp, A. Håvelsrud, et al. October 2007. "A Televised, Web-Based Randomised Trial of an Herbal Remedy (Valerian) for Insomnia." *PLoS ONE* 2(10): e1040.

Rezvani, Mohammad Ebrahim, Ali Roohbakhsh, Mohammad Allahtavakoli, and Ali Shamsizadeh. February 2010. "Anticonvulsant Effect of Aqueous Extract of *Valeriana officinalis* in Amygdala-Kindled Rats: Possible Involvement of Adenosine." *Journal of Ethnopharmacology* 127(2): 313–318.

Sego, Sherril. March 2007. "Valerian." *Clinical Advisor* 10(3): 171–172.

Taibi, Diana M., Michael V. Vitiello, Suzanne Barsness, et al. March 2009. "A Randomized, Clinical Trial of Valerian Fails to Improve Self-Reported, Polysomnographic, and Actigraphic Sleep in Older Women with Insomnia." *Sleep Medicine* 10(3): 319–328.

Website

National Center for Complementary and Alternative Medicine. www.nccam.nih.gov.

Watercress 🌱

Like so many herbs, watercress has ancient roots. The Greeks thought that it increased intellect and stamina. Hippocrates, the father of medicine, is believed to have located his hospital near a stream so that his patients could eat the freshest watercress. Watercress was also said to be used by the Egyptian pharaohs to increase the productivity of their slaves. Supposedly, the slaves drank freshly squeezed watercress juice in the morning and afternoon.[1]

Like the other cruciferous vegetables, such as broccoli and cauliflower, watercress, scientifically known as *Nasturtium officinale,* is filled with vitamins and nutrients. These include vitamins B1, B6, C, K, iron, calcium, magnesium, manganese, zinc, and potassium. It also contains large amount of isothiocyanates, sulfur-containing compounds found in cruciferous vegetables that have been found to destroy cancer cells. One of the most well-known isothiocyanates is sulforaphane. But, what have the researchers learned?

Cancer
In a single-blind, randomized, crossover study published in 2007 in *The American Journal of Clinical Nutrition,* researchers from the United Kingdom wanted to determine the effects of watercress supplementation on biomarkers related to the risk of cancer in healthy adults. The cohort consisted of 30 men and 30 women (30 smokers and 30 nonsmokers) between the ages of 19 and 55 (with a mean age of 33 years). In addition to their usual diets, for eight weeks the subjects ate 85-g raw watercress each day. Although the benefits were more apparent in the smokers than

the nonsmokers, when compared to the control phase, the subjects eating watercress were found to have "reductions in basal DNA damage." That means that the watercress actually reduced their risk of developing cancer.[2]

Breast Cancer

In a study published in 2010 in the *British Journal of Nutrition,* researchers from the United Kingdom and Amherst, New York, organized a small group of women who had previously been treated for breast cancer. All the women underwent a period of fasting before eating 80 g (about the amount in a full cereal bowl) of watercress. During the following 24-hour period, the women had a number of different blood tests. The researchers found that a plant compound (phenylethyl isothiocyanate—PEITC) in watercress appeared to have the ability to suppress the growth of breast cancer cells. Apparently, the compound interferes with the functioning of a protein (hypoxia inducible factor—HIF) that plays a vital role in the development of cancer. Following the watercress meal, the researchers found significant levels of PEITC in the blood of the volunteers. They also determined that the functioning of the protein HIF was measurably affected. While acknowledging that their results need to be replicated in a larger group of women, the researchers wrote that "dietary intake of watercress may be sufficient to modulate this potential anti-cancer pathway."[3]

In a study published in 2008 in *The American Journal of Clinical Nutrition,* researchers from Tennessee and China reviewed the intake of cruciferous vegetables among more than 6,000 Chinese women. The researchers found that high consumption of cruciferous vegetables was associated with a moderately lower breast cancer risk. But, the benefit appeared to be strongest among the women who carried two copies of a particular variant of a gene called *GSTP1,* which increased their risk of breast cancer. Among these women, when compared to the women who ate the least amount of cruciferous vegetables, those who ate the highest amounts of cruciferous vegetables had half the risk of breast cancer. The researchers concluded that "cruciferous vegetable intake consistent with high isothiocyanate exposure may reduce breast cancer risk. Cruciferous vegetable intake also may ameliorate the effects of the *GSTP1* genotype."[4]

Prostate Cancer

In a study published in 2009 in *Cancer Research,* researchers from Pennsylvania examined the ability of sulforaphane to impair the growth of prostate cancer that routinely develops in TRAMP (transgenic adenocarcinoma of the mouse prostate) mice following the onset of puberty. From their extensive investigations, the researchers determined that the oral administration of sulforaphane both killed prostate cancer cells and "inhibited prostate cancer progression in TRAMP mice." The sulforaphane also decreased cell proliferation and "inhibited pulmonary metastasis," a common cause of death in men with prostate cancer. And, sulforaphane accomplishes these goals without harmful side effects.[5]

Colorectal and Colon Cancer

In a study published in 2008 in *Cancer Epidemiology Biomarkers & Prevention,* researchers from China, Minnesota, Washington DC, and California examined the association between the amount of isothiocyanates in the urine and the risk of colorectal cancer in men. The cohort consisted of 18,244 men who lived in Shanghai, China, and were followed for 16 years. During this time, urinary total isothiocyanates were quantified on 225 incident cases of colorectal cancer and 1,119 matched controls. The researchers found a statistically significant inverse association between levels of isothiocyanates in the urine and the risk of developing colorectal cancer. The people who ate higher amounts of foods with isothiocyanates, such as watercress, had a lower risk of developing colorectal cancer.[6]

In a study published in 2008 in *The Journal of Nutrition,* researchers from Minnesota evaluated the association between the consumption of cruciferous vegetables (watercress, green cabbage, red cabbage, or broccoli) and the risk of colon cancer. In the first trial, they compared rats fed a basal diet (vegetable-free diet) to those fed a diet of different freeze-dried cruciferous vegetables in concentrations between 4% and 10%. These diets began two weeks before and seven weeks after the administration of a carcinogen to induce colon cancer. In the second trial, rats were fed either a basal diet or diets containing 10%–22.6% fresh cruciferous vegetables. These second trial diets began 3 weeks before and 12 weeks after the administration of the same carcinogen. Rats fed fresh vegetables were also injected with a low dose of the carcinogen 18 to 24 hours prior to termination. The researchers found that while the freeze-dried vegetables did not alter markers of colon cancer, the consumption of the fresh cruciferous vegetables did. They concluded that "fresh but not lyophilized [freeze dried] cruciferous vegetables reduce colon cancer risk in rats."[7]

Treats Chronic Urinary Tract Infections

In a study published in 2007 in *Current Medical Research & Opinion,* researchers from Germany wanted to determine if an herbal medication containing watercress and horseradish would be useful for people who deal with chronically recurring urinary tract infections. The trial began with the screening of 219 adults between the ages of 18 and 75. While the initial cohort included 174 subjects, only 131 completed the 90-day trial, which required the ingestion of the medication or a placebo twice daily. The vast majority of the subjects were female. All subjects were required to have a history of three recurrent urinary tract infections—at least two of which had occurred within the past six months. The researchers found that there was a statistical difference in the number of urinary tract infections experienced by those taking the herbal medication (0.43) and those on the placebo (0.77). And, they concluded that their findings "demonstrated the efficacy and safety of the herbal medicinal product . . . in the prophylactic treatment of chronically recurrent UTIs [urinary tract infections]."[8]

Is Watercress Beneficial?

Watercress appears to be an amazingly healthful herb. Is it as useful as some of the studies indicate? Quite possibly, yes. It is certainly packed with vitamins and nutrients. Since watercress is relatively inexpensive and available throughout the year, it is probably a good idea to add some to salads, soups, and other frequently consumed foods several times a week.

Notes

1. The Watercress Alliance Website. www.watercress.com.uk/about/watercress-alliance.
2. Gill, Chris I.R., Sumanto Haldar, Lindsay A. Boyd, et al. February 2007. "Watercress Supplementation in Diet Reduces Lymphocyte DNA Damage and Alters Blood Antioxidant Status in Healthy Adults." *The American Journal of Clinical Nutrition* 85(2): 504–509.
3. Syed Alwi, Sharifah S., Breeze E. Cavell, Urvi Telang, et al. November 2010. "In Vivo Modulation of 4E Binding Protein 1 (4E–BP1) Phosphorylation by Watercress: A Pilot Study." *British Journal of Nutrition* 104(9): 1288–1296.
4. Lee, Sang-Ah, Jay H. Fowke, Wei Lu, et al. March 2008. "Cruciferous Vegetables, the *GSTP1 Ile*[105]*Val* Genetic Polymorphism, and Breast Cancer Risk." *The American Journal of Clinical Nutrition* 87(3): 753–760.

5. Singh, Shivendra, Renaud Warin, Dong Xiao, et al. March 2009. "Sulforaphane Inhibits Prostate Carcinogenesis and Pulmonary Metastasis in TRAMP Mice in Association with Increased Cytotoxicity of Natural Killer Cells." *Cancer Research* 69(5): 2117–2125.
6. Moy, Kristin A., Jian-Min Yuan, Fung-Lung Chung, et al. June 2008. "Urinary Total Isothiocyanates and Colorectal Cancer: A Prospective Study of Men in Shanghai, China." *Cancer Epidemiology Biomarkers & Prevention* 17(60): 1354–1359.
7. Arikawa, Andrea Y. and Daniel D. Gallaher. March 2008. "Cruciferous Vegetables Reduce Morphological Markers of Colon Cancer Risk in Dimethylhydrazine-Treated Rats." *The Journal of Nutrition* 138: 526–532.
8. Albrecht, U., K.H. Goos, and B. Schneider. October 2007. "A Randomised, Double-Blind, Placebo-Controlled Trial of a Herbal Medicinal Product Containing *Tropaeoli majoris* herba (Nasturtium) and *Armoraciae rusticanae* radix (Horseradish) for the Prophylactic Treatment of Patients with Chronically Recurrent Lower Urinary Tract Infections." *Current Medical Research & Opinion* 23(10): 2415–2422.

References and Resources

Magazines, Journals, and Newspapers

Albrecht, U., K.H. Goos, and B. Schneider. October 2007. "A Randomised, Double-Blind, Placebo-Controlled Trial of a Herbal Medicinal Product Containing *Tropaeoli majoris* herba (Nasturtium) and *Armoraciae rusticanae* radix (Horseradish) for the Prophylactic Treatment of Patients with Chronically Recurrent Lower Urinary Tract Infections." *Current Medical Research & Opinion* 23(10): 2415–2422.

Arikawa, Andrea Y. and Daniel D. Gallaher. March 2008. "Cruciferous Vegetables Reduce Morphological Markers of Colon Cancer Risk in Dimethylhydrazine-Treated Rats." *The Journal of Nutrition* 138: 526–532.

Gill, Chris I.R., Sumanto Haldar, Lindsay A. Boyd, et al. February 2007. "Watercress Supplementation in Diet Reduces Lymphocyte DNA Damage and Alters Blood Antioxidant Status in Healthy Adults." *The American Journal of Clinical Nutrition* 85(2): 504–509.

Lee, Sang-Ah, Jay H. Fowke, Wei Lu, et al. March 2008. "Cruciferous Vegetables, the *GSTP*1 *Ile*[105]*Val* Genetic Polymorphism, and Breast Cancer Risk." *The American Journal of Clinical Nutrition* 87(3): 753–760.

Moy, Kristin A., Jian-Min Yuan, Fung-Lung Chung, et al. June 2008. "Urinary Total Isothiocyanates and Colorectal Cancer—A Prospective Study of Men in Shanghai, China." *Cancer Epidemiology Biomarkers & Prevention* 17(6): 1354–1359.

Singh, Shivendra V., Renaud Warin, Dong Xiao, et al. March 2009. "Sulforaphane Inhibits Prostate Carcinogenesis and Pulmonary Metastasis in TRAMP Mice in Association with Increased Cytotoxicity of Natural Killer Cells." *Cancer Research* 69(5): 2117–2125.

Syed Alwi, Sharifah S., Breeze E. Cavell, Urvi Telang, et al. November 2010. "In Vivo Modulation of 4E Binding Protein 1(4E-BP1) Phosphorylation by Watercress: A Pilot Study." *British Journal of Nutrition* 104(9): 1288–1296.

Website
The Watercress Alliance. www.watercress.com.uk/about/watercress-alliance.

Glossary

Allergic rhinitis—a medical condition caused by an allergy that has symptoms including runny nose and itchy eyes.

Amyloid plaques—a pathologic lesion of amyloid protein in brains of people with Alzheimer's disease.

Anaphylaxis—life-threatening systemic allergic reaction.

Anthocyanin—antioxidant flavonoids found in fruits that protect many body systems.

Antiandrogen—a substance that reduces levels of androgens (male hormones).

Antihyperglycemic—pertains to a substance that lowers glucose levels in the blood.

Antimycotic—an agent that inhibits the growth of fungus.

Antinociceptive—reducing sensitivity to painful stimuli.

Anxiolytic—preventing or reducing anxiety.

Apoptosis—a pattern of cell death.

Aspartate transaminase—an enzyme that is released into the blood when the liver or heart is injured.

Ayurveda—the ancient Hindu science of health and medicine.

Benign prostatic hyperplasia—an enlarged prostate gland, a common condition as men age. Also known as benign prostatic hypertrophy.

Biofilm–thin layer of microorganisms adhering to the surface of a structure.

Blepharoplasty—plastic surgery on the eyelids.

Bradycardia—a regular but slower than normal heart rate.

C-reactive protein—a substance in the blood that is a measure of inflammation; higher amounts may be seen in individuals at risk for cardiovascular disease.

Carotenoid—class of high unsaturated yellow to red pigments found widely in plants and animals.

Cell apoptosis—cell death.

Central nervous system—the part of the nervous system consisting of the brain and the spinal cord.

Chlorhexidine—chemical antiseptic.

Chronic venous insufficiency—a syndrome that includes leg swelling, enlarged veins, leg pain, itching, and skin ulcers.

Colic—persistent unexplained crying in an infant.

Collagenous colitis—a type of colitis that occurs primarily in middle-aged women.

Cutaneous—relating to the skin.

Cytotoxic—toxic to cells.

Cytotoxicity—the degree to which something is toxic to living cells.

Desquamation—shedding of the outer layer of skin.

Diabesity—a popular term denoting type 2 diabetes caused by overweight or obesity.

Diuretics—medications designed to reduce the amount of water in the body.

DOI–Digital Object Identifier.

Dorsal—pertaining to or situated on the back.

Dyslipidemia—high levels of lipids such as cholesterol and triglycerides in the blood.

Dysplasia—a pathological term meaning an appearance of abnormal cells.

Ecchymosis—blood under the skin such as bruising.

Echinacea—an herb that some believe boosts the body's immune system.

Emetogenic–capacity to induce vomiting, as in some forms of chemotherapy.

Erythema—a skin condition characterized by redness

Erythrocytes—red blood cells.

Exudate—fluid rich in protein and other cellular elements that oozes out of blood vessels usually due to inflammation and is deposited in nearby tissue.

Fibroblasts—cells that give rise to connective tissue.

Furosemide—a diuretic medication used to reduce swelling and fluid retention in the body.

Gentamicin—a broad spectrum antibiotic.

Glaucoma—a condition in which fluid pressure builds up inside the eye.

Glycemia—the normal presence of sugar in the blood.

Hepatitis—inflammation of the liver.

Hepatotoxicity—damage to the liver caused by drugs, chemicals, or other agents.

Hot plate test—a test used to evaluate the pain responses in animals; by observing the reaction to pain caused by heat, it determines the effectiveness of analgesics.

Hypercholesterolemia—higher than normal levels of cholesterol in the blood.

Hyperglycemia—higher than normal levels of glucose in the blood.

Hyperinsulinemia—excess levels of insulin circulating in the blood.

Hyperphagia—an abnormally increased appetite for food and its consumption.

Hypersomnia—excessive sleepiness.

Hypertension—high blood pressure.

Hypoglycemia—concentrations of glucose in the blood are lower than normal.

Ibuprofen—a nonsteroidal anti-inflammation medication that is used to alleviate mild to moderate pain.

Insulin resistance—a condition where one needs relatively more insulin to maintain blood glucose in a normal range.

Ischemic—insufficient supply of blood.

Isothiocyanates—sulfur containing compounds found in cruciferous vegetables.

Lactation—secretion of milk from mammary glands.

Leptin—a hormone that affects feeding behavior and hunger.

Lidocaine—a local anesthetic that works by stopping nerves from sending pain signals.

Linalool—a liquid commonly found in essential oils such as lavender.

Lisinopril—a medication used to treat high blood pressure.

Lorazepam—in a group of drugs known as benzodiazepines, this medication, which is also known as Ativan, is used to treat anxiety.

Lumbago—nonspecific lower back pain.

Lymphedema—swelling caused by lymph fluid accumulating in the tissue.

Metabolic syndrome—a cluster of health problems that include insulin resistance, abnormal blood fats, and borderline or elevated blood pressure. These problems have been associated with chronic diseases such as cardiovascular disease and diabetes.

Metformin—a medication used to treat type 2 diabetes.

Methimazole—a medication used to treat hyperthyroidism, where the thyroid releases excessive amounts of thyroid hormones.

Microangiopathy—development of lesions in small blood vessels.

Mometasone furoate ointment—topical steroid used to reduce skin inflammation.

Monoaminergic system—neurons that secrete monoamine neurotransmitters such as serotonin or dopamine.

Mucilage—a sticky substance often produced by plants.

Myocyte—a type of cell found in muscles.

Nephrotoxicity—a substance that is toxic to the kidney.

Nonalcoholic steatohepatitis (NASH)—a progressive liver disease related to the metabolic syndrome, obesity, and diabetes.

Nootropic—memory/cognitive enhancers.

Normotensive—normal blood pressure.

Nosocomial pathogens—microorganisms causing infections in a hospital or other health care facility.

Nutrients—foods or chemical humans need to grow and metabolize. They must be taken in from the environment.

Occlusion—blockage of passageway such as an artery.

Open field test—a common measure of general activity and exploratory behavior in mice and rats.

Osteoarthritis—a type of degenerative arthritis that is caused by the breakdown and eventual loss of cartilage in one or more joints.

Ovariectomy—surgical removal of one or both ovaries.

Oxidized LDL—LDL that is bombarded by free radicals, a process that is thought to cause atherosclerosis.

Palpitation—irregular beating or pulsation of the heart.

Pathogenic oral microflora—disease-causing bacteria in the mouth.

Perfusion—pumping a liquid into an organ or tissue.

Periodontitis—chronic inflammatory disease of the gums and bones around the teeth.

Phenethyl isothiocyanate (PEITC)—a naturally occurring substance in vegetables such as broccoli and kale.

Phonophobia—a fear of loud noises.

Photophobia—abnormal sensitivity to or intolerance of lights.

Platelets—cellular fragments in the blood that assist in blood clotting.

Polyphenols—a group of chemicals found in many fruits and other foods. As antioxidants, they remove free radicals from the body.

Prepubertal gynecomastia—a rare condition in which boys or girls develop enlarged breast tissue prior to puberty.

Prostatitis—infection or inflammation of the prostate gland.

Psoriasis—chronic autoimmune skin condition that can be characterized by dry red patches covered with scales.

Psoriasis vulgaris—also known as plaque psoriasis, it is the most common type of psoriasis.

Psycholeptic drugs—medications that have a calming effect.

Quercetin—a plant-derived flavonoid found in fruits, vegetables, leaves, and grains.

Re-epithelialization—regrowth of the epithelium over the surface of a wound. It marks the final stage of healing.

Rhinorrhea—runny nose.

Salmonella enteritidis—a bacterium that infects the ovaries of hens that appear healthy and contaminates the eggs before the shells are formed.

Salmonella typhimurium—a bacterium that causes typhoid fever. It is uncommon in the United States.

Saponins—phytochemicals found in most vegetables, beans, and herbs.

Sesquiterpene lactone—a substance found in some plants that may have anti-inflammatory and anticancer effects.

Silver sulfadiazine—a topical medicine used to prevent and treat bacterial or fungal infections especially useful in burn treatment.

Simvastatin—a statin medication used to lower levels of LDL (bad) cholesterol and triglycerides and to raise levels of HDL (good) cholesterol in the blood.

Sleep latency—the amount of time it takes to fall asleep.

Somatization—physical symptoms caused by psychological problems.

Steatosis—the abnormal retention of fats in a cell; also fatty liver disease.

Streptococcus mutans—a bacterium that lives in the mouth and causes tooth decay.

Syncope—fainting.

Thrombosis—formation, presence, or development of a thrombus—blood clot.

Titratable acidity—a food-processing metric.

Tonsillectomy—surgical removal of the tonsils.

Tramadol—synthetic opiate pain medication used to relieve moderate to severe pain.

Triamcinolone acetonide—used for a variety of skin conditions, this topical steroid medication reduces swelling, redness, and itching.

Triglycerides—chemical form in which most fat exists in food and the body.

Troxerutin—a natural bioflavonoid reported to have many benefits and medicinal properties.

Venereology—branch of medicine dealing with venereal (sexually transmitted) infections.

Venous—relating to the veins, the blood vessels that carry blood toward the heart.

Wound slough—layer or mass of dead tissue separated from surrounding living tissue.

Xenograft—tissue graft from one species to an unrelated species.

Index

About the Authors

MYRNA CHANDLER GOLDSTEIN, M.A., has been a freelance writer and independent scholar for two decades. She is the author of *Boys into Men, Controversies in the Practice of Medicine, Food and Nutrition Controversies Today,* and *Healthy Foods: Fact versus Fiction* with Greenwood Press.

MARK A. GOLDSTEIN, M.D., is the founding Chief of the Division of Adolescent and Young Adult Medicine at Massachusetts General Hospital. Dr. Goldstein, a member of the Harvard Medical School faculty, is author or editor of numerous professional and lay publications. His research interests include studying the effects of eating disorders and malnutrition on bone mineralization in adolescents and young adults.

DISCARDED